UNDERSTANDING INFECTIOUS DISEASE

Understanding Infectious Disease

Paul D. Ellner, Ph.D.
Professor Emeritus of Microbiology and Pathology
Columbia University, College of Physicians and Surgeons
New York, New York

Harold C. Neu, M.D.
Professor of Medicine and Pharmacology
Chief, Division of Infectious Disease
Columbia University, College of Physicians and Surgeons
New York, New York

Marie T. Dauenheimer, Illustrator

616.9
E47U

3/94

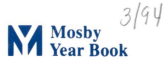

Mosby
Year Book

St. Louis   Baltimore   Boston   Chicago   London   Philadelphia   Sydney   Toronto

CUYAHOGA COMMUNITY COLLEGE
METRO CAMPUS LIBRARY

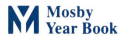
Mosby
Year Book
Dedicated to Publishing Excellence

Sponsoring Editor: Kim Kist
Assistant Editor: Penny Rudolph
Assistant Director, Manuscript Services:
    Frances M. Perveiler
Production Supervisor: Karen Halm
Proofroom Manager: Barbara Kelly

1 2 3 4 5 6 7 8 9 0 CL MV 96 95 94 93 92

Library of Congress Cataloging-in-Publication Data
Ellner, Paul D. (Paul Daniel), 1925-
        Understanding infectious disease / Paul D. Ellner,
Harold C. Neu,
            p.   cm.
        Includes bibliographical references and index.
        ISBN 0-8016-1892-4
        1. Communicable diseases.   I. Neu, Harold C., 1934-.
    II. Title.
        [DNLM: 1. Communicable Diseases.   WC 100 E47u]
    RC111.E33 1992   91-46179
    616.9—dc20   CIP
    DNLM/DLC
    for Library of Congress

To Connie, Diane, David, and Jonathan
P.D.E.

To Carmen, Maria, Natalie, and Harold
H.C.N.

PREFACE

This book is largely based upon lectures given to medical and dental students for the past 26 years at the College of Physicians and Surgeons of Columbia University. It presents in concise form the basic information required by the student physician to understand the epidemiology, pathogenesis, and host response to commonly encountered microbial infections.

The medical student approaching the study of infectious disease needs to be aware of the etiologic possibilities; for each of the agents he should have some knowledge of its source and means of transmission to man, the mechanism by which tissue damage is produced, its susceptibility to antimicrobial agents, and the host response to the microbial challenge. This essential information must usually be gleaned during the preclinical years from courses in microbiology where organism by organism, and immunology is presented; the antimicrobial drugs may be taught in a pharmacology course, while courses in infectious diseases are generally taught by organ system.

We have organized the above material and presented it in a compact format based upon organ systems. Starting with an illustrative case, the possible etiologic agents are listed in the order of frequency with which they cause that particular infection, and the appropriate differential diagnostic procedures are given. For each listed organism the reader is referred to a section of the book where its characteristics, source and transmission, and pathogenetic mechanisms are briefly described.

This book was written for the medical and dental student and presumes a basic knowledge of biology, chemistry, and immunology. There are a number of excellent encyclopedic tomes available dealing with microbiology and infectious disease. These books contain far more information than can be digested by beginning students who usually do not have the time to consult such sources until later in their careers.

The present book should be useful as a supplement to lectures in microbiology and infectious disease. The clinical organization and the material on the use of the diagnostic laboratory will extend its utility to students starting their clinical rotation. The applied aspects of infectious disease are best learned at the bedside of the patients.

PAUL D. ELLNER, PH.D.

INTRODUCTION

The medical student starting his clinical rotation soon recognizes that significant numbers of the patients he encounters suffer from infectious diseases—those ailments that are caused by transmissible microscopic life forms. These agents of disease represent a very small fraction of the myriad species of microorganisms in the world; indeed, animal and plant life on this planet would not be possible without the multiplicity of microbial life.

From ancient times infectious diseases have had a tremendous impact on culture, religion, wars, social organization, and virtually every aspect of daily life. These diseases accounted for a large part of medical practice. As recently as 1990, 4 million children died from acute respiratory infection and another 4 million died from diarrheal disease. Tuberculosis is still responsible for 3 million deaths annually. There are 200 million cases of schistosomiasis and 100 million cases of malaria every year. Five percent of adolescents and young adults contract sexually transmitted diseases each year and 5 to 10 million are infected with the AIDS virus. In the United States there are about 50 million acute infections per year.

When Louis Pasteur advanced the germ theory of disease in 1878, he noted, "if it is a terrifying thought that life is at the mercy of the multiplication of these minute bodies, it is a consoling hope that Science will not always remain powerless before such enemies. . . ."

To a great extent Pasteur's hope has been realized. By the early 18th century, as a result of the pioneering work of Jenner and Pasteur, it was recognized that a growing number of these diseases could be prevented by artificial immunization, and that the spread of many of these diseases could be controlled by improving the living conditions, particularly sanitation. By the end of the 19th century the microbial causes of many infectious diseases had been discovered, and many specific vaccines and antisera had become available. Despite these advances, 4.5 million children died in 1983 in developing countries from vaccine preventable diseases; more than 2.5 million from measles, over 1 million from neonatal tetanus, and 840,000 from pertussis.

Celsus, perhaps the greatest of Latin medical writers who lived in Rome about A.D. 25, remarked that to determine the cause of a disease often leads to the remedy.* The cause of some diseases, e.g., multiple sclerosis, Hashimoto's syndrome, and Alzheimer's disease—suspected of being due to infectious agents—is still not known. We are just beginning to learn about AIDS and Cat Scratch disease, and there is still

---

*"Et causae quoque estimatio saepe morbum solvit."

much we don't know about Legionnaires' disease, Lyme disease, and toxic shock syndrome.

Paul Ehrlich conceived of "magic bullets"—drugs that would kill the microorganism responsible for a disease while being innocuous to the host, and many of the antimicrobial agents we have today approach that concept. Nevertheless, to use these drugs effectively the physician must determine which microbe has infected his patient.

In order to effectively and rationally deal with infectious disease, the physician needs to become familiar with the characteristics of the pathogenic microorganisms. He must know the source and the means of their transmission to the human host, the mechanisms by which these microorganisms produce tissue damage, and the host's response to the infection. This knowledge is the basis for understanding the epidemiology of infectious diseases, the pathogenesis of the various infections, the immune mechanism involved, and the principles of specific therapy.

PAUL D. ELLNER, PH.D

CONTENTS

PART I

Dynamics of Infection

CHAPTER 1

Characteristics of Pathogenic Microorganisms

MICROBIAL DRAMATIS PERSONAE

Single-celled microscopic organisms are classified into two large groups: eukaryotic cells and prokaryotic cells.

Eukaryotic cells are characterized by containing a nucleus with a distinct nuclear membrane and distinguishable membrane-bound organelles such as mitochondria. Eukaryotic cells contain both RNA and DNA. Examples of eukaryotic cells are protozoa and fungi.

Prokaryotic cells also contain both types of nucleic acid but lack a nuclear membrane and distinct organelles. The prokaryotes include most bacteria, mycelial organisms (*Mycobacterium, Actinomyces, Nocardia*), spirochetes, and intracellular parasites such as *Mycoplasma, Chlamydia*, and *Rickettsia*.

Bacteria are classified primarily on three characteristics: shape (rods or cocci), reaction to the Gram stain* (positive or negative), and their ability to grow in the presence of atmospheric oxygen (aerobic or anaerobic). Facultative bacteria are those that can grow under aerobic or anaerobic conditions. Using the criteria of shape, Gram stain reaction and ability to grow in air, bacteria can be separated into eight groups (Table 1–1). Other characteristics that are considered in bacterial taxonomy are the ability to form spores, the presence of various enzymes (catalase, urease, oxidase, etc.), specific surface antigens (flagella, cell wall), and their DNA relatedness to other bacteria.

Viruses are submicroscopic forms that contain a single type of nucleic acid in a protein coat. They are obligate intracellular parasites that replicate by assembling newly synthesized subunits. Viruses are classified by their size, type of nucleic acid (RNA or DNA), the presence or absence of an envelope, and the arrangement of the protein coat subunits (capsomeres) (Table 1–2).

Recent studies have revealed a disease-causing agent that is still smaller and less complex than viruses. These rod-shaped agents, termed *prions*, have been shown to be associated with slowly progressive degenerative disorders of the central nervous system. These diseases—kuru

*The Gram stain consists of treating the fixed bacterial cells on a slide with a purple dye (crystal violet), followed by an iodine mordant. The smear is then decolorized with alcohol or acetone and counterstained with a red dye (safranin or fuchsin). Bacteria that retain the purple dye despite decolorization and appear purple when examined with the microscope are called *gram-positive*. Organisms that are decolorized, take up the counterstain, and appear red when visualized microscopically are termed *gram-negative*.

TABLE 1-1.

Characteristics of Some Clinically Significant Bacteria

	Cocci		Bacilli	
	Gram-Positive	Gram-Negative	Gram-Positive	Gram-Negative
Aerobic	Staphylococcus	Neisseria	Corynebacterium	Enterobacteriaceae
	Streptococcus		Bacillus	(*E. coli,* Shigella,
			Mycobacterium	Salmonella, Proteus
			Nocardia	Klebsiella,
				Enterobacter)
				Pseudomonas
				Hemophilus
				Legionella
				Bordetella
Anaerobic	Peptococcus	Veillonella	Clostridium	Bacteroides
	Peptostreptococcus		Propionibacterium	Fusobacterium
			Lactobacillus	

TABLE 1-2.

Characteristics of the Major Groups of Viruses

Virus Group	Nucleic Acid Strands	Envelope*	Capsomere Arrangement	Size (nm)
DNA viruses				
Poxviruses	Double	+	Complex	240-300
Herpesviruses	Double	+	Icosahedral	150
Adenoviruses	Double	-	Icosahedral	75
Papovaviruses	Double	-	Icosahedral	45-55
Hepatitis B	Double	-	Icosahedral	42
Parvoviruses	Single	-	Icosahedral	20
RNA viruses				
Paramyxoviruses	Single	+	Helical	120-150
Orthomyxoviruses	Single	+	Helical	90-120
Coronaviruses	Single	+	Helical	80-120
Arenaviruses	Single	+	Helical(?)	80-300
Bunyaviruses	Single	+	Helical	80-100
Rhabdoviruses	Single	+	Helical	70-170
Togaviruses	Single	+	Icosahedral	50-70
Retroviruses	Single	+	Icosahedral	100-120
Hepatitis A	Single	-	Icosahedral	18-30
Picornaviruses	Single	-	Icosahedral	25-30
Reoviruses	Double	-	Icosahedral	70-80

*+ = present; - = absent.

and Creutzfeldt-Jakob disease—are transmissible to animals. Prions are similar to the agent that causes scrapie, a neurologic disease of sheep and goats. Scrapie prions contain a single major protein, designated "Pr P" which is required for infectivity. No nucleic acid genome has been found in prions, but a single Pr P–related gene has been detected in human and marine DNA. The mechanism of replication is unknown.

DISTRIBUTION OF MICROBES

Microorganisms are widely distributed throughout the world. They are present in the soil, and in fresh and sea water. Many microbes are free-living; others exist in association with higher plants or animals. This parasitism may be benign, beneficial, or harmful to the host. Organisms causing tissue damage or disease are termed **pathogens.** A very small number of species of the total microbial world are pathogenic for man.

More than 100 years ago Robert Koch attempted to relate a specific microbial species with a particular disease by three criteria which have come to be known as Koch's postulates. They state that the organism should be recovered from all patients with the disease in question, from anatomic areas corresponding to observed lesions; the organisms should be cultivated in pure culture outside the host for several generations; and the organism should reproduce the same disease when introduced into other animals.

TYPES OF PATHOGENS

Theoretically, any organism that can survive in the body has the potential for disease production. However, there are marked differences in the ability of microorganisms to invade and produce tissue damage. **Virulence** is the term used to quantitate pathogenicity; i.e., a highly virulent organism has a much greater potential for producing disease than an organism of low viru-

lence. Virulence is often expressed as the minimum infective dose—the lowest number of organisms required to produce infection or death in a specified experimental animal within a defined time.

Highly virulent organisms that can produce disease in relatively low numbers in an otherwise intact and healthy host are referred to as **primary pathogens.** Organisms of low virulence that require a disruption in one or more host defenses or a large dose to initiate infection are referred to as **opportunists** (Fig 1–1). Opportunists are often components of the indigenous flora or are occasionally acquired from the nonliving environment. The distinction between primary pathogens and opportunists is not clear-cut, and there are many organisms that fall into a gray area between these two definitions.

It is also useful to recognize microbial pathogens by the type of parasitism they exhibit. Extracellular parasites are promptly ingested and killed by phagocytic cells. Infections by extracellular parasites are usually characterized by acute inflammation. Intracellular parasites can survive and multiply within the phagocytic cells. Such organisms are often associated with chronic granulomatous diseases. Viruses, rickettsia, and chlamydia are obligate intracellular parasites and require the intracellular environment for growth and reproduction.

TRANSMISSION OF PATHOGENS

Infection acquired from organisms whose natural reservoir is outside the body are termed **exogenous;** infections caused by a member(s) of the indigenous flora are designated **endogenous.**

Pathogens may be transmitted to the host by direct contact (respiratory aerosol of an infected person), by an insect vector, by contaminated food or water, or by contaminated inanimate objects (fomites). The pathogen may enter the host's body by inhalation, ingestion, or injection (trauma, sexual contact, insect or animal bite) (Fig 1–2).

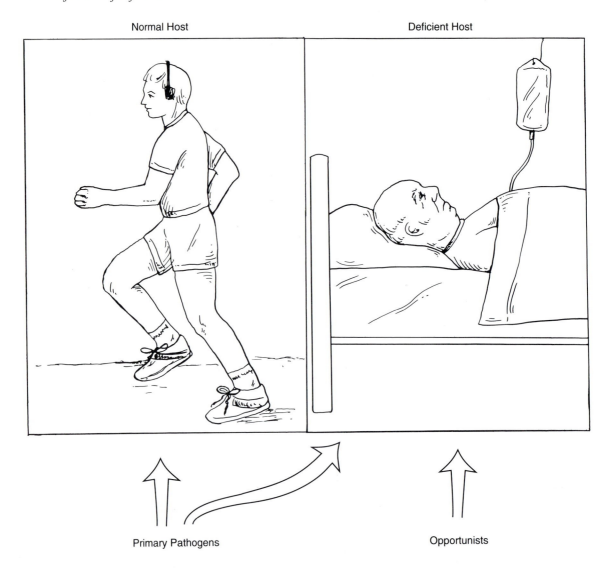

Normal Host   Deficient Host

Primary Pathogens   Opportunists

MICROORGANISMS

FIG 1–1.
Primary pathogens vs. opportunists.

Some microorganisms have specific mechanisms for attaching to or penetrating the body surfaces of the host. Under some circumstances the organism is introduced by a biting arthropod (fly, flea, tick, mite, mosquito). In endogenous infections the organism is already in the body (Fig 1–3).

INDIGENOUS BACTERIAL FLORA

While the majority of microorganisms have remained free-living, a number of species have opted for various degrees of symbiosis with higher forms. These dependent life styles range from commensalism, wherein the microorganism

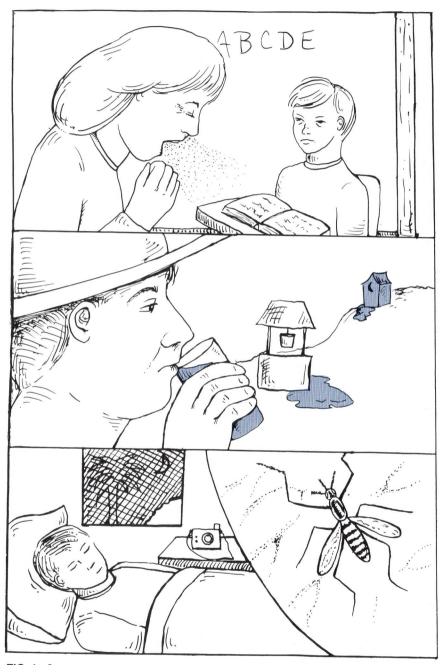

FIG 1–2.
Pathways of infection: inhalation, ingestion, injection.

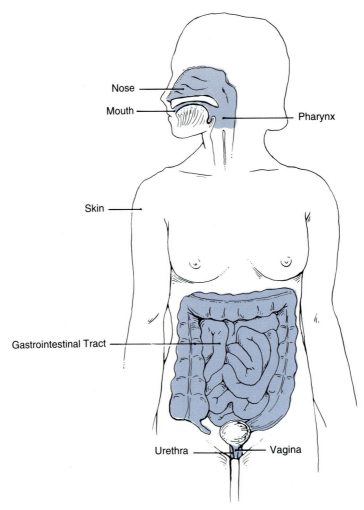

FIG 1–3.
Body sites with indigenous microflora.

merely derives food or other benefits from the host but retains its potential for independent existence, to strict parasitism, in which the parasite cannot exist outside of the host. Man has not been exempt from playing host to germs, and every human carries a complex resident microbial flora from the cradle to the grave.*

*This was succinctly stated in a bit of doggerel entitled "On the Antiquity of Microbes": "Adam had 'em" (Strickland Gillilan, 1912).

This resident indigenous flora consists of fixed types of microorganisms regularly found in an anatomic site. Other microorganisms may transiently inhabit the skin or mucous membranes for a few hours, days, or weeks, but do not produce disease as long as the resident indigenous flora remains intact.

The fetus remains sterile as long as it resides in the uterus, the intact placenta providing a barrier to the entry of microorganisms. The first exposure to microorganisms comes during passage of the fetus through the vagina. Immediately after delivery the infant becomes exposed to other organisms in its environment, some of which become permanently established in or on its body. By the end of the first week or two the infant has acquired most of the organisms found in the adult.

Each anatomic area is selective in the species that colonize it; only certain species become established, others are rejected. For example, in the mouth and throat viridans streptococci appear by the third to the fifth day and protect against colonization by *Staphylococcus aureus.* In the gastrointestinal tract bacteria appear in a few days; the source is food. Breast-fed infants have a distinctly different intestinal flora from that of bottle-fed babies. In breast-fed infants lactobacilli predominate with a few coliforms, enterococci, and micrococci present; in bottle-fed infants the intestinal flora is composed of coliforms, enterococci, clostridia, diphtheroids, and a few lactobacilli.

Local host factors exert a marked effect in selecting the colonizing species. These involve the blood supply, moisture, temperature, pH, the degree of oxidation or reduction, and the presence of enzymes and specific antibodies, such as IgA. In some cases colonizing organisms are selected by the nature of their exopolysaccharides, and organ- or tissue-specific receptors.

There is a flora characteristic for each site. The indigenous flora of the skin, conjunctiva, nose, throat, and urethra is predominantly gram-positive; the flora of the colon is predominantly gram-negative, while that of the small intestine, vagina, and mouth is a mixture of gram-positive and gram-negative species.

Once established, the normal flora is difficult to alter. Under normal circumstances, if the indigenous flora is disturbed it promptly reestablishes itself. Qualitative changes in the flora occur in hospitalized patients, particularly in their pharynx, vagina, skin, and intestine.

The indigenous flora have a variety of activities, some of which may be viewed as beneficial to the host, while others are potentially detrimental. The bowel flora is metabolically active and deaminates amino acids to aldehydes, and ammonia to alcohol and alpha-hydroxy acids. Forty percent of the urea synthesized by the liver is deaminated to ammonia*; the bile acids are degraded and disaccharides such as lactose are split. The bowel flora may alter potential carcinogens associated with the diet. Intestinal microorganisms synthesize vitamin K, riboflavin, pantothenic acid, pyridoxine, and biotin. (While this activity is clearly supplementary rather than indispensable, it may explain why some patients on long-term antimicrobial therapy develop symptoms suggestive of vitamin B deficiency.) It has been suggested that kwashiorkor, a severe form of protein malnutrition, may be due in part to a disturbance of the intestinal flora.

One of the most important activities of the indigenous flora is their involvement in host defense mechanisms. These organisms help protect the host from colonization by more virulent bacteria. One mechanism is competitive exclusion; the adherence of indigenous bacteria blocks the attachment of pathogens to epithelial cells. The indigenous flora also play a major role in stimulating the immunologic tissues of the body. Certain members of the normal microflora appear to activate macrophages nonspecifically, and stimulate the development and function of lymphoid tissue. The indigenous flora may at times be a liability rather than an asset. Indigenous organisms may behave as opportunists in situations in which the host's defenses are compromised. These opportunistic infections are seen in the newborn, in persons with diabetes, sickle cell anemia, neutropenia, and agammaglobulinemia, and in patients with prosthetic devices. In some instances, the resident organisms appear to assist pathogens in penetrating the host or in avoiding destruction during therapy.

Familiarization with the nature of the indigenous flora provides insight into the types of infection associated with tissue injury at inhabited

---

*This is the rationale for antibiotic therapy of hepatic coma, which is associated with increased blood ammonia levels.

TABLE 1–3.

Principal Indigenous Flora*

	Skin and Conjunctiva	Upper Respiratory Tract	Mouth	Small Intestine	Colon	Vagina	Urethra
Gram positive							
Staphylococci	X	X	X	–	–	X	X
Corynebacteria (diphtheroids)	X	X	X	–	–	X	X
Propionibacteria	X	–	–	–	–	–	–
Streptococci viridans group	–	X	X	X	–	X	X
Pneumococci	–	X	X	–	–	–	–
Nonhemolytic	–	X	X	–	–	X	–
Hemolytic Non-Group A	–	X	X	–	–	X	–
Enterococci	–	–	X	X	X	X	–
Anaerobic	–	–	X	X	X	X	–
Lactobacilli	–	–	X	X	–	X	–
Clostridia	–	–	–	X	X	X	–
Gram negative							
Neisseria	–	X	X	–	–	X	X
Aerobic bacilli (E. coli, Klebsiella, Enterobacter, Proteus, Pseudomonas, etc.)	–	–	X	–	X	–	X
Hemophilus	–	X	X	–	–	–	–
Bacteroides and Fusobacteria	–	X	X	–	X	–	–
Candida	–	X	X	X	X	X	–

*X = organism present.

anatomic sites, provides recognition of the consequences of suppression or overgrowth of these organisms, and facilitates the interpretation of the significance of these organisms when they are recovered from clinical infections. The distribution of the principal indigenous flora is given in Table 1–3 and illustrated in Figure 1–4.

PATHOGENIC MECHANISMS

BACTERIAL SURFACE COMPONENTS

Some bacteria produce extracellular polymeric material that may be variously categorized as a capsule, slime layer, or glycocalyx. These materials are usually polysaccharides that surround the bacterial cell and cling to its surface. Capsules have a distinct outer margin, and exclude recognition by host factors. The capsule also acts to impede phagocytosis by host cells. Slime and glycocalyces are exopolysaccharides with indistinct margins. The glycocalyx is a mass of long polysaccharide fibers generated from sugar molecules by polymerases on the bacterial surface. Slime and glycocalyces are important in mediating the adherence of bacteria to surfaces within the body of the host. Additionally, a glycocalyx can also function as a food reservoir for the bacteria.

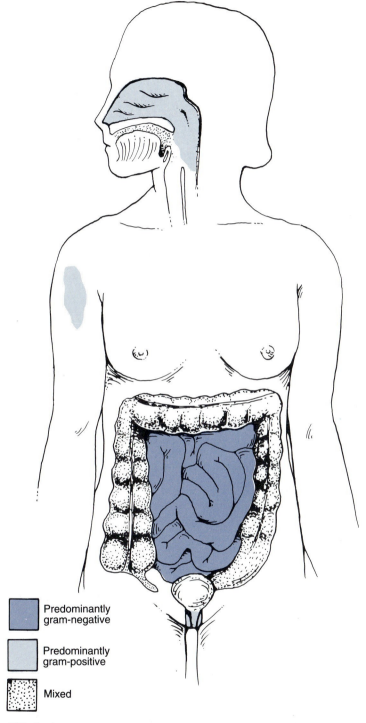

FIG 1–4.
Types of indigenous bacterial flora.

Predominantly
gram-negative

Predominantly
gram-positive

Mixed

The bacterial envelope consists of the cell wall and the cytoplasmic membrane. The cell wall of gram-positive bacteria is composed of layers of peptidoglycan, a polymer of amino acids and sugars, and chains of ribitol or glycerol lipoteichoic acids. The peptidoglycan provides rigidity to the bacterial cell, and can induce chronic granulomatous inflammatory lesions of dermal connective tissue, fever, and shock. The lipoteichoic acids project beyond the cell wall and are involved in the attachment of gram-positive organisms to the epithelial cells of the host. The gram-positive cell surface may also contain hydrolytic enzymes such as IgAl protease that may play a role in facilitating the colonization of mucosal surfaces.

The cell wall of gram-negative bacteria is thinner than in gram-positive species, contains peptidoglycan and is separated from the cytoplasmic membrane by a periplasmic space. The bilayered outer membrane contains phospholipids, proteins, and lipopolysaccharides. The outer membrane protein is the most exposed region of the bacterial cell structure and is involved in most of the specific recognition processes of the host—bacteria interaction. In some instances the outer membrane protein may contribute to the organism's ability to resist killing by host serum. The lipopolysaccharide portion of the gram-negative cell is known as **endotoxin.** Endotoxin can produce fever, shock, and intravascular coagulation, as well as effects on host defense mechanisms. A comparison of the structure of gram-positive and gram-negative bacteria is shown in Figure 1–5.

The cell envelope of mycobacteria is composed of wax, lipids, and polysaccharides in addition to peptidoglycan. Some of these substances play a role in the development of delayed-type hypersensitivity to the organism and in the production of granulomatous lesions.

Some bacteria have some microscopic hairlike fibrils projecting from the surface of the organism. These structures are termed **pili** or **fimbriae** and are important in mediating the adherence of bacteria to surfaces. Additionally, pili may potentiate the delivery of toxins to host cells.

ELABORATION OF TOXIC SUBSTANCES

These materials include the potent exotoxins, other extracellular products, and endotoxin.

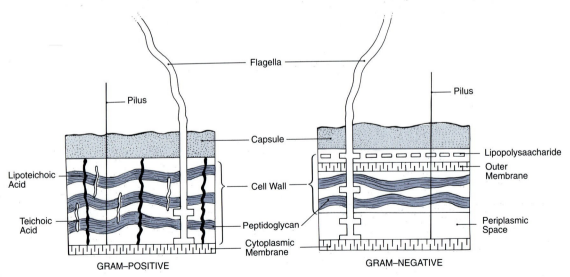

FIG 1–5.
Comparison of Gram positive and Gram negative envelopes.

Exotoxins are soluble proteins secreted by some bacterial species. They include some of the most poisonous substances known; a single microgram of botulinum A toxin contains 1,200 lethal mouse doses. Each exotoxin has a specific action that in many cases accounts for the symptoms of a disease. Examples of exotoxins that cause the major manifestations of disease entities are diphtheria, botulinum, tetanus, and cholera toxins and the enterotoxins of *Clostridium perfringens* and *S. aureus*. Other toxins, e.g., *Pseudomonas* exotoxin A, contribute to the pathogenesis of a disease. Still other toxins such as pertussis toxin, Shiga toxin, streptolysin O, and staphylococcal toxic shock toxin (TSST-1) probably have a role in disease production but their importance remains to be proved.

Exotoxins produce tissue damage by various mechanisms such as cell lysis, increasing cyclic adenosine monophosphate (AMP) production, inhibition of protein synthesis, or blockage of nerve function. Toxins are categorized by the tissues or organ systems they affect; neurotoxins act on the nervous system, enterotoxins on the gastrointestinal tract, cytotoxins or histotoxins damage cells and tissues.

Many of the exotoxins conform to the A-B model in which the toxin is composed of A and B subunits. The A and B subunits are initially synthesized as a single polypeptide chain which is partially hydrolyzed during or after secretion into light (A) and heavy (B) chains joined by disulfide bridges. The A subunit is enzymatically active and is responsible for toxic activity once inside the cell; the B subunits bind to the target cells but are nontoxic by themselves. Target cell receptors are often glycoproteins or gangliosides.

The exotoxins are antigenic and the antibodies they elicit are termed **antitoxins.** Antitoxins specifically combine with toxins and neutralize their toxic activity. Toxin-antitoxin complexes may dissociate and release active toxin. Because the amount of toxin needed to elicit an immune response often greatly exceeds the quantity that produces tissue damage, toxins are not used as immunizing agents. Treating protein toxins with formaldehyde produces **toxoid,** a product that has lost toxicity but retains immunogenicity. Toxoids are used to actively immunize against toxigenic diseases such as tetanus, diphtheria, and botulism.

Other extracellular products of bacteria may contribute indirectly to pathogenesis. Hemolysins that lyse erythrocytes, leukocidins that injure leukocytes, and enzymes such as hyaluronidase, lipase, collagenase, protease, and DNAse that can damage tissue and facilitate the spread of bacteria are examples of these products.

Many pathogenic bacteria require iron for growth or toxin production and host proteins such as lactoferrin and transferrin keep free ionic iron at levels too low for bacterial growth. Many gram-negative bacteria secrete low-molecular-weight iron-binding compounds called **siderophores,** which compete with the host and scavenge the required iron.

Endotoxins are lipopolysaccharide constituents of the gram-negative cell envelope. The lipopolysaccharide consists of three components: lipid A, essential for toxicity; a core polysaccharide containing an unusual sugar, ketodeoxyoctanoic acid (KDO); and a long carbohydrate chain unique to the species, called the O antigen. Whereas the protein exotoxins are usually inactivated by heating at 56° C for 30 minutes, endotoxin is very heat-stable, and retains its activity even after exposure to 120° C for 30 minutes or longer. Endotoxin elicits a variety of pathophysiologic effects, the most important of which are the production of fever, shock, and disseminated intravascular coagulation. In small amounts endotoxin activates B lymphocytes to increase antibody synthesis; acts on macrophages and monocytes to produce interleukin-1 and tumor necrosis factor (cachectin) which results in fever; and activates complement by the alternative pathway leading to the inflammatory response. In larger amounts endotoxin produces shock, and acts on platelets causing the release of clotting factors leading to disseminated intra-vascular coagulation.

IMMUNOMODULATION

Microorganisms may produce symptoms or tissue damage by affecting the immune response. Rhinoviruses induce local anaphylaxis with histamine release that is largely responsible for the nasal congestion and rhinorrhea associated with the common cold. In poststreptococcal glomerulonephritis, damage to the basement membrane of the glomerulus is due to the deposition of immune complexes resulting in an Arthus-type reaction. In tuberculosis, tertiary syphilis, and certain fungus infections, lesion production is associated with the development of delayed-type hypersensitivity. The human immunodeficiency virus HIV-1 primarily infects T lymphocytes, causing the acquired immunodeficiency syndrome (AIDS).

Other pathogenetic mechanisms include the damage to vascular endothelium by rickettsia and some viruses, and the ability of some viruses to induce hyperplasia—sometimes benign as with some papillomaviruses, and sometimes malignant, causing the transformation to cancer cells by herpesviruses and possibly other papillomaviruses.

GENETIC CONTROL OF VIRULENCE

The expression of many of the previously mentioned virulence factors is controlled by specific genes. Genes that regulate toxin production and release may be chromosomal or plasmid-mediated and in at least one case (diphtheria toxin) are carried by a bacteriophage. Similarly, the expression of capsules, pili, and certain outer membrane proteins is often plasmid-mediated.

ADDITIONAL READING

Berkowitz FE: Bacterial exotoxins: How they work. *Pediatr Infect Dis J* 1989; 8:42–47.

Isenberg HD: Pathogenicity and virulence: Another view. *Clin Microbiol Rev* 1988; 1:40–53.

CHAPTER 2

Microbe-Host Interaction

ESTABLISHMENT OF INFECTION

COLONIZATION AND INVASION

Infection may be defined as the invasion of the tissues of the body by pathogenic microorganisms resulting in injury and disease. Encounters with microorganisms by inhalation, ingestion, or injection are a daily occurrence beginning at birth and continuing throughout life. In many of these encounters the microbial presence in or on the tissues is transitory and the microorganism is unable to replicate or is destroyed by host defense mechanisms. In other instances the microorganism is able to successfully attach to host tissues and begin to grow.

The infectivity of bacteria is related to their ability to attach to tissue; adherence to host cells is an essential step in pathogenesis. Initial contact between bacteria and the host cell is the result of nonspecific electrostatic forces which bring the microbe close to the cell surface. Firm irreversible chemical bonds then form between bacterial surface structures (adhesins) and complementary receptor molecules on host cell surfaces. Bacterial adhesins may be extracellular polysaccharides that act as a slime layer, or lectinlike proteins with a high affinity for carbohydrates on the host cell surface. Pili (fimbriae) are filamentous structures projecting from the bacterial cell wall and containing lipoteichoic acid or protein. The adherence of many species of bacteria to host cells is mediated by pili. Many host cells have a coating of glycoproteins such as laminin or fibronectin that are involved in the binding of some bacterial species to the cell surface. Viruses, fungi, and mycoplasmas have special mechanisms for attachment to cells. These are described in detail in chapters devoted to those organisms.

The establishment of replicating microorganisms in or on the tissues of the host without producing tissue damage is called **colonization.** Infants are colonized at the time of birth. Colonization may be permanent or periodic, the colonizing species persisting for weeks or months. Colonization may be influenced by environmental and personal contacts such as admission to a hospital or membership in a closed population, like a military training camp. Although colonization does not always proceed to clinical infection, it is invariably the first stage in the development of a clinical infection. Various factors in the resistance of the host determine the consequence of colonization.

LOCALIZATION AND DISSEMINATION

Some microorganisms are confined to the epithelial surfaces, unable to penetrate into the deeper tissues. Certain species are unable to replicate at 37° C. Rhinoviruses are limited to the surface membranes of the upper respiratory tract where the temperature is about 33° C. Similarly, *Mycobacterium marinum* and *M. ulcerans* grow at 31° C and consequently the lesions they produce are limited to the skin. The dermatophytic fungi are restricted to the cornified epithelium by their dependence upon keratin. Other species can pass the epithelial layer, penetrate the basement membrane, and reach the subepithelial tissues. This ability to penetrate and spread is often due to the production of extracellular enzymes (lipase, collagenase, DNAse, IgA protease, hyaluronidase) by the microbial invader.

In the subepithelial tissues the organism becomes exposed to host defenses such as phagocytic cells, tissue fluids, and specific immunoglobulins. Subsequent spread of the microorganism throughout the tissues may be by direct extension to adjacent structures, or the microbes might reach distant body sites via the lymphatics or bloodstream.

Certain organisms demonstrate distinct tissue tropisms. *Neisseria meningitidis* has a predilection for the meninges; *Bordetella pertussis* grows only in the ciliated epithelium of the tracheobronchial tree.

BACTERIAL GROWTH IN THE HOST

Bacteria replicating within the body of the host exhibit significantly different behavior than when growing in the laboratory in broth or on agar. In laboratory media there is an abundance of nutrients, and growth is planktonic (cells freely suspended in the medium) and rapid. In the body nutrients are not as readily available, e.g., one limiting factor in in vivo growth may be the availability of free ionic iron. Under these conditions of limited nutrition, many bacteria produce a mass of tangled fibers of polysaccharides that form a matrix surrounding the bacterial cell. This matrix or glycocalyx adheres to other bacteria and to surfaces of tissues to form a

biofilm. Sessile (attached) bacteria growing within the biofilm grow more slowly than in vitro, and their morphology and chemical composition differ from the same species growing in laboratory media. The biofilm tends to concentrate nutrients and the bacteria enjoy protection from the host's phagocytic cells, antibodies, and even antimicrobial agents. Some bacteria lose their virulence when cultivated repeatedly on laboratory media; in many cases virulence is regained when the organism is transferred from mammalian host to host. In certain cases the loss of virulence is associated with the loss of a protective capsule on prolonged subculture on laboratory media.

PATHOGENETIC MECHANISMS

Microorganisms can produce tissue damage expressed as disease affecting one or more organ systems. Tissue damage may occur by several means, including inflammation, alterations in cellular function or metabolism, or immunomodulation.

INDUCTION OF INFLAMMATION

Microorganisms and microbial products such as toxins can activate the production of white blood cells, primarily neutrophils, via interleukin-1, a potent hormonelike polypeptide. The local inflammatory reaction is characterized by redness, swelling, heat, and pain. Pus, a mixture of exudate, bacteria, and living and dead white blood cells, is often present. The pus may be present as a walled-off collection (abscess). Inflammation may lead to scar formation and organ destruction or dysfunction. Interleukin-1 can also stimulate prostaglandins and other interleukins which act on the thermoregulatory center producing fever. Other actions of interleukin-1 include shock, intravascular coagulation, and other pathophysiologic activities (Fig 2–1).

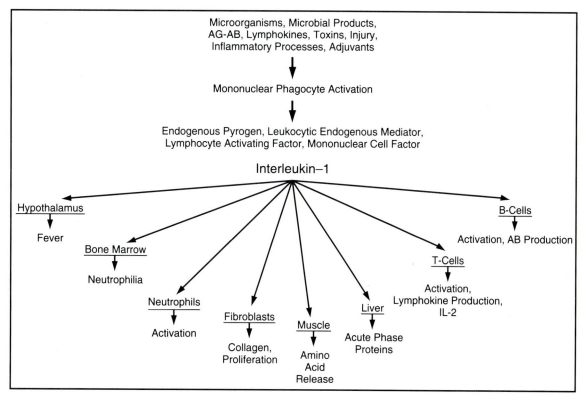

FIG 2–1.
Biological activities of interleukin = 1. (Redrawn from Dinarello CA: *N Engl J Med* 1984; 311:1413. Used by permission.)

ALTERATION OF CELLULAR FUNCTION OR METABOLISM

Intracellular organisms such as viruses, rickettsia or chlamydia, or toxins can cause direct damage to cells leading to organ dysfunction. The enterotoxins of *Vibrio cholerae* and *Escherichia coli* act on adenylate cyclase causing altered water and electrolyte excretion resulting in acute diarrhea.

IMMUNOMODULATION

Rhinoviruses, frequent agents of the common cold, induce local anaphylaxis in the nasal mucosa, causing the well-known symptoms. Delayed-type hypersensitivity occurs in tuberculosis, syphilis, and fungal infections and is responsible for some of the lesions characteristic of those diseases. Formation of immune complexes and their deposition on the basement membrane of the glomerulus is the pathogenetic mechanism of poststreptococcal glomerulonephritis. Severe immunodeficiency is the result of infection with the human immunodeficiency virus HIV-1 in the acquired immunodeficiency syndrome (AIDS).

HOST RESISTANCE TO INFECTION

Most infections in normal persons are self-limited, owing to a constellation of immune mechanisms that constitute the resistance of the host. These defenses are of two types: **innate im-**

munity, in which host resistance is not influenced by repeated infection; and **adaptive immunity,** characterized by increasingly effective resistance following repeated exposure to a microbe or its products.

INNATE MECHANISMS OF HOST RESISTANCE

The first lines of defense against the establishment of pathogenic microbes in the host are the mechanical barriers provided by the intact skin and mucous membranes, and the specialized mechanisms that have evolved in the eyes and the respiratory, gastrointestinal, and genitourinary tracts, where the mucocutaneous junction provides a possible pathway for infection. The flushing action of tears, urine, and saliva, the stickiness of mucus which entraps bacteria, and the expulsive mechanisms of the cilia of the respiratory tract, coupled with the cough reflex, all provide impediments to the entrance of microorganisms.

The indigenous microflora of the skin, vagina, and gastrointestinal tract has been described in Chapter 1. These organisms discourage adherence and colonization by pathogens by occupying available sites, competing for nutrients, and by exerting one or more forms of bacterial interference that inhibit the pathogen. This interference may involve the production of antibiotic substances or the elaboration of bacteriocins (proteins produced by one species that inhibit other strains of the same species). On the skin some pathogens are inhibited by toxic fatty acids produced by the action of the indigenous cutaneous bacteria on skin lipids. The predominantly gram-negative bowel flora further contribute to host defenses by providing an endotoxin pool in the intestine, which helps to maintain the lymphoid tissue and the reticuloendothelial system in an active state. It has recently been shown that indigenous bacteria from cervical, vaginal, and urethral surfaces adhere to uroepithelial cells and competitively exclude uropathogens by blocking their attachment.

Numerous biochemical factors also play an important role in the primary defense against infection. Bile and the low pH of the stomach and vagina are markedly inhibitory to the growth of many pathogens. Tears, saliva, and other secretions contain lysozyme, a basic protein enzyme that dissolves the cell wall of some gram-positive bacteria. Tissues contain several basic peptides, heme compounds, and polyamines that have bactericidal properties.

The complement system is involved in the bactericidal property of blood, resistance to viruses and parasites, the action of opsonins, and the initiation of the acute inflammatory response. This system consists of a number of proteins normally present in serum in an inactive state. When activated, these proteins are involved in a series of reactions, resulting in the production of a number of biologically active products. The complement system may be activated by two major pathways: the classic pathway and the alternative pathway. The classic pathway is typically activated by the reaction of antibody and antigen, while the alternative pathway may be activated by surface constituents of certain bacteria and fungi. An important end product of both pathways is complement fragment C3b (heat-labile opsonin), which provokes phagocytosis and promotes the attachment of phagocytic leukocytes to sensitized particles.

Microbial invasion provokes a cluster of responses known collectively as the **acute phase response.** One of the first reactions is a rapid migration of phagocytic cells of the reticuloendothelial system, derived from bone marrow stem cells, to the infection site. A fundamental event in the initiation of the acute phase response is the production of the mediator molecule **interleukin-1,** a polypeptide produced from macrophages, lymphocytes, monocytes, fibroblasts, and other cells. Interleukin-1 enters the circulation and acts as a hormone, mediating the host's responses to infection and inflammation (see Fig 2–1). The migration of phagocytic cells into an inflammatory site is directed by a variety of chemotactic factors present in serum and activated by microbial products, antigen-antibody complexes, or enzymes from platelets or lymphocytes, mediated by interleukin-1.

The primary phagocytic cell is the polymorphonuclear neutrophil, which represents about 70% of the total white blood cells. These cells, which have a short life (6–7 hours), rush to the site of inflammation and ingest the invading bacteria. Phagocytosis is facilitated by specific antibodies called **opsonins,** as well as by nonspecific factors, such as certain components of complement. Phagocytosis via the activation of C3b is the critical factor; specific antibody is only needed when bacteria are protected with polysaccharide capsules. Ingestion of bacteria or other particulate material coated with C3b or specific antibody is promoted by fibronectin, a high-molecular-weight glycoprotein present on cell surfaces and in plasma.

Once bacteria or other particles are bound to the surface of the neutrophil, they are ingested into a vacuole called the **phagosome.** Following ingestion, the metabolism of the neutrophil is markedly increased with the consumption of molecular oxygen and the production of lactic acid and carbon dioxide. This respiratory burst is associated with oxidative intracellular killing mechanisms; the generation of superoxide anion by NADPH oxidase, followed by the production of bactericidal hydrogen peroxide by superoxide dismutase, and the oxidation of chloride and iodide anions by myeloperoxidase to form hypochlorite ions, which are also bactericidal. The phagocytic vacuole fuses with lysosomal granules of the neutrophil to produce a **phagolysosome** in which microorganisms are subjected to additional nonoxidative killing mechanisms that include acid production to pH 3.0; lysozyme, which degrades the bacterial cell wall; lactoferrin, which binds iron required for bacterial

growth; bactericidal cationic proteins; and several cysteine-rich peptides (defensins) with a broad spectrum of antimicrobial action against bacteria, fungi, and some viruses.

The neutrophil response is followed by a migration of lymphoid cells, predominantly lymphocytes and monocytes, from blood vessels. Monocytes develop into macrophages, which are relatively long-lived and multiply in the tissues, actively engulfing and digesting bacteria. If large bodies or "indigestible" bacteria are present, these cells may fuse to form foreign body giant cells. These cells not only ingest and kill microorganisms but are also capable of producing a variety of substances such as complement components, interferons, transferrin, etc., that contribute to microbial destruction.

The lymphoid cells and macrophages may eventually develop into fibroblasts, which in turn wall off foreign bodies. Regional lymph nodes tend to filter out bacteria seeking to enter the bloodstream. Should microorganisms succeed in reaching the bloodstream they are rapidly cleared by the activities of the reticuloendothelial system in spleen, liver, bone marrow, and to some extent by the lungs and kidneys.

In addition to leukocytosis, other manifestations of the acute phase response include fever, depressed levels of serum iron and zinc, elevation of serum copper, and increased synthesis of acute phase proteins by the liver. One of these proteins, **C-reactive protein,** is important in the binding of bacteria and fungi to phagocytic cells, facilitates phagocytosis, and activates complement.

Interferons are antiviral glycoproteins produced by monocytes, lymphocytes, epithelial cells, and other cell types in response to viral infection. Other factors, such as bacterial products, endotoxin, and RNA, can also stimulate these cells to produce interferons. Interferons induce virus-infected cells to synthesize a protein that inhibits the synthesis of viral protein. In addition to inhibiting viral replication in infected cells, interferons protect uninfected cells against the virus. Interferons may also activate **natural killer cells**—leukocytes that can recognize viral-infected cells by alterations in their cell surface, bind to these target cells, and kill them.

Fever is another manifestation of the acute phase response and is initiated by the activation of macrophages by infection, various bacterial products and toxins, and by immunologic reactions. The activated macrophages produce interleukin-1, which acts on the anterior hypothalamic endothelium, causing increased synthesis of prostaglandin E and other metabolites of arachidonic acid. These substances affect the thermoregulatory neurons, resulting in muscle contraction and increased heat production, but more importantly, vasoconstriction and heat conservation.

Another innate defense mechanism against infection is **iron withholding.** Host defense iron-binding proteins, transferrin and lactoferrin, are produced in response to acute or chronic infection and limit the availability of free iron to pathogenic microorganisms, limiting the growth of these species.

ADAPTIVE IMMUNE MECHANISMS

Specific immunity can be categorized into two components: the **B lymphocyte system,** associated with the production of specific immunoglobulins; and the **T lymphocyte system,** associated with cell-mediated immunity. Both systems are activated by the antigenic stimulus of infection or artificial immunization and play an active role in immunity. Both components are interdependent. In brief, antigens are "processed" in monocytes or macrophages. Accessory T cells recognize the antigen and become T helper cells which activate B cells. B cells are produced in the bone marrow and migrate to lymph nodes, spleen, and other organs. The activated B lymphocytes differentiate into plasma cells which produce the various classes of immunoglobulins.

These include: IgG, the major antibody of the secondary response, accounting for 70% to 75% of the total immunoglobulins and capable of crossing the placental barrier; IgM, composing 10% of immunoglobulins, the first antibody formed and the most effective in activating complement and phagocytosis; and IgA, representing 15% to 20% of immunoglobulins, and the class that predominates in saliva, colostrum, milk, and is present on mucous membranes as secretory IgA. Induction of secretory IgA (SIgA) occurs when B lymphocytes are stimulated by antigen presented to the lymphoid tissue of the mucosa. SIgA is produced by plasma cells of the submucosa and glandular stroma and is largely responsible for the immune protection of large areas of mucosal surfaces. SIgA limits the entrance and adherence of microorganisms to the mucosa, and neutralizes toxins and viruses. IgD accounts for less than 1% of the antibody pool, but its function is not known. IgE is present in trace amounts and triggers eosinophils and basophils to release histamine and enzymes. This antibody may be involved in eliminating helminthic parasites, and is associated with immediate hypersensitivity reactions.

HOST FACTORS PREDISPOSING TO INFECTION

Breaks in the intact skin or mucous membrane following trauma (accidental or surgical) or extensive burns provide a means whereby microorganisms can gain entrance to normally sterile tissues.

The flushing action of urine may be impeded by prostatic hypertrophy, renal calculi, or congenital abnormalities; tears and saliva may be decreased in Sjögren's syndrome (a condition characterized by chronic arthritis, "dry" mouth and eyes). Prolonged high-dose antimicrobial therapy can eliminate much of the indigenous flora and predispose to infection by resistant bacteria or fungi.

Agranulocytosis associated with bone marrow failure, which may be secondary to radiation, corticosteroid therapy, or treatment with the cytotoxic or antimetabolite agents used in neoplastic disease, results in impaired response of phagocytic cells. Persons whose white blood cell count falls below 1,000/mm^3 are severely at risk for infection.* The most common infections in these neutropenic patients are bacterial. A decrease in the numbers of functional leukocytes is also seen in acute leukemia and Hodgkin's disease. Impaired microbiocidal activity of neutrophils may be seen in patients with chronic granulomatous disease of childhood, Chédiak-Higashi syndrome, or deficiencies of myeloperoxidase. A poor immune response is seen in hypogammaglobulinemia, altered splenic function secondary to splenectomy or sickle cell anemia; nephrotic syndrome; neoplastic diseases such as lymphatic leukemia, lymphosarcoma, or multiple myeloma; or therapy with antineoplastic drugs. These patients are particularly susceptible to recurrent infections due to encapsulated pyogenic cocci and *Haemophilus influenzae.* Diminished cell-mediated immunity occurs in allograft recipients (kidney, heart, bone marrow, etc.). Infections that occur in this group of patients are often caused by intracellular organisms such as *Listeria, Salmonella, Brucella, Mycobacterium tuberculosis, Candida, Toxoplasma, Pneumocystis carinii,* and the herpes group of viruses.

Chilling, interference with the blood supply by vascular occlusion, or exsanguination, all tend to depress the inflammatory reaction, and consequently increase the susceptibility to infection. Certain underlying diseases, such as cirrhosis, diabetes, alcoholism, and AIDS, predispose to infection by impairment of multiple defense mechanisms.

Foreign bodies, such as splinters, bullets, sutures, indwelling urinary or vascular catheters, prostheses, and other implanted medical devices, are targets for infection. These metal or plastic materials often undergo some degree of surface decomposition releasing breakdown products such as metallic ions or plasticizers that stimulate irritative tissue reactions resulting in some degree of chronic inflammation. Body fluids such as fibrin and fibronectin are deposited on the surface of these objects forming a biofilm. These substances as well as the surface charge, hydrophobicity, and degree of roughness provide receptors for bacterial adherence. These devices are readily colonized during placement or by a subsequent bacteremic episode. Bacteria attach by mechanisms previously described, and grow in and on the biofilm which protects the bacteria from serum bactericidal substances and even antimicrobial agents. Foreign bodies are covered with macrophages, but these cells are unable to ingest the bacteria within the biofilm. Bacterial microcolonies develop, break off from the device, and cause infection of the adjacent tissue.

CONSEQUENCES OF MICROBE-HOST INTERACTION

Every attempt by a microorganism to infect the host is not necessarily successful. In many cases the microorganism fails to penetrate the outer defenses of the host, and in other cases where penetration is achieved the microorganism is rapidly eliminated. In those cases where infection is accomplished the outcome is not always disease. The infecting organism can enter into a symbiotic relationship with the host and may elicit an immune response. As a result of this immune response the organism may be eliminated, or the extent of the infection curtailed, resulting in attenuated infection. Should the infection become progressive, reversible or irreversible pathologic changes in the host may follow, resulting in chronic disease or death of the host. Reversible pathologic changes may also

*Normal white blood cell (WBC) count is 5,000 to 10,000/mm^3.

induce attenuation of the infection, eradication of the infection, immunity, or any combination of these. Thus, it can be seen that interaction between host and parasite usually results in attenuated infection; this is the rule in nature and progressive infection and disease are comparatively rare.

From the standpoint of the infecting agent, there are considerably more advantages in establishing an attenuated infection than a lethal infection. As long as the host remains healthy, food and living space are available and reproduction can proceed, although on a limited scale. Should reproduction proceed unchecked and progressive infection occur, the death of the host invariably results in the death of the parasite.

Possible outcomes of the host's encounter with a microorganism include:

1. No infection: The organism lacks sufficient virulence or numbers to cause infection and is promptly shed or eliminated.

2. Colonization: The organism is able to become established in the body but cannot invade or produce pathologic tissue changes because of the host defenses.

3. Inapparent infection: The host never becomes clinically ill, but antibody synthesis occurs with resultant immunity, or the host becomes an asymptomatic carrier.

4. Clinical (overt) infection, the result of which may be recovery with immunity or susceptibility to reinfection.

5. Death may be due to the infection itself, to noninfectious sequelae of infectious disease, or to associated underlying illness.

Death due to the infection itself may be classified as early—occurring within the first 48 hours—and late. Early deaths are associated with a sudden acute onset of disease and are known to occur in acute fulminant meningococcemia, septicemia due to gram-negative bacteria, staphylococci, pneumococci, or hemolytic streptococci. Acute fulminant death has also been associated with disseminated tuberculosis, pneumonic plague, pulmonary anthrax, and melioidosis. Such deaths are usually assumed to be due to an overwhelming toxemia, although in most cases the actual toxins have yet to be isolated and characterized.

Late deaths in infection are essentially the result of organ destruction or dysfunction. Renal function may be markedly impaired in shock due to clostridial or gram-negative infections; chronic renal insufficiency may develop in pyelonephritis; cardiac insufficiency in bacterial endocarditis; tamponade in tuberculous pericarditis; hepatic failure in hepatitis or leptospirosis; electrolyte imbalance in cholera or staphylococcal enteritis; and pulmonary insufficiency in massive pneumonia.

Death due to noninfectious sequelae of infectious disease may be due to amyloidosis, postinfectious encephalomyelitis, rheumatic heart disease, or hemorrhagic glomerulonephritis. Examples of death due to underlying associated illnesses are pneumonia in patients with emphysema, or infections in patients with diabetes or Addison's disease.

FACTORS INFLUENCING THE MICROBE-HOST RELATIONSHIP

A dynamic equilibrium can be considered to exist between the microorganisms in the environment (including the normal resident flora) and the varying state of resistance of the host. This equilibrium may be upset in two ways: the host may come into contact with a primary pathogen of considerable virulence, or the resistance of the host may become impaired, permitting infection by opportunists. It is important to emphasize that neither the host factors nor the microbial factors described are stable. Both are subject to change, and indeed, both are constantly changing. The microbe-host relationship is a balanced state, and changes in the characteristics of the microorganism or in the resistance of the host can disturb this delicately poised balance.

Microorganisms may undergo phenotypic or genotypic changes. These changes may be in host range, growth requirements, pathogenicity, and virulence toward a particular host, or changes in the site of preferential multiplication and organ tropism. Rapid passage, as in epidemics, frequently is responsible for an increase in virulence. Immunologic stress can influence strain variation. In the latter stages of an epidemic with the emergence of an immune population, the trend is for the infection to become attenuated and to produce progressively milder disease. Thus, the variation in the susceptibility of the population involves changes in both the host and the microbe.

With respect to the host, the genetic constitution is extremely important. Persons with blood group P are more susceptible to pyelonephritis caused by *E. coli* strains possessing P fimbriae than persons with other blood groups. There is a continuous selective process by which a species ultimately acquires immunity to a specific infection. These considerations are more significant in populations than in individuals. For example, people with the sickle cell trait have a marked resistance to malaria.

The physiologic state of the host is an important consideration in resistance. Factors include:

1. Age: Most infectious diseases are more severe at the extremes of life. The immature infant appears to be more susceptible to peritonitis, partly because of the relative shortness of the omentum. Antibody production is relatively inefficient and does not reach the adult level until about 6 years of age. Changes in the blood-brain barrier and the cerebral blood vessels occur with increasing age, and these changes are correlated to some extent with increased resistance to bacterial meningitis.

2. Nutritional state: In malnutrition with its attendant avitaminoses and decreased protein intake, antibody production may be inadequate. While little precise data are available concerning the role of altered nutritional states, the general observation is that affected persons show a decreased resistance to certain bacterial infections.

Hormonal factors that occur during pregnancy or prolonged exposure to the crowding and stress associated with war or natural disasters may also predispose to decreased resistance to infectious diseases.

ADDITIONAL READING

Roth JA (ed): *Virulence Mechanisms of Bacterial Pathogens.* Washington, DC, American Society for Microbiology, 1988.

Urbaschek B (ed): *Perspectives on Bacterial Pathogenesis and Host Defense.* Chicago, University of Chicago Press, 1988.

PART II

Respiratory Tract Infections

CHAPTER 3

Overview of Upper Respiratory Tract Infections

The upper respiratory tract includes the nose, pharynx, sinuses, middle ear, and larynx. The nose and throat are normally colonized with an indigenous flora that is primarily gram-positive (diphtheroids) and coagulase-negative staphylococci. Pneumococci, *Staphylococcus aureus*, *Moraxella*, and *Haemophilus* species may also be present. Anaerobic bacteria (*Bacteroides*, fusobacteria, anaerobic cocci) outnumber the aerobic flora by 10:1. The nasal sinuses, middle ear, larynx, and trachea are usually sterile.

The majority of nose and throat infections are acquired from exogenous sources: sick persons or healthy carriers. Transmission is via infected secretions transferred by direct hand-to-hand contact or by respiratory aerosols produced by sneezing, coughing, etc. and result from the intrusion of pharyngeal organisms into those normally sterile sites.

Important defense mechanisms of the upper respiratory tract are the tonsillar and adenoidal lymphoid tissue (Waldeyer's ring) and the presence of secretory IgA (SIgA) on the pharyngeal mucosa. Infections of the upper respiratory tract include the common cold (coryza, rhinitis), pharyngitis, sinusitis, and otitis media (middle ear in-

fection). They are summarized in Table 3–1. Frequently, several sites are simultaneously infected, e.g., nose, throat, and sinuses.

COLDS

Colds are caused by a variety of viruses, the most common being rhinoviruses (25%–30%) and coronaviruses (10%). There are more than 100 different serotypes of rhinoviruses. Other viral agents are influenza and parainfluenza (10%–15%), respiratory syncytial, echo-, adeno-, and coxsackieviruses. There is a distinct seasonal variation in viral etiology; spring, summer, and fall colds are usually rhino-, echo-, and coxsackievirus infections, while colds occurring in the late fall and winter are frequently due to influenza, parainfluenza, and respiratory syncytial viruses. The main reservoir of these organisms is in young children.

Transmission, once thought to be exclusively by respiratory droplet infection, is now known to also occur via hand-to-hand transmission of infected nasal secretions. After an incubation period of 2 to 3 days there is the onset of

TABLE 3–1.

Summary of Upper Respiratory Infections

Infection	Etiology	Source	Transmission	Diagnostic Procedure
Common cold	Rhinovirus Corona viruses	Exogenous (young children)	Respiratory aerosols hand to hand	Clinical
Pharyngitis	Respiratory viruses Group A streptococcus *Mycoplasma pneumoniae* Other bacteria	Exogenous (asymptomatic carriers and sick persons)	Respiratory aerosols hand to hand	Throat culture Direct antigen detection for group A streptococcus
Sinusitis	*Streptococcus pneumoniae* Nontypable *Haemophilus influenzae* *Moraxella*	Endogenous (nasopharyngeal flora)	—	Clinical
Otitis media	*S. pneumoniae* Nontypable *H. influenzae* *Moraxella*	Endogenous (nasopharyngeal flora)	—	Clinical
Epiglottitis	*H. influenzae* type b	Exogenous	Respiratory aerosols?	Clinical
Croup	Parainfluenza viruses	Exogenous	Respiratory aerosols?	Clinical

the characteristic symptoms of sneezing, nasal discharge, and obstruction and coughing, which last 1 to 2 weeks.

In the United States the highest incidence is during the colder months. Adults average two to four colds per year; children average six to eight. Immunity is serotype-specific. Colds are usually self-limited, but bacterial superinfection is common and often leads to the development of sinusitis or otitis media. Specific antibiotic treatment for uncomplicated colds is not indicated unless there is evidence of a bacterial infection.

PHARYNGITIS

About half of all cases of pharyngitis are caused by respiratory viruses (adenoviruses, 25%; rhinoviruses, 20%; echo-, coxsackie-, Epstein-Barr, and cytomegalovirus, less than 1% each). Group A streptococci are responsible for 15% to 30% of cases. There is both an age and a seasonal variation in the incidence of streptococ-

cal pharyngitis; streptococci account for 5% to 10% of cases of pharyngitis in the summer, and for 25% of cases in the winter and early spring. Streptococcal pharyngitis is uncommon in children under 3 years of age; the peak incidence is in 3- to 18-year-olds. Other less common causes of pharyngitis are *Mycoplasma pneumoniae, Corynebacterium diphtheriae; Neisseria gonorrhoeae, Arcanobacterium hemolyticum, Chlamydia pneumoniae,* and the mixed anaerobic bacteria associated with Vincent's angina. It is important to distinguish streptococcal pharyngitis since treatment can prevent extension of the infection to adjacent tissues, shorten the course of the disease, reduce the possibility of rheumatic fever, and deter the spread to other persons. Rapid diagnosis of streptococcal pharyngitis can often be made in a few minutes by direct antigen detection from a throat swab. If the test is positive, treatment can be initiated immediately. A negative direct antigen test should be confirmed by a throat culture when clinical suspicion exists.

SINUSITIS

Sinusitis refers to inflammation within the paranasal sinuses (Fig 3–1). Sinus infection is associated with headache, facial pain, and a mucopurulent nasal discharge. The maxillary sinus is most frequently involved, the frontal and ethmoidal sinuses less frequently; the sphenoidal sinus is seldom infected. Sinusitis may follow viral infections (colds), allergic rhinitis, diving, all of which interfere with drainage and cause bacte-

rial contamination of the sinuses with bacteria normally present in the healthy throat. Other predisposing factors may be congenital or acquired obstruction or facial fractures.

Acute sinusitis is predominantly bacterial with *Streptococcus pneumoniae* or nontypable *Haemophilus influenzae* causing almost half of all infections. Other organisms occasionally recovered are *Moraxella (Branhamella) catarrhalis*, group A streptococci, and *S. aureus*. Viruses (rhinoviruses, influenza and parainfluenza vi-

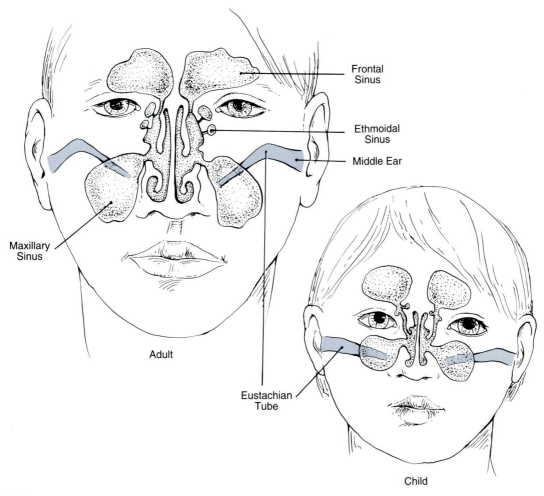

Frontal Sinus

Ethmoidal Sinus

Middle Ear

Maxillary Sinus

Adult

Eustachian Tube

Child

FIG 3–1.
The paranasal sinuses.

ruses) are found in about 20% of cases, often together with bacteria. Chronic sinusitis is usually polymicrobial, with one or more anaerobic species recovered. The diagnosis of sinusitis is clinical, based upon physical examination, transillumination, and x-ray studies. Treatment is empirical, utilizing antibiotics effective against the common causative bacterial agents.

OTITIS MEDIA

Otitis media is the most common disease for which infants and children seek health care. Approximately 10% of infants have an episode of middle ear infection by 3 months of age; the peak incidence is between 6 and 36 months, but the infection is also seen in adults. Otitis media occurs when organisms from the nasopharynx enter the middle ear compartment via the eustachian tube. Symptoms are ear pain, decreased auditory activity, and fever. Otoscopic examination often reveals a red bulging tympanic membrane.

The microbiology of otitis media is predominantly bacterial and resembles that of sinusitis. The major organisms are *S. pneumoniae* (30%) and nontypable *H. influenzae* (20%). *Moraxella (Branhamella) catarrhalis* is recovered from about 10% to 15% of cases, and S. *aureus* and group A streptococci from about 2% each. Viruses have been isolated from about 30% of cases, often together with bacteria. The inflammatory reaction provoked within the middle ear results in the production of exudate which obstructs the eustachian tube. Chronic otitis media

is invariably polymicrobic with *S. aureus*, *Pseudomonas aeruginosa*, and several anaerobic species such as *Peptococcus* and *Bacteroides*. Complications of otitis media include mastoiditis, labyrinthitis leading to vertigo or hearing loss, and meningitis. As in the case of sinusitis, the diagnosis of otitis media is based upon clinical examination, and treatment is the empirical use of antibiotics directed against the common bacterial agents of this infection. In refractory cases, fluid may be aspirated by tympanocentesis and cultured to determine the antimicrobial susceptibility of the organism(s) present.

EPIGLOTTITIS

Epiglottitis is an uncommon acute infection of the supraglottic area in young children, causing respiratory obstruction. It rarely occurs in elderly males with chronic lung disease. The most common cause is *H. influenzae* type b. The organisms probably reach the epiglottis by direct extension from the nasopharynx, but are also present in the bloodstream. The resulting inflammatory response of the supraglottic tissue is accompanied by edema. The onset of acute epiglottitis is abrupt, symptoms occurring within a few hours. The diagnosis is based upon physical examination. *Haemophilus influenzae* is usually recovered from blood cultures. Treatment consists of establishing an airway and administering an antibiotic effective against *H. influenzae*. *Croup* is a similar infection, usually caused by parainfluenza viruses.

CHAPTER 4

Respiratory Viruses

A 35-year-old salesman became ill the day after attending his office Christmas party. He had previously been in good health, but awoke with fever of 38.8° C, a severe headache, and aching muscles, especially in his back. Later that day he developed a "runny" nose, mild sore throat, and a dry cough. Over the next few days his fever gradually decreased but his cough worsened. After a week he returned to work, but complained of feeling weak and tired for the next 2 weeks. Since there were reports of influenza in the community, it was assumed to be the diagnosis in his case. By the third week he had completely recovered.

The common respiratory viruses include the influenza viruses, parainfluenza viruses, respiratory syncytial virus, rhinoviruses, coronaviruses, and adenoviruses. Other viruses such as echoviruses, coxsackieviruses, and measles virus may also cause respiratory infection; they are described later.

INFLUENZA VIRUSES

Influenza is an acute respiratory infection characterized by fever, chills, headache, myalgia, coryza, sore throat, and severe and protracted cough. Retro-orbital pain is a common symptom. Recovery is in 2 to 7 days in uncomplicated cases. Secondary bacterial pneumonia is a serious complication. Influenza virus can also cause common colds, croup, or pneumonia in children.

Influenza viruses are members of the orthomyxovirus group. The genome is composed of eight different negative (−)-strand molecules of RNA, associated with nucleoprotein. The genome is enclosed in an M protein matrix surrounded by a glycolipid envelope. This lipid bilayer is derived from the host cell membrane. Projecting from the surface of the virus particle are glycoprotein spikes, each spike consisting of several peptide chains. These spikes have two distinct activities, hemagglutinin* and neuraminidase, which determine the antigenic speci-

*Hemagglutinin has the ability to agglutinate chicken and guinea pig erythrocytes.

ficity of the virus, and also play a role in viral attachment to host cells.

There are three types of influenza viruses: A, B, and C. Type A is associated with pandemics and epidemics, type B causes more limited epidemics, and type C is seen in sporadic cases. New subtypes frequently appear, owing in part to the multiplicity of the RNA molecules. Subtypes (strains) of type A are described by the type of hemagglutinin (H) and neuraminidase (N) antigens, and by the country and year of origin. An example would be A/Hong Kong/1/68 ($H_3 N_2$). The appearance of these new subtypes is referred to as **antigenic shift** or **drift.** In recent years pandemics have occurred, in 1947, 1957, and 1968. In the United States epidemics of type A influenza occur every 1 to 3 years. The attack rate may reach 25%.

Although the influenza virus can attack horses, swine, and birds, man is the main reservoir of human infection. Transmission is by the transfer of respiratory secretions by direct hand-to-hand contact or via the inhalation of respiratory aerosols produced by sneezing, coughing, etc.

Upon reaching the respiratory mucosa, the viral particles bind to host cell surface receptors via the hemagglutinin. The virus enters the columnar epithelial cells and is enclosed in the phagosome where the envelope is digested. The acidic environment of the phagosome alters the peptide sequence of the hemagglutinin and the viral membrane fuses with the lysosomal membrane permitting release of the nucleocapsid into the cytoplasm. Viral replication occurs in the nucleus, but final virus assembly takes place at the plasma membrane. The nucleocapsid is enveloped by the plasma membrane containing the hemagglutinin and neuraminidase, and intact virus is formed and "buds" off of the cell surface. Neuraminidase appears to function in mediating viral envelope and host membrane fusion, and also facilitates the release of viral particles from the infected cell.

Infected cells lyse releasing enzymes that provide an inflammatory response that is predominantly mononuclear. These cells in turn release interferon and interleukin-1 which are responsible for some of the generalized symptoms of influenza.

Antibodies (IgG and IgA) directed against the hemagglutinin, neuraminidase, and ribonucleoprotein appear within a few days. The hemagglutinin antibody is the most protective, since it is able to neutralize viral infectivity. However antibodies are of relatively short duration (1–2 years) and are specific for the subtype. Vaccines are available, but new vaccine must be formulated each year as a result of antigenic shift. Influenza A may be treated with amantidine hydrochloride or simantidine, drugs which act by inhibiting viral uncoating or transcription of viral RNA.

A serious complication of influenza (and many other viral infections) is Reye's syndrome, which is characterized by neurologic manifestations such as obtundation, seizures or coma, and respiratory arrest, preceded by nausea and vomiting. The mortality is 10% to 40%. The pathophysiology of Reye's syndrome is not yet understood but it has been postulated that the viral infection may trigger some unknown toxic reaction.

The laboratory diagnosis of influenza can be made by isolating virus in cell culture, and by detecting rises in hemagglutinin inhibition antibody.

PARAINFLUENZA VIRUSES

Parainfluenza viruses are important causes of respiratory disease, especially in infants and young children. These viruses are responsible for 15% of childhood colds, croup, bronchitis, and pneumonia. The average duration of illness is 7 to 10 days.

Parainfluenza viruses are members of the

paramyxovirus group which also includes mumps, measles, and respiratory syncytial virus. Paramyxoviruses are characterized by a nucleocapsid containing RNA enclosed within a lipid-containing envelope derived from host cell membrane. Two different glycoproteins, HN and F, form spikelike projections from the surface of the envelope. There are five antigenic types of parainfluenza viruses; 1, 2, 3, 4A, and B. Types 1 and 2 cause colds, bronchitis, and croup in infants; type 3 can cause bronchitis, pneumonia, croup, and colds; types 4A and B cause mild disease in older children.

Parainfluenza infections peak in the fall and winter months. The reservoir is in infected persons and transmission is by transfer of infected respiratory secretions by direct hand-to-hand contact or by inhalation of respiratory aerosols.

Parainfluenza viruses attach to ciliated columnar epithelial cells by means of the neuraminidase activity of the HN spike which binds to a glycoprotein cell receptor. Penetration into the cell is mediated by the F spike which fuses viral and cell membranes. Viral replication is in the cytoplasm. The incubation time from entrance of the virus to the occurrence of symptoms is 3 days. Most adults have high levels of antibody to all types of parainfluenza virus, but low concentrations of IgA in respiratory secretions. Reinfection is common but usually is of a milder nature.

RESPIRATORY SYNCYTIAL VIRUS

Respiratory syncytial virus (RSV) is the most frequent cause of serious respiratory disease of infants and young children, expressed as bronchiolitis, pneumonia, or upper respiratory infections. RSV can also cause severe disease in adults, especially the elderly and the immunocompromised. Patients with underlying cardiac or pulmonary disease are also at risk. These infections are usually self-limited and last 10 to 14 days, but severe cases may require hospitalization as a result of cardiorespiratory failure or secondary bacterial pneumonia.

RSV is a paramyxovirus with a single-stranded negative-sense RNA genome enclosed in a protein envelope. There are two surface glycoproteins, G and F; G mediates attachment to host cell receptors, and F induces viral penetration and fusion of the envelope with the host surface membrane. The F glycoprotein also induces fusion of viral-infected cells resulting in syncytium formation characterized by multinucleated giant cells.

The reservoir of RSV is in older children. Transmission of infected respiratory secretions to the mouth, the eyes, or nose is primarily by direct hand-to-hand contact. The virus survives on surfaces. Outbreaks of RSV infection typically occur during fall, winter, and early spring in families with children and persist for 2 to 3 months. Nosocomial outbreaks in pediatric areas or nurseries are a major problem. The incubation period is about 5 days.

The virus replicates in ciliated epithelial cells and is generally confined to the middle and lower respiratory tract. The virus disrupts protein and nucleic acid synthesis leading to cell death and the release of various enzymes which activate complement and initiate a local inflammatory response. Necrotic cells, desquamate and together with mucus and fibrin, plug small airways. Otitis media is a common complication of RSV infection, particularly in infants, and may be due to the virus itself, or in combination with *Streptococcus pneumoniae* or other bacterial pathogens.

IgG and IgA antibodies are formed to the F and G proteins, but immunity is incomplete and repeated infections are common but less severe than the initial episode. Laboratory diagnosis of RSV may be made by isolating the virus in cell culture or by detection of viral antigens in a nasopharyngeal swab by rapid ELISA (*e*nzyme-*l*inked *i*mmunosorbent *a*ssay) or immunofluorescent methods.

RHINOVIRUSES

Rhinoviruses cause 25% to 30% of colds. They are members of the picornavirus group and are icosahedral in shape with four structural proteins and one positive (+)-strand RNA molecule. There is a cleft on the capsid surface believed to be the site of viral attachment to host cells. The optimal temperature for viral replication is 33 to 35° C, the ambient temperature of the nose and large airways. Very little growth occurs at 37° C and consequently disease is limited to the upper respiratory tract. There are more than 100 immunotypes of rhinoviruses.

The main reservoir of rhinoviruses is in school-children. Transmission is primarily via direct hand-to-hand transfer of infected nasal secretions. The recipient then inoculates his or her own nasal or conjunctival mucosa. Transmission can also occur by the inhalation of respiratory droplet aerosols from infected persons.

The virus binds to the epithelial cells of the nasal and conjunctival mucosa and spreads by direct extension. Viral synthesis takes place in the cytoplasm. Infected cells of the nasal mucosa release bradykinin and histamine, chemical mediators that cause the nasal mucosa to become edematous and hyperemic resulting in the thin watery discharge characteristic of early colds. The incubation period is about 2 days. The nasal discharge later becomes mucopurulent and contains many neutrophils. Infections last 7 to 10 days, and are more common in the fall and spring.

Immunity is type-specific and is associated with neutralizing antibodies (IgG and IgA) in the nasal secretions. All infections do not necessarily result in an antibody response.

CORONAVIRUSES

Coronaviruses attack a wide variety of animals including man. Human strains can cause acute respiratory disease, and gastroenteritis in infants. Coronaviruses may be responsible for 10% to 15% of colds, and can also cause pneumonia. The viral capsid contains three proteins: a surface glycoprotein thought to stimulate neutralizing antibody, a membrane glycoprotein, and an RNA protein complex. Viral synthesis occurs in the cytoplasm of host cells. Coronavirus infections occur more often in the winter and spring. The incubation period is about 3 days, and the duration of the illness is about 7 days. Reinfection is common, especially in children.

ADENOVIRUSES

Adenoviruses are the cause of 2% to 10% of acute febrile respiratory infections ranging from pharyngitis, sometimes accompanied by conjunctivitis, croup, or bronchiolitis in infants and young children, to acute respiratory disease and pneumonia in young adults.

Adenoviruses are naked, icosahedral, with a genome of double-stranded DNA. Fiberlike projections (pentons) are present at each of the 12 corners of the virus. There are more than 40 serotypes of adenoviruses that affect humans, classified into five subgroups (A–E). The reservoir of adenoviruses is in sick persons or asymptomatic carriers. Transmission may be by transfer of respiratory secretions or via the fecal-oral route.

Adenoviruses replicate in epithelial cells resulting in cell death and an inflammatory response of predominantly mononuclear cells. Viremia occurs with viral localization in lymphoid tissues (tonsils, Peyer's patches). The virus is latent in these tissues, but may be reactivated and shed at a later time. Immunity is serotype-specific and long-lasting.

CHAPTER 5

Streptococci

A 10-year-old boy presented with a sore throat of 2 days' duration and fever to 40° C. He had previously enjoyed good health until 2 days before being seen by the pediatrician. On that day he had no appetite for lunch or dinner; he said he felt weak and tired, and went to bed. He awoke the following morning complaining of a very sore throat, pain on swallowing, and a headache. His mother persuaded him to eat a little breakfast, but he complained of nausea and vomited shortly thereafter. On physical examination the pharynx, tonsils, and uvula were found to be "beefy-red" and edematous, and the tonsils were covered with exudate. The anterior cervical lymph nodes were swollen and tender. A throat culture was taken which grew out a hemolytic streptococcus, subsequently identified as group A. A 2-week course of oral penicillin was prescribed.

Streptococci are gram-positive cocci that typically occur in pairs or in chains, and lack the ability to produce the enzyme catalase (Fig 5–1). They are categorized by the type of hemolysis produced on blood agar (Fig 5–2), the na-ture of their cell wall antigens, and their biochemical characteristics.

Like Caesar's Gaul, streptococci are divided into three groups. The groups are based upon the appearance of the medium around the colonies when grown on blood agar. Colonies surrounded by a greenish zone are designated as *alpha* (α-hemolytic) streptococci; they include the viridans group and *Streptococcus pneumoniae.* Colonies of *beta* (β-hemolytic) streptococci are surrounded by a clear zone of complete hemolysis; this group includes the important pathogen *S. pyogenes* (Lancefield group A). Nonhemolytic *(gamma)* streptococci do not produce any apparent change in the medium surrounding their colonies. Some streptococci, particularly groups B and D, are difficult to classify by the above criteria because their reaction on blood agar is dependent upon the species of animal blood used to prepare the medium.

The β-hemolytic streptococci are classified into serologic Lancefield groups based upon the chemical nature of the cell wall carbohydrate (group-specific C carbohydrate). There are 15 groups, designated A–O; some of these groups are further subdivided into types (1, 2, 3, etc.) based upon cell wall protein antigens. Biochemical reactions are sometimes useful in characterizing some streptococci. Group A streptococci and enterococci produce the enzyme pyrogluta-

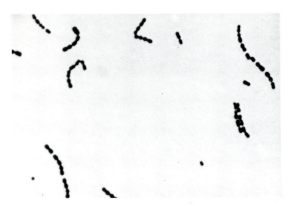

FIG 5–1.
Streptococci.

mate aminopeptidase; group B streptococci can hydrolyze hippurate; group D streptococci hydrolyze esculin and can grow in the presence of 40% bile.

The streptococci obtain energy by the fermentation of glucose to lactic acid. They are facultative anaerobes. Many species require a medium enriched by the addition of blood or serum. The optimal temperature for growth is 35 to 37° C. Colonies appear in about 24 hours and are relatively small (0.5–1.0 mm in diameter). The clinically important streptococci are summarized in Table 5–1.

With the exception of group A streptococci, all of the streptococci are members of the nor-

mal indigenous flora of mucous membranes of the upper respiratory, genitourinary, and gastrointestinal tracts. They are opportunists and only cause disease following some defect in the host's defenses. The group A streptococcus is a primary pathogen; otherwise healthy, immunocompetent persons exposed to this organism frequently become infected.

GROUP A STREPTOCOCCUS

The group A streptococcus (*S. pyogenes*) is primarily a human pathogen and is rarely associated with animal infections, excepting acute mastitis in cattle. The most common infections caused by this organism are pharyngitis and skin infections. Group A streptococcal infections are sometimes followed by nonsuppurative diseases (acute rheumatic fever or glomerulonephritis). The virulence and certain aspects of the pathogenesis of group A streptococcal infections are associated with some of the structural components of the organism and certain soluble toxic metabolites it produces.

STRUCTURAL COMPONENTS OF GROUP A STREPTOCOCCI

Freshly isolated strains of group A streptococci are covered with a hyaluronic acid capsule. While this capsular material is not antigenic (it resembles host hyaluronic acid), it contributes to the virulence of the organism by interfering with phagocytosis. Beneath the capsule is the cell wall, composed of a mosaic of proteins and a complex of peptidoglycan and the group-specific carbohydrate.

The most important protein is the **M protein**, since the virulence of group A streptococci is primarily related to this substance. The primary action of M protein is the inhibition of ingestion of the organism by phagocytic cells. M proteins have also been shown to exert an immunotoxic effect on platelets and polymor-

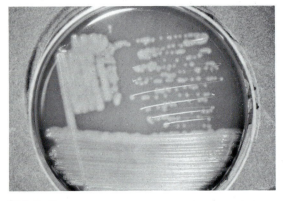

FIG 5–2.
Group A *streptococci* on blood agar.

TABLE 5–1.

Clinically Important Streptococci and Their Infections

Group A (*S. pyogenes*)	Pharyngitis, erysipelas, impetigo, septicemia, tissue and wound infections, rheumatic fever, glomerulonephritis
Group B	Neonatal, maternal, and cutaneous infections in diabetes
Groups C and G	Respiratory (pneumonia), puerperal sepsis, cutaneous infections
Group D (*S. bovis*) E. faecalis	Bacteremia associated with gastrointestinal cancer, urinary tract infections, bacteremia, endocarditis
S. pneumoniae (pneumococcus)	Pneumonia, sinusitis, otitis media, meningitis
Viridans group streptococci	Endocarditis, dental caries, liver, and brain abscesses

phonuclear neutrophils. The M proteins show a structural resemblance to alpha tropomyosin and show immunologic cross-reactivity with mammalian muscle. Hydrolysis of M protein reveals it to be composed of seven peptides, each with a type-specific determinant group. There are 60 serotypes of group A streptococci based upon the M protein. Groups C and G streptococci may have an M protein identical to the M protein of type 12 group A streptococcus. The production of M protein may be under extrachromosomal control (plasmid or prophage DNA).

The peptidoglycan group-specific carbohydrate complex makes up the remainder of the cell wall. The group-specific carbohydrate (C carbohydrate) is a simple polysaccharide composed of rhamnose and *N*-acetylglucosamine. This polysaccharide has been shown to cross-react with the glycoprotein present in heart valves. The peptidoglycan induces chronic granulomatous inflammatory lesions of dermal connective tissue; the polysaccharide component protects the peptidoglycan from digestion by tissue lysozyme. The peptidoglycan has many of the biologic features of the endotoxin of gram-negative bacteria; both materials induce fever

and shock, produce the Shwartzman reaction, and enhance nonspecific resistance to infection. The peptidoglycan-carbohydrate complex has been shown to cause suppression of specific and nonspecific stimulation of T cells in rats.

Another component of the cell wall is **lipoteichoic acid.** Filamentous structures (fimbriae), composed of lipoteichoic acid and M protein, extend from the cell wall through the hyaluronic acid capsule to the cell surface. These hairlike fibrils are involved in the attachment of group A streptococci to the epithelial cells of the host. The binding of lipoteichoic acid to host cells is mediated by the glycolipid end of the molecule, which can form ionic complexes with streptococcal surface protein (M protein), permitting the reorientation of the lipoteichoic acid to expose its lipid end toward the surface of the organism and free to interact with host cell membrane receptors. These cell membrane receptors appear to consist of a lipid-binding region on fibronectin, a glycoprotein on host cell membranes. Lipoteichoic acid also produces tissue injury, and specifically stimulates T lymphocytes. Beneath the cell wall is the cytoplasmic membrane. This material can suppress immature B cells in bone marrow.

EXTRACELLULAR PRODUCTS

Group A streptococci secrete at least 20 distinct antigens, some of which are toxins and enzymes, and may be involved in one or more aspects of disease production.

The pyrogenic exotoxins or **erythrogenic toxins** are proteins with a molecular weight of 29,000 daltons. Three erythrogenic toxins have been described, each immunologically distinct. About 90% of group A strains produce one or more of these toxins. Certain bacteriophages have the capacity to convert nontoxigenic strains to toxin producers. The erythrogenic toxins are rather potent; as little as 0.001 ng will produce local erythema in a sensitive person. The toxin enters the circulation and localizes in skin cells, producing the erythematous rash characteristic of scarlet fever.* In addition to skin reactivity, fever, and shock, tissue damage (particularly liver and myocardium) is produced. Other effects of the pyrogenic exotoxin are altered permeability of the blood-brain barrier, enhanced susceptibility to endotoxin shock, and modification of the immune response through an effect on T suppressor cells.

The cytolytic toxins or hemolysins include **streptolysin S,** which is produced in the presence of serum and is oxygen-stable, and **streptolysin O,** which does not require serum and is oxygen-labile. Streptolysin S is an unstable polypeptide associated with various carrier molecules. The carrier molecules induce the release of the active hemolysin from its cell-bound state. Streptolysin S is irreversibly bound to phospholipids of the red cell membrane, inducing cell lysis. Streptolysin S is also responsible for the leukotoxic properties of group A streptococci, in which neutrophils are killed after ingesting streptococci. Streptolysin S is produced by almost all strains of group A streptococci, as well as by groups C and B. Streptolysin S is nonimmunogenic. Despite the cytolytic effects of streptolysin S, there is no evidence that it is essential for virulence, nor is it involved in the pathogenesis of rheumatic fever.

Streptolysin O is one of a group of oxygen-labile hemolysins produced by gram-positive bacteria including *S. pneumoniae* (pneumolysin), *Clostridium perfringens* (theta toxin), and *Listeria monocytogenes*. They are single polypeptide chains, reversibly inactivated by atmospheric oxygen and requiring the presence of a thiol reducing agent for maximal expression of biologic activity. They produce membrane damage after binding to surface-exposed membrane cholesterol to form toxin-cholesterol complexes. In the case of streptolysin O, damaged membranes have been shown to exhibit large functional holes that allow for the passage of very large molecules. Streptolysin O lyses a wide range of mammalian cells, including erythrocytes, neutrophils, platelets, lysosomes, mitochondria, and various fixed tissue cells. When neutrophils are exposed to streptolysin O, the granules explode and discharge their contents into the cytoplasm which liquefies, resulting in cell death. Streptolysin O suppresses chemotaxis and the mobility of neutrophils and inhibits phagocytosis by macrophages. Streptolysin O is cardiotoxic, producing focal myocardial necrosis. Electrocardiographic changes indicate disruption of the conduction system. Streptolysin O may play a role in the pathogenesis of rheumatic fever by providing the initial injury to the myocardial cells, to be followed by immunologic damage. Most strains of group A streptococci produce streptolysin O. Patients with streptococcal pharyngitis develop a strong antibody response to streptolysin O, while persons with streptococcal skin infections have a weak or absent antistreptolysin O response. This difference may be explained by the large amounts of free cholesterol present in epidermal tissues.

Other nontoxic antigens elaborated by group

---

*Erythrogenic toxins are antigenic and are neutralized by specific antibodies. In vivo neutralization, i.e., blanching of the skin rash following intradermal injection of antiserum, is known as the Schultz-Charlton phenomenon (a risky procedure considering the potential for transfer of hepatitis B or HIV).

A streptococci include hyaluronidase, streptokinase, DNAses, and NADase. Hyaluronidase liquifies the hyaluronic acid component of the connective tissue matrix and facilitates the rapid spread of the infectious process through the dermis. Streptokinase and the DNAses may account for the serosanguineous nature of exudate, characteristic of group A streptococcal infections.

The reservoir of group A streptococci is largely in humans who are either infected with the organism or who are carriers. Many normal people are transient asymptomatic carriers of group A streptococci and harbor the organism in low numbers in their pharynx, vagina, anus, or in otherwise insignificant skin lesions. Transmission is by direct contact with a patient or carrier. Anal carriers have been responsible for nosocomial wound infections. Outbreaks of streptococcal pharyngitis may follow the ingestion of contaminated milk, milk products, or eggs. The incubation period is 1 to 3 days.

GROUP A INFECTIONS

Pharyngitis

About 25% of sore throats are due to hemolytic streptococcal infection. Invariably, group A streptococcus is the etiologic agent, rarely other groups, e.g., B, C, and G. These nongroup A streptococci are often recovered from the throats of normal persons or from patients with nonbacterial (viral) pharyngitis. Similarly, the presence of group A streptococci in the throat may represent clinical or subclinical infection, transitory colonization, or a chronic carrier state.* Streptococcal pharyngitis is more frequent during the winter and early spring months. In infants 6 months old or younger, upper respiratory streptococcal infections tend to be more generalized, with mild or absent pharyngeal involvement but with middle ear infection and sometimes bacteremia. In older children and adults the charac-

teristic clinical picture is one of redness and edema of the throat and tonsils, which are frequently covered with exudate (Fig 5–3), and fever. The anterior cervical nodes are swollen and tender, and the white blood cell count is often elevated. Malaise, headache, abdominal pain, and nausea and vomiting often occur. In order to produce pharyngitis, group A streptococci must compete with the indigenous flora, adhere to the epithelial cells of the pharynx or tonsils, and elude the host defense mechanisms. Some degree of protection is provided by the indigenous flora of the throat, in particular, streptococci of the viridans group and staphylococci, which produce bacteriocins which tend to inhibit colonization by group A streptococci.

Attachment of group A streptococci to pharyngeal epithelial cells occurs via the fimbriae, composed of lipoteichoic acid and M protein (Fig 5–4). After attachment, tissue damage is produced by the pyrogenic exotoxins and the hemolysins. The infection commonly extends to involve the anterior cervical lymph nodes where the organisms may persist for many months after the acute infection has resolved.

Scarlet fever is a syndrome in which the symptoms of pharyngitis are accompanied by a generalized skin rash that persists for about a week. The skin eventually becomes branny and desquamates. It was believed until recently that

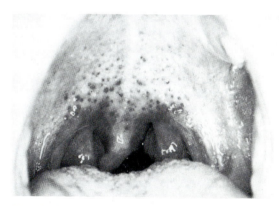

FIG 5–3.
Streptococcal pharyngitis.

---

*Group A streptococci may be cultured intermittently from 20% of asymptomatic persons.

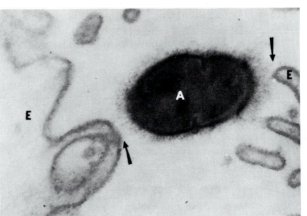

FIG 5–4.
Electron micrograph of group A streptococcus **(A)** attached to pharyngeal epithelial cells *(E)*. Attachment is mediated by fimbriae (arrow) composed of streptococcal lipoteichoic acid and M protein. *(From J Exper Med 1976; 143:759. Used by permission of Experimental Med of the Rockerfeller University Press.)*

scarlet fever occurred when the infecting group A strain produced an erythrogenic toxin to which the patient had no antibodies. However, it is difficult to accept this concept in view of the marked decrease in the incidence of scarlet fever and the high prevalence of erythrogenic toxin-producing strains. These observations have led to a revised view that scarlet fever is due to the enhancement of pyrogenic exotoxin or acquired hypersensitivity to the same or different erythrogenic toxin or some unrelated streptococcal product.

Other Group A Infections

Streptococcus pyogenes infection may complicate surgical wounds, leading to fasciitis or myonecrosis. The organism tends to disseminate via the lymphatics (lymphangitis), which may lead to septicemia. Streptococcal septicemia occasionally follows a surgical procedure; a local tissue infection becomes edematous and painful, the entire process spreads very rapidly, and the patient appears extremely ill. Thrombocytopenia is common and shock may supervene.

Nonsuppurative Poststreptococcal Sequelae

Rheumatic Fever.—About 3 weeks following streptococcal pharyngitis there is the onset of fever, accompanied by multiple painful and swollen joints. The peak age incidence of rheumatic fever is 5 to 14 years, the same as for streptococcal pharyngitis. About half of the affected persons develop cardiac complications—valvulitis, especially mitral stenosis or pericarditis—and 6% develop neurologic symptoms characterized by involuntary movements, i.e., chorea ("St. Vitus' dance"). About 20% of these patients still have throat cultures positive for group A streptococci, and all show a higher titer of streptococcal antibodies (antistreptolysin O, anti-DNAse B, antihyaluronidase) than do "normal" persons recovering from streptococcal infections.

The pathogenesis of rheumatic fever is still not completely understood. Certain facts emerge however: group A streptococci must have been present in the upper respiratory tract and have persisted for some time, and streptococcal antibodies must be produced. Recent studies have shown that rheumatic fever (RF) strains adhere more tightly to epithelial cells than do other non-RF strains. Furthermore, pharyngeal cells from donors with RF have a greater avidity for RF-associated strains than cells from normal control donors. This may be a reflection of a genetic predisposition, since only 2% to 3% of the population appears to be susceptible to RF. The effect of this unusually prolonged and "tight" adherence of the streptococci via the fimbriae may permit the lipoteichoic acid to act as a carrier of various streptococcal antigens, binding them to organ tissues where they may provoke immunocytotoxic effects. Certain streptococcal antigens such as M protein share chemical moieties with tissue antigens of cardiac muscle and valves and cross-react with them. In experimental animals administration of M protein and streptococcal proteases can cause subendocardial lesions, and streptolysin O exhibits cardiotoxicity.

Glomerulonephritis.—About a week after a streptococcal skin infection such as impetigo, a few patients develop transient elevations in their blood pressure, generalized edema, and their urine is found to contain increased amounts of albumin and red blood cells. This form of glomerulonephritis is associated with infections by nephritogenic types of group A streptococci (types 4, 12, and others). Glomerulonephritis is thought to be an autoimmune disease that results from the deposition of streptococcal antigen-antibody-complement complexes on the glomerular basement membrane, producing a local inflammatory Arthus-like reaction in the glomerulus (these persons typically have low serum complement levels).

The injection of lipoteichoic acid into experimental animals can produce arthritis or nephritis, presumably by binding to tissue cell membranes and provoking local immunotoxic effects.

IMMUNITY TO GROUP A STREPTOCOCCAL INFECTIONS

The immune response to streptococcal infections is M type–specific and is characterized by the appearance of antibodies to the M protein, streptolysin O, DNAse B, hyaluronidase, etc.

The development of a streptococcal vaccine has been hampered by the presence of antigens, thought to be M protein, that cross-react with heart tissue. (The M proteins show a close structural relationship with tropomyosin, a muscle protein.) More recently, peptic digests of M protein have been found to be highly immunogenic and to elicit type-specific, protective opsonic antibodies.

The frequency and severity of streptococcal infections and their sequelae have declined sharply in the past 80 years, although the prevalence of streptococcal infections is still high and there have been major outbreaks in the past few years. This decline may be related to host resistance, virulence of the organism, and environmental factors. This decline in morbidity and mortality began long before penicillin became available.

GROUP B STREPTOCOCCUS

Group B streptococci are among the normal indigenous flora of the upper respiratory, gastrointestinal, and female genitourinary tracts. They are opportunists whose pathogenicity depends upon lowered host resistance. There are five major serotypes (Ia, Ib, Ic, II, and III). Serotype III accounts for about two thirds of all invasive infections, mostly maternal and neonatal.

In the United States 20% of postpartum endometritis, amnionitis, and associated bacteremia are caused by group B streptococci. The organism colonizes the genitalia of approximately 20% of women and appears to infect the uterus and membranes through ascending spread from the vagina.

Although up to 70% of infants born vaginally to mothers genitally colonized with group B streptococci acquire mucous membrane colonization, only 1% to 2% develop disseminated infection. Disease may occur during the first 5 days of life and present as septicemia, pneumonia, or meningitis, individually or severally. Risk factors are intrapartum fever, prolonged rupture of membranes, and low birth weight. Mortality is about 25% and almost half of the survivors have permanent neurologic damage. Meningitis may also appear after about 3 weeks. Group B streptococci also produce cutaneous infection similar to those of Group A streptococci, particularly in diabetic patients.

ANTIBIOTIC SUSCEPTIBILITY OF STREPTOCOCCI

Most streptococci have remained susceptible to penicillin, and this is the drug of choice in nonallergic patients. Resistance of group A streptococci to erythromycin and clindamycin has been reported, but such strains are uncommon in the U.S. Resistance to both of these agents is plasmid-mediated.

LABORATORY DIAGNOSIS

Streptococci are readily cultured from throat, wound, or genital swabs on tryptic soy, heart infusion, or Columbia agar containing 5% sheep erythrocytes. Colonies appear after 24 hours at 35° C. Rapid diagnosis of streptococcal pharyngitis can be performed by extracting throat swabs with acid or enzyme and testing the extract by latex agglutination.

CHAPTER 6

Haemophilus influenzae

> A 2-year-old boy developed difficulty in swallowing. His temperature rose rapidly to 39.4° C and within a few hours he showed signs of acute inspiratory obstruction (stridor). On physical examination the child exhibited suprasternal retraction and was markedly apprehensive. His epiglottis was observed to be red and swollen. Cultures of the epiglottis, nasopharynx, and blood were obtained. Nasotracheal intubation was performed and the child was treated with sedation, humidified oxygen, and an antibiotic. All cultures subsequently grew *Haemophilus influenzae* type a.

Haemophilus influenzae is one of the commonest causes of acute life-threatening infections of infancy and early childhood. *Haemophilus influenzae* type b is the leading cause of meningitis in the United States, resulting in an estimated 8,000 to 11,000 cases every year. Age-specific incidence rates are highest among children less than 1 year of age and decrease steadily thereafter. The mortality is approximately 3% to 7% and neurologic complications are common. In addition, *H. influenzae* type b

causes an estimated 6,000 cases a year of other invasive diseases, including epiglottitis, pneumonia, and septic arthritis. The organism is also a common cause of sinusitis, otitis media, and acute conjunctivitis. In adults *H. influenzae* can cause meningitis, pneumonia, chronic bronchitis, and postpartum infections.

Haemophilus species are small, facultative, nonmotile, gram-negative coccobacilli that require blood or blood constituents for growth. Some species (*H. influenzae*) require hemin (X factor) and NAD (V factor) for growth; other species may need only X or V factor. Both X and V factors may be supplied by the addition of horse or rabbit blood to the basal medium. Sheep blood agar will not support the growth of *H. influenzae* because the sheep erythrocytes contain NADase. This deficiency may be overcome by growing a colony of *Staphylococcus aureus* on the agar that has been inoculated with *H. influenzae*, which grow as satellite colonies around the staphylococcal colony. Alternatively, the sheep blood agar may be heated to inactivate the NADase. This heated blood (chocolate) agar is commonly used to cultivate *H. influenzae*. Pathogenic species besides *H. influenzae* include *H. parainfluenzae* and *H. ducreyi*. Other species, such as *H. aphrophilus*, *H. paraphrophilus*, *H, haemolyticus*, and *H. parahaemolyti-*

cus, are normal commensals indigenous to the mouth and upper respiratory tract. They can cause endocarditis and brain abscess.

The virulence of *H. influenzae* is related to the presence of a polysaccharide capsule which acts to impede phagocytosis. Six antigenically distinct capsular polysaccharides are recognized, designated types a through f. *Haemophilus influenzae* type b is the most common type involved in invasive disease in children. The type b capsule is a polymer of ribosyl-ribitol-phosphate; other types have capsules of other sugar phosphates. There is no clear explanation of why type b appears to be the most pathogenic.

A subtyping system based on the outer membrane protein (OMP) has been described for nonencapsulated *H. influenzae*. The OMP composition of *H. influenzae* is typical for that of gram-negative bacteria in that about 20 proteins are present in the outer membrane with four to six proteins accounting for most of the protein content. There is no clear relationship between biotype and OMP subtype. Some OMP subtypes are more pathogenic than others.

Man is the only reservoir of *H. influenzae*. Transmission occurs by airborne droplet infections or direct contact with respiratory secretions. Exposure to the organism begins at birth and up to 80% of the population are carriers. Invasive *H. influenzae* infection is usually preceded by nasopharyngeal colonization, followed by bacteremia and metastatic spread, with localization to the meninges, lungs, joints, etc. Nasopharyngeal carrier rates of encapsulated type b decrease with increasing age: under 1 year, the rate is 38% to 70%; at 1 to 4 years, 12%; and at 5 to 15 years, 0% to 3%. Nonencapsulated (nontypable) strains are found in the nasopharynx of normal adults and children, where they may produce localized infection such as sinusitis, otitis media, and bacterial exacerbations of bronchitis. About 75% of respiratory isolates from adults or children with nonbacteremic lower respiratory disease are nontypable. Nonserotypable *H. influenzae* is an important cause of nonbacte-

remic (and usually nonfatal) pneumonia in elderly men. Patients with lower respiratory tract infection caused by nonserotypable strains have a 7% mortality as compared to a 50% mortality in patients with similar infections caused by serotypable strains.

Most strains of *H. influenzae*, both encapsulated and nonencapsulated, produce IgAl protease. (IgAl protease is also produced by *H. parainfluenzae*, *H. parahaemolyticus*, pneumococcus, meningococcus, and gonococcus.) Anticapsular mucosal antibody is present in the nasopharyngeal secretions and saliva of most adults. While the production of IgAl protease may facilitate the establishment of *H. influenzae* in the respiratory tract, it cannot account for the increased pathogenicity of type b strains (occasional type b strains do not produce IgA protease), the high rate of nasopharyngeal colonization with nontypable strains, or the low colonization rate seen with encapsulated strains. The group most susceptible to invasive *H. influenzae* infection are children aged 3 months to 5 years. Susceptibility then declines through age 12. Susceptibility appears to correlate with the lack of specific antibody to the capsular polysaccharide. The only other type of note is type f which causes bacteremia.

Immunity to *H. influenzae* type b infection is associated with bactericidal antibody directed against the polyribose phosphate capsule, which appears to prevent bloodstream invasion and dissemination. The antibody is acquired passively in neonates; the majority of lactating women have the anticapsular antibody in their colostrum and breast milk, primarily as IgA. Older children and adults gradually acquire active immunity from inapparent or low-grade infections.

The capsular polysaccharide of *H. influenzae* type b is clearly a virulence determinant, and passive immunization with the corresponding antibody was the mainstay of treatment prior to the advent of antibiotics. The purified polyribose phosphate is highly immunogenic in adults and older children and elicits antibodies that are bactericidal, opsonic, and protective. Children under 6 years of age, particularly infants during the first year of life, respond poorly or not at all to this antigen. The majority of children aged 3 to 25 months fail to produce antibody following *H. influenzae* meningitis. Preliminary studies have shown that combining the polyribose phosphate with OMP results in a more effective immunogen for infants.

The demonstration of biotypes and OMP subtypes suggests that there may be virulence factors other than the presence of the capsules. It is possible that OMPs of nonencapsulated *H. influenzae* are important in virulence. While the role of nonencapsulated *H. influenzae* in patients with chronic obstructive pulmonary diseases is unclear, it has been shown that nonencapsulated *H. influenza* produces a substance (an OMP?) that inhibits ciliary activity and damages respiratory epithelial cells. This substance could prolong infections caused by *H. influenzae* in patients with chronic bronchitis.

It is becoming apparent that antibodies directed against noncapsular somatic antigens including OMPs are important in immunity to *H. influenzae*. Antibodies to OMPs are widely prevalent among healthy adults and have recently been detected in infants after systemic disease due to *H. influenzae* type b. Currently a conjugate vaccine consisting of *H. influenzae* capsular polysaccharide covalently linked to diphtheria toxoid has been found to be an effective immunogen in children 18 to 23 months old.

The laboratory diagnosis of *H. influenzae* infection is readily accomplished by culture of the organism from cerebrospinal fluid, blood, joint aspirates, etc. Rapid diagnosis of meningitis may be done by direct antigen detection in spinal fluid using sensitized latex particles.

Ampicillin was initially effective against *H. influenzae*, but at present 10% to 35% of strains are ampicillin-resistant. There is considerable geographic variation in the distribution of resistant strains. Resistance to ampicillin is due to plasmid-mediated production of one or more β-lactamase. Plasmid resistance to chloramphenicol and trimethoprim/sulfamethoxazole also occurs but is less common. Several of the cephalosporins are presently used in treatment.

CHAPTER 7

Moraxella (Branhamella) catarrhalis

An 18-month-old infant awoke crying in the middle of the night because of ear pain. The pediatrician diagnosed otitis media and prescribed ampicillin. After 5 days of treatment there was no clinical improvement and reexamination of the affected ear revealed a red, bulging tympanic membrane. Cloudy fluid aspirated by tympanocentesis grew out a pure culture of *Moraxella catarrhalis*, resistant to ampicillin.

Moraxella catarrhalis, previously regarded as a harmless inhabitant of the pharynx, is now recognized as an important cause of otitis media as well as an etiologic agent of acute maxillary sinusitis and lower respiratory tract infections that include tracheitis, pneumonia, exacerbations of chronic bronchitis, and empyema. The organism has also been known to cause conjunctivitis, urethritis, meningitis, and endocarditis.

Previously called *Neisseria catarrhalis* and *Branhamella catarrhalis*, the organism is a gram-negative diplococcus that is easily mistaken for the meningococcus or gonococcus on a Gram stain. Like these organisms *M. catarrhalis* is oxidase-positive, but fails to ferment carbohydrates.

The outer membrane of the cell wall contains outer membrane proteins (OMPs), lipooligosaccharide (LOS), phospholipid, and pili (fimbriae). Eight major OMPs have been identified, some of which may function as porins, forming channels through the outer membrane for passive diffusion of small molecular nutrients and antibiotics. LOS may be a virulence factor; LOS lacks the surface-exposed polysaccharide typical of the lipopolysaccharide O antigen of enteric bacteria. The absence of this antigen increases outer membrane permeability, enhancing the susceptibility of this organism to hydrophobic antimicrobial agents such as rifampin and some macrolides. Pili play a role in adherence and colonization of mucosal surfaces.

Many strains of *M. catarrhalis* produce β-lactamase, but susceptibility has been demonstrated to erythromycin, tetracycline, chloramphenicol, trimethoprim-sulfamethoxazole, certain cephalosporins, and ampicillin–clavulanic acid.

CHAPTER 8

Corynebacterium diphtheriae

A 4-year-old child had been ill for 4 days with sore throat, mild cough, and other symptoms of an upper respiratory infection, but on the evening of the fifth day, he became weak, limp, and lethargic. He was taken to a hospital where he developed respiratory distress and died in the emergency room. At autopsy, a pharyngeal membrane was noted, cultures of which were positive for virulent *Corynebacterium diphtheriae.*

Diphtheria is a disease produced by infection with *Corynebacterium diphtheriae*, characterized by local inflammation of mucous membranes—usually of the upper respiratory tract—and systemic effects of the potent exotoxin produced by the organism. In the early 1900s the case rate of diphtheria in the United States was 1,500/100,000 population with a fatality rate of 8% to 10%. In recent years the number of cases in this country has markedly decreased to about 200 annually, partially as a result of widespread immunization. Diphtheria is representative of a group of diseases called **toxemias** that include tetanus and botulism. The bacterial agents causing these diseases are not highly invasive and generally remain at a local site, e.g.,

in a wound, where they elaborate a soluble toxin. The toxin diffuses into the surrounding tissue where it may produce local damage, but it also enters the circulation causing systemic effects.

The corynebacteria are a group of gram-positive bacilli that are among the indigenous flora that colonize the skin and mucous membranes. They are facultative, nonmotile, non-spore-forming, rod-shaped bacteria that share a basic cell wall composition with their cousins *Nocardia* and *Mycobacterium*. The cell wall contains a peptidoglycan bonded to polysaccharides, and branched, long-chain fatty acids. Characteristics of corynebacteria are their pleomorphism (the organisms vary in width, tend to be club- or wedge-shaped, and even slightly curved); the presence of so-called metachromatic granules within the cells (the lack of uniform staining is due to the accumulation of polyphosphates); their microscopic appearance as "Chinese letters"; and their ability to reduce potassium tellurite incorporated into the agar medium to telluride, resulting in grayish or black colonies. The single primary pathogen in the group is *C. diphtheriae;* the other species of indigenous corynebacteria are referred to as diphtheroids, and are rarely pathogenic in immunocompetent persons.

Corynebacterium diphtheriae is able to grow on relatively simple media that supply essential amino acids, vitamins, and glucose. It prefers a carbon dioxide–rich atmosphere at 37° C. Five strains or types (*gravis, intermedius, mitis, ulcerans,* and *pseudotuberculosis*) can be distinguished, based upon colony appearance, biochemical reactions, and toxin production.

The most important characteristic of *C. diphtheriae* is its capacity to produce an extremely potent exotoxin. All strains of *C. diphtheriae* do not produce toxin; the genetic information controlling toxin production is carried by certain temperate corynebacteriophages as the gene *tox*. Toxin is produced only by strains of *C. diphtheriae* carrying the tox gene. Nontoxigenic strains may be converted to toxin production by being infected with a beta corynebacteriophage carrying the tox^+ gene, and becoming lysogenic. Toxigenic conversion can occur if the beta phage is growing vegetatively producing lysis, as a prophage, or as a nonreplicating piece of DNA in lysogenic cells. All toxigenic strains contain prophages closely related to prophage beta tox^+.

There are several ways in which the tox gene may spread among the population after being introduced into a community by a tox^+ carrier: lysogenic, toxigenic strains of *C. diphtheriae* may be brought in from an endemic area by an immune carrier and spread by droplet infection. Alternatively, when a person carrying a tox^+ bacillus arrives in an immunized community, the spread of the tox gene may be via phage conversion of tox^- *C. diphtheriae* already present in the nasopharyngeal flora of the local population rather than colonization with the tox^+ strain itself.

Several phage mutants have been isolated which code for antigenically similar but nontoxic proteins (crm proteins). *Escherichia coli* can be programmed to produce toxin by DNA from the beta phage. Under optimal conditions, 75% of all the protein that is secreted by the cell is toxin. Toxin production can be blocked by antibiotics such as chloramphenicol or rifampin.

An important factor in toxin production is the availability of inorganic iron; no toxin will be produced until the iron in the culture medium or environment has been depleted and the concentration of the iron in the bacteria is low. This suggests that there is an iron-containing protein that acts as a repressor of the tox gene.

DIPHTHERIA TOXIN

Diphtheria toxin is a protein with a molecular weight of 62,000. It is released from the bacterium as a single polypeptide chain with two cystine bridges. If the protein is treated with trypsin or similar proteases, it is split into two large peptides connected by a disulfide bridge: an amino-terminal fragment (A), and a carboxy-terminal fragment (B). The A fragment is highly active, whereas the B fragment shows no enzymatic activity. Neither fragment alone produces toxicity toward intact cells; both the A and B fragments are necessary to produce cellular damage. However, if isolated A fragment is injected into any eukaryotic cell, even a cell resistant to diphtheria toxin, cell death ensues.

The toxin enters the cell by a process called receptor-mediated endocytosis. The first step is the binding of the B fragment of the toxin to a cell membrane receptor. The toxin and receptor are then engulfed in a vesicle formed by an invagination of the plasma membrane called a coated vesicle. The vesicle is acidified, and the A fragment is split off and penetrates the bilayer membrane of the vesicle to enter the cytoplasm.

It is believed that the A fragment is toxic only after it has entered the cell. In the cell the A fragment interferes with protein synthesis. Specifically, the diphtheria toxin inactivates the enzyme translocase (elongation factor 2, or EF-2) by catalyzing the reaction that results in the union of the enzyme with adenosine diphosphate (ADP) ribose in the presence of NAD, producing a ribosylated translocase which is inactive. This is an unusual amino acid named **diphthamide**, a modification of a histidine residue. Without active translocase, the movement of peptidyl transfer RNA is prevented, and amino acids cannot be added to the forming peptide chain and its elongation stops. Nothing longer than a dipeptide can be made and protein synthesis ceases. A single molecule of the toxin is enough to inactivate all of the translocase in an entire cell within a few hours, leading to cell death.

Diphtheria toxin is highly antigenic, and antibodies produced against the toxin (antitoxin) are capable of competing with receptor sites on the cell surface and neutralizing its lethal action. Its extreme toxicity (3.5 guinea pig lethal doses per microgram) limit its usefulness as an immunogen. If diphtheria toxin (like other protein exotoxins) is treated with formalin, it is converted into **toxoid.** Toxoid retains the antigenic specificity of the toxin, but does not damage cells. Since toxoid elicits specific antitoxin, it can be used to actively immunize against diphtheria toxin. Toxoid also contains other corynebacterial antigens.

PATHOGENESIS OF DIPHTHERIA

Man is the only natural host of *C. diphtheriae* and thus the only reservoir of infection. The organisms primarily inhabit the upper respiratory tract and person-to-person transmission is by means of respiratory aerosols. Skin lesions such as impetigo, pyoderma, ecthyma, etc., caused by hemolytic streptococci or *Staphylococcus aureus*, may also be colonized by *C. diphtheriae* and infective skin exudate may also be involved in person-to-person spread.

Persons may be colonized by toxinogenic or nontoxinogenic strains. The invasiveness of a strain (its capacity to colonize) is related to the production of **trehalose dimycolate** (cord factor)* which damages the mitochondria of the host cells. Other factors that may also be involved in the invasiveness of *C. diphtheriae* are a **neura-**

*A similar cord factor is present in virulent strains of *Mycobacterium tuberculosis.*

minidase, which splits *N*-acetylneuraminic acid (NAN) from mucins and from cell surfaces; *NAN lyase,* which hydrolyzes NAN into mannosamine and pyruvate; and diphthin, a protease said to hydrolyze certain immunoglobulins. Levels of circulating antitoxin have no bearing on colonization or the establishment of the carrier state.

One percent to 5% of healthy people are carriers of *C. diphtheriae.* The organism is an efficient colonizer of the tonsillar crypts and people with tonsils harbor the organism longer. Efforts to eliminate the carrier state by treatment with penicillin or erythromycin have met with limited success; the duration of the carriage of corynebacteria may be shortened, but recolonization often occurs when antibiotic treatment is discontinued.

CLINICAL ASPECTS

The incubation period of diphtheria is usually 2 to 5 days, during which time the organism becomes established on the epithelial cells of the upper respiratory tract. Diphtheria has two distinct components: (1) a local infection characterized by edema, and the formation of a pseudomembrane composed of fibrin, leukocytic exudate, red blood cells, and bacteria (Fig 8–1), and (2) a profound toxemia which affects the heart and peripheral nerves. The local infection may involve the anterior nares, the tonsils, the pharynx, or the larynx and bronchi. Diphtheritic infection of the skin or wounds is more common in the tropics. The pseudomembrane is often thick and very adherent, and can cause respiratory obstruction in infants and young children.*

Typical severe diphtheria is caused by toxin-producing strains, and the local lesions are accompanied by marked prostration and severe toxemia. The principal organs affected by the

*Removal of the pseudomembrane increases the absorption of toxin and should not be done prior to the administration of antitoxin unless necessary to maintain an airway.

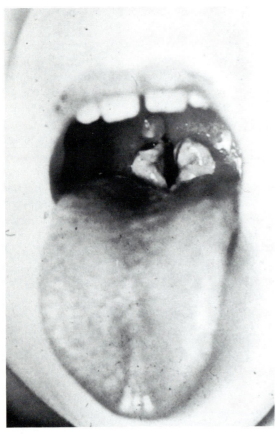

FIG 8-1.
Diphtheria.

gia; spinal nerve involvement can cause weakness, paralysis, or paresthesias of the neck, abdomen, or extremities. Some form of paralysis occurs in 10% to 20% of all patients with diphtheria.

Severe, often fatal, cases of hypertoxic (malignant or "bull neck") diphtheria occur, especially in young children. There is an abrupt onset with a rapidly developing and spreading pseudomembrane and extensive swelling of the cervical lymph nodes and edema of the neck and upper chest. There is a possibility that bull neck diphtheria may be due in part to the production of large amounts of hyaluronidase (spreading factor) by the diphtheria bacillus. Outbreaks of mild diphtheria are sometimes caused by nontoxicogenic strains of *C. diphtheriae*, or by tox[+] strains in immune persons.

The rational treatment of toxemia involves two principles: neutralization of circulating toxin before it becomes bound to tissue, and elimination of the source of additional toxin. Neutralization of toxin is generally accomplished by the administration of specific antitoxin. Eliminating the source of additional toxin may require surgical debridement or extirpation of infected tissues and the administration of appropriate antibiotics.

In diphtheria the prompt administration of antitoxin is important because the toxin binds very rapidly and irreversibly to tissue sites. For example, if a mixture of 1 unit of toxin and 1 unit of antitoxin is injected intradermally, no lesion is produced. If however, 1 unit of toxin is injected intradermally and after only a 5-minute delay 1,000 units of antitoxin are injected into the area, a necrotic lesion develops. The incidence of paralysis, myocarditis, and fatalities increases markedly with delay in therapy (Table 8-1): **antitoxin treatment cannot wait for laboratory confirmation.** Erythromycin should also be given, but this is secondary in importance to antitoxin.

Active immunity to diphtheria can be produced by the administration of diphtheria toxoid. Diphtheria toxoid is a component of the

toxin are the heart and peripheral nerves.

Toxic myocarditis occurs in 10% to 20% of cases, resulting in arrhythmias and conduction defects, and sometimes sudden death due to ventricular fibrillation. Some degree of cardiac impairment is detectable in about 50% of patients suffering from diphtheria. Myocardial damage due to diphtheria toxin varies from cloudy swelling with loss of striation to complete degeneration of muscle fibers. Neuritis occurs after the second week of disease. In the spinal cord, lesions are seen in the anterior horn ganglion cells and in the posterior root ganglia. Common manifestations of cranial nerve involvement are paralysis of the soft palate and dyspha-

TABLE 8–1.

Effect of Delay in Administration of Antitoxin in Diphtheria

Antitoxin Given on Day	Percent of Cases Resulting in		
	Myocarditis	Paralysis	Case Fatality
1	4.7	0.4	0
2	6.0	2.0	4.2
3	10.3	2.0	11.1
4	10.3	1.0	17.3
5+	12.1	2.5	18.7

DPT (diphtheria-pertussis-tetanus) vaccine used to immunize children. (Patients who recover from diphtheria should also be actively immunized with toxoid.) The immune status of an individual to diphtheria toxin may be determined by the Schick test, which consists of the intradermal injection of a minute quantity of toxin. The appearance of a necrotic lesion at the injection site within 48 to 96 hours that persists for several days indicates insufficient circulating antitoxin (Schick-positive). The absence of a lesion indicates adequate antitoxin in the circulation (Schick-negative). Some persons, including those with or without circulating antitoxin, may give an immediate hypersensitivity reaction (pseudoreaction) within 20 to 45 minutes, indicating an allergy to other corynebacterial antigens also present in the toxoid. These persons usually give a positive reaction when skin-tested with heated toxin or toxoid (Moloney test). Combined reactions, consisting of immediate hypersensitivity and a Schick-positive lesion, also occur.

CHAPTER 9

Overview of Lower Respiratory Tract Infections

The lower respiratory tract includes the trachea, bronchi, and lungs. Microorganisms can gain access to the respiratory tract via the airway, the bloodstream, or by direct penetration into the chest cavity. Entry into the lungs via the airway can occur by inhalation of aerosol droplets or dust, or by aspiration of fluids from the nasopharynx.

Exogenously acquired infection originates from sick persons, carriers, or the environment; but at least one third of healthy persons harbor potential pathogens in their pharynx. During the winter months, up to 40% of normal persons have pneumococci in their throats, and many people are also colonized with *Staphylococcus aureus*, *Haemophilus influenzae*, and group A streptococci.

Host defense mechanisms against respiratory infection include the epiglottal reflex, which helps guard against aspiration of secretions containing bacteria; bronchial mucus, which traps bacteria; ciliated tracheal epithelial cells, which sweep mucus-trapped organisms toward the pharynx; the cough reflex which expels bacteria-laden mucus; alveolar macrophages, which phagocytose infecting organisms; and lymphatic drainage, which removes phagocytosed organisms (Fig 9–1).

Factors that suppress pulmonary defenses and predispose to infection include air pollutants and irritants such as cigarette smoke, ethanol, general anesthesia, narcotics, aspiration of vomitus, and chilling.

The pathogenesis of pulmonary infection is initiated when bacteria reach the alveoli. Only inhaled particles of 0.5 to 2.0 μm can reach the terminal airway, but aspirated fluid can reach the alveoli. Less commonly, microorganisms may reach the lungs hematogenously via the pulmonary circulation. The primary response is an outpouring of edema, which facilitates the spread of the infection to neighboring alveoli via Kohn's pores. Bacteria multiply in the edema fluid, and there is local alveolar hemorrhage. This phase is followed by an influx of polymorphonuclear neutrophils which attempt to engulf the bacteria. Encapsulated species such as pneumococci and *H. influenzae* resist phagocytosis until the appearance of anticapsular antibodies which promote opsonization. Eventually the neutrophils are replaced by macrophages and healing or consolidation occurs. In lobar pneumonia the lesion expands centripetally, so that tissue sections demonstrate the various phases of the infection: consolidation in the center, surrounded by an area of tissue infiltrated by neu-

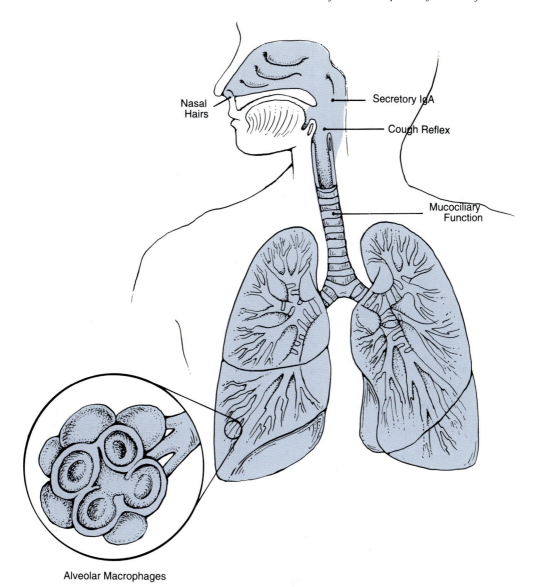

FIG 9–1.
Host defense mechanisms against respiratory infection.

trophils and macrophages (gray hepatization), which in turn is enclosed by an area of hemorrhage and edema (red hepatization). Depending on the species of microorganisms and the degree of tissue destruction, lung tissue may be replaced with normal functioning cells or by fibrotic scar tissue.

Infection may involve the trachea (tracheitis), the bronchi (bronchiolitis or bronchitis), or the lungs (pneumonia, pneumonitis, or lung abscess). Tracheitis is an uncommon infection resembling epiglottitis, with an acute onset marked by high fever and respiratory obstruction. The pathogenesis of this infection is not clear, but *S. aureus*, group A streptococci, and *H. influenzae* type b are commonly recovered from the respiratory exudate in these patients. Herpesvirus can cause tracheobronchitis in immunocompromised and elderly immunocompetent patients.

Bronchiolitis is seen in children younger than 2 years of age. Most cases of bronchiolitis are caused by respiratory syncytial virus. Acute bronchitis in older children and adults is usually caused by influenza virus, adenovirus, rhinovirus, coronavirus, parainfluenza virus, or *Mycoplasma pneumoniae*. Chronic bronchitis may also be due to respiratory viruses, nontypable *H. influenzae*, or the pneumococcus.

Pneumonia may be caused by viruses, *M. pneumoniae*, bacteria, fungi, chlamydia, *Coxiella burnetii*, or *Pneuomcystis carinii* (a protozoan). Viral pneumonias in adults are caused primarily by influenza and adenovirus, and usually occur in the winter and early spring. Varicella, measles virus, enteroviruses, and cytomegalovirus can also cause pneumonia. *Mycoplasma pneumoniae* infection most frequently occurs in adolescents and young adults in the fall, and is characterized by a dry nonproductive cough, low-grade fever, and headache.

A large number of bacteria can cause acute pneumonia. The commonly encountered species are *Streptococcus pneumoniae* (pneumococcus), *H. influenzae*, *Bordetella pertussis*, *Bacteroides* and anaerobic streptococci, *S. aureus*, *Klebsiella pneumoniae* and other enteric gram-negative bacilli, *Chlamydia pneumoniae* (TWAR agent), and *Legionella pneumophila*. Less common bacterial agents that can cause pneumonia are *Streptococcus pyogenes* (group A streptococcus), *Bacillus anthracis*, brucella, *Yersinia*, *Neisseria meningitidis* group Y, *Chlamydia psittaci*, and *Moraxella catarrhalis*. Pulmonary tuberculosis, a common protracted lung infection, is caused by *Mycobacterium tuberculosis;* other mycobacterial species can also cause lung disease. The common fungi causing pneumonitis are *Coccidioides immitis*, *Histoplasma capsulatum*, *Blastomyces dermatitidis*, and *Aspergillus fumigatus*.

Lung abscess may be due to *Actinomyces*, *Nocardia*, *Bacteroides*, and anaerobic streptococci, or may be a complication of pneumococcal, gram-negative bacillary, staphylococcal, or fungal pneumonitis. Other complications of pneumonia are empyema (a localized accumulation of pus), bronchiectasis (chronic dilation of the bronchi), or fibrosis (scarring).

The laboratory diagnosis involves the Gram stain and cultures of sputum or exudate obtained by transtracheal aspiration, fiberoptic bronchoscopy, or lung biopsy. Blood cultures should also be obtained since up to one third of patients with bacterial pneumonias also have the organism in their blood.

CHAPTER 10

Streptococcus pneumoniae (Pneumococcus)

A 75-year-old retired woman with known congestive heart failure presented with a chief complaint of cough and chest pain for the past 24 hours. Two days prior to admission, the patient developed a mild cough productive of purulent sputum. The afternoon of admission, she experienced sudden pleuritic chest pain on the right side, followed by increased cough. She had a shaking chill and developed a fever. Because of the severe chest pain, she sought medical attention. On physical examination, she had a temperature of 40° C, the respiratory rate was 28, pulse 120, and she was in moderate respiratory distress. Examination of her chest revealed dullness to percussion and rales at the right base. A radiograph showed a right lower lobe infiltrate. Her white blood cell count was 26,500. A Gram stain of her sputum revealed large numbers of polymorphonuclear neutrophils with many gram-positive diplococci (Fig 10–1), and the patient was diagnosed as having pneumococcal pneumonia. Specimens of sputum and blood were sent to the laboratory for culture, both of which grew out *Streptococcus pneumoniae*.

Pneumonia is the fifth leading cause of death in the United States. About half of all pneumonias are bacterial, the remainder being caused by mycoplasmas (10%) and viruses (40%). Seventy-five percent of outpatient bacterial pneumonias are caused by pneumococci.

Pneumococci are normal inhabitants of the upper respiratory tract and are present in 20% to 70% of adults. They invade when the defense mechanisms of the host have been weakened. They are extracellular parasites that produce disease while growing and multiplying outside of phagocytic cells. When pneumococci are ingested by neutrophils and macrophages, they are rapidly destroyed by these cells.

In common with other streptococci, *S.*

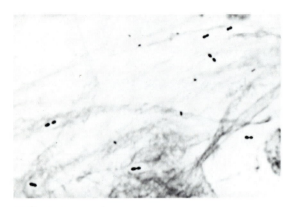

FIG 10–1.
Pneumococci in sputum.

pneumoniae is gram-positive and grows in pairs or short chains. Pneumococci tend to be elongated, and the pairs typically appear with the pointed ends opposing each other. They require an enriched medium, usually supplied by the addition of blood or serum to the broth or agar. Some strains require additional carbon dioxide and better growth occurs under anaerobic conditions. When grown on blood agar, tiny colonies appear after 18 to 24 hours at 35° C. The colonies are surrounded by a green zone of alpha hemolysis. Pneumococci ferment glucose to lactic acid. During the fermentation, hydrogen peroxide accumulates, and since pneumococci lack catalase, the culture dies. During growth, particularly in broth, an endogenous autolytic enzyme may be activated that splits L-alanine from the muramic acid in the peptidoglycan of the cell wall and the organisms lyse. This enzyme may be activated by surface-active agents and is the basis of the bile solubility test. This susceptibility to lysis by bile or sodium deoxycholate is a method used in the laboratory to distinguish pneumococci from other α-hemolytic streptococci.

The cell walls of pneumococci contain a carbohydrate (C) that reacts with a beta globulin present in the blood of persons with inflammatory disease. This globulin is designated **C-reactive protein** and is not an antibody; its detection is a useful diagnostic test for acute inflammation. One of the characteristic features of the pneumococcus is its capsule. The capsule is composed of polysaccharide, which is antigenic in man. There are about 80 types of pneumococci, each with its own polysaccharide capsule, and each capsule having a different chemical composition and being immunologically distinct.*

About 80% of pneumococcal strains causing lobar pneumonia involve certain types: 1, 3, 4, 7, 8, and 12 in adults, and higher types (14, 18, 19, and 23) in children. About 20% to 25% of the population carries these more virulent types in the nasopharynx. Type 3 is the most virulent and carries the highest mortality, presumably because of its extremely large capsule. Nasopharyngeal carriage of type 3 is very common.

Pneumococci that have been freshly isolated from clinical material are encapsulated and the colonies are glistening and "smooth." On repeated transfer on laboratory media, the organisms tend to lose their capsules; the colonies become more granular, and are termed "rough." This transition from smooth to rough can be reversed by animal passage; i.e., the injection of rough strains into mice eventually can result in the selection of smooth variants.

The mouse is particularly susceptible to the pneumococcus (except type 14). As few as one to ten encapsulated pneumococci injected intraperitoneally into a mouse can produce overwhelming infection and death within 18 to 24 hours. The same organism in its rough form (lacking the capsule) may require a dose of 10^3 to 10^6 organisms to initiate infection. This demonstrates the role of the capsule in the virulence of the organism.

Griffith† demonstrated that pneumococci could be transformed from one type to another. If he injected live rough type 2 pneumococci into a mouse, the mouse would survive. If, on

*Pneumococci may be identified and typed utilizing the quellung reaction. The capsules of the organisms are observed to swell when mixed with type-specific antiserum.
†Griffith F: *J Hyg* 1928; 27:113–159.

the other hand, he injected the same dose of live rough type 2 mixed with killed smooth type 1 into a mouse, the mouse would die, and from the heart blood he could isolate live smooth type 1. Avery and co-workers‡ showed that the transforming principal was DNA from the dead smooth type 1. This experiment opened the door to molecular genetics.

The capsule permits the pneumococcus to survive and grow extracellularly by interfering with ingestion by phagocytic cells. The capsular material inhibits phagocytosis by preventing the attachment of the bacteria to the cell membrane of the phagocyte. Phagocytosis takes place more readily when the bacterial surface has been coated with specific antibody (opsonization). Persons with agammaglobulinemia suffer repeated infections with pneumococci and other encapsulated bacteria because their neutrophils are unable to phagocytose the organisms in the absence of opsonizing antibody. Large quantities of polysaccharide produced by certain strains of *S. pneumoniae* can bind all available antibody— a possible explanation for the virulence of type 3. Phagocytosis can occur in the absence of antibody on solid surfaces such as the lining of a lymphatic vessel or an alveolus.

Complement appears to play an important role in pneumococcal disease by facilitating the clearance of *S. pneumoniae* from the bloodstream and its subsequent phagocytosis. Clearance occurs primarily in the spleen and liver. In the presence of specific IgG anticapsular antibody, encapsulated strains of pneumococci activate the classic complement pathway and become coated with C3b. All pneumococci— whether encapsulated or not—can activate the alternative complement pathway. There is some evidence that the cell wall teichoic acid may be the activating factor. Regardless of the pathway, the result is cleavage of C3 and fixation of C3b to the bacterial surface. Organisms coated with C3b are efficiently ingested and killed by poly-

morphonuclear neutrophils. Even in the absence of specific antibody, pneumococci coated with C3b are phagocytosed and killed, a possible explanation for the resistance of nonimmune hosts to pneumococcal infection.* While the capsule is clearly an important determinant of the ability of the pneumococcus to produce disease, there are a number of other factors that also may be involved in the pathogenesis of infection.

Streptococcus pneumoniae produces an IgA protease specific for the IgA 1 subclass, and capable of splitting this immunoglobulin. Serum IgA is the primary mediator of specific immunity on human mucosal surface and is the predominant immunoglobulin in colostrum and parotid fluid, and is also present in genital and nasal secretions. IgA maintains the integrity of mucous membranes by inhibiting colonization, neutralizing viruses and toxins, and preventing penetration of microbial antigens. Although the exact role of pneumococcal IgA protease in the pathogenesis of infection is unclear, it is probable that this enzyme is involved in the ability of the pneumococcus to colonize and invade mucous membranes. Systemic or local disease is always preceded by nasopharyngeal colonization.

Pneumococcal strains vary in their ability to attach to epithelial cells. In vitro experiments have shown that pneumococci isolated from the nasopharynx of children with otitis media adhered strongly to pharyngeal epithelial cells while encapsulated strains recovered from the bloodstream of patients with pneumococcal infections adhered poorly.

It has long been known that persons with overwhelming pneumococcal disease associated with bacteremia such as pneumonia or meningitis, if not treated within a certain time die regardless of treatment. Cultures taken from these

---

‡Avery OT, et al: *J Exp Med* 1944; 79:137–158.

*Phagocytic cells have specific surface receptors for the Fc portion of IgG and IgM molecules and also for C3. This ensures that bacteria coated with antibody and complement are effectively attached to the phagocytic cell.

patients during the agonal stages of disease or at autopsy are invariably sterile.

Pneumococci produce a purpura-producing principle which causes skin and internal hemorrhage when injected into rabbits. A toxic neuraminidase is also produced, which may be involved in the neurotoxicity of meningeal infections. On autolysis, pneumococci release a cell-bound hemolytic toxin antigenically related to streptolysin O and other oxygen-labile hemolysins. The role of these substances in disease is not known, and the cause of death in overwhelming pneumococcal infection is undoubtably due to activities of Il1, TNF, etc., and a cardiodepressant which are not adequately characterized.

PNEUMOCOCCAL DISEASE

The incidence of pneumococcal pneumonia is greatest in children under 5 years of age and in adults over 50. *Streptococcus pneumoniae* is the most frequent cause of pneumonia, otitis media, and septicemia in infants 1 to 6 months of age. This susceptibility to pneumococcal infection can be related to deficiencies in complement function, lack of specific antibody, and lack of "natural antibodies" associated with pathogenic bacteria that cross-react with pneumococci. In children 7 to 12 months of age, occult pneumococcal bacteremia may occur in association with minimal respiratory symptoms and progress to meningitis if untreated.

In all age groups, pneumococci are a common cause of upper respiratory infections such as sinusitis and otitis media, but not pharyngitis or tonsillitis. These infections can extend to involve the meninges. *Streptococcus pneumoniae* is the most frequent cause of bacterial meningitis. Older people, particularly those with underlying diseases (heart failure, malignancy, or chronic liver, kidney, or pulmonary disease), have a higher incidence of bacteremia (33%) associated with pneumococcal infections than do

children (5%), and a significantly higher mortality.

Other immunodeficiency states that can predispose to pneumococcal infection are hypogammaglobulinemia, sickle cell anemia, lack of a functional spleen, or Wiskott-Aldrich syndrome.* Pneumococcal peritonitis occurs in persons with cirrhosis or carcinoma of the liver, and in children with ascites secondary to nephrosis.

Pneumococcal pneumonia is more common in chronic alcoholics than in any other patient group. Alcohol is known to interfere with mucociliary function and the cough reflex, and it also depresses the migration and function of phagocytic cells. Aspiration of vomitus or mucus containing pneumococci may occur during episodes of profound unconsciousness. Predisposing factors are those that cause an accumulation of alveolar fluid. These include pulmonary virus infection, cardiac failure, trauma to the thorax, and prolonged immobilization.

The introduction of aspirated pneumococci into an alveolus is promptly followed by edema. This fluid is a good culture medium and facilitates the spread of pneumococci to adjacent alveoli with rapid multiplication of the bacteria, accompanied by edema and hemorrhage. There is a tremendous accumulation of polymorphonuclear neutrophils, followed later by macrophages, and the infection spreads peripherally until the entire lobe or several lobes are involved.

The infection may extend to involve the pleura and lead to the development of pleuritis or empyema (an accumulation of pus in the pleural space). With the involvement of the hilar nodes the organisms may spread to the lymphatics and then enter the bloodstream, leading to metastatic lesions in distant tissues such as the heart valves, joints, meninges, and peritoneum. Bacteremia occurs in about 30% of cases of pneumococcal pneumonia. In the lung tissue the inflammatory cells phagocytose the pneumococci

---

*This syndrome is an immunodeficiency state characterized by eczema and thrombocytopenia and the inability to produce antibodies to polysaccharide antigens.

until the organisms are removed and killed, with resolution of the infection and complete healing. Phagocytosis is relatively inefficient in fluid-filled cavities such as the pleura, the pericardium, and the subarachnoid space.

Five percent to 20% of persons with pneumococcal pneumonia will die if untreated or if treatment is delayed for more than 3 days. The death rate is higher with bacteremia; in the aged; in people with diabetes; in splenectomized children; in those with sickle cell disease; in patients with chronic cardiac, pulmonary, hepatic, or renal disease; and in the presence of a lymphoproliferative disorder such as Hodgkin's disease. Eighty-five percent of patients who die from pneumococcal pneumonia have some underlying disease.

Streptococcus pneumoniae is the leading cause of bacterial meningitis in adults, and the second most frequent agent in meningitis in children over 2 years old. The organisms that colonize the oropharynx reach the central nervous system via the bloodstream. Pneumococcal bacteremia may be associated with pneumonia, endocarditis, a local infection such as sinusitis or mastoiditis, or have no apparent source. Once the blood-brain barrier has been penetrated, the organisms produce an acute inflammatory reaction of the leptomeninges. The bacterial cell wall appears to be the most potent pneumococcal surface component in inducing the inflammation by a mechanism that is still unclear. However, the pneumococcal cell wall is known to activate the alternative pathway of complement, which in turn could damage the blood-brain barrier and initiate the inflammatory reaction. Recovery from pneumococcal disease is due to the immune response. Antibodies that neutralize capsular polysaccharide appear by the fifth or sixth day and facilitate opsonization.

Protection against pneumococcal infection depends upon opsonic antibody and complement, a functioning spleen, and competent phagocytic leukocytes. Humans injected with 30 to 60 μg of polysaccharide produce protective antibodies. A vaccine is now available that contains polysaccharides from the 23 types of pneumococci that cause 80% of the bacteremic pneumococcal disease in the United States. Immunization seems to reduce nasopharyngeal colonization with the types represented in the vaccine. Vaccination is recommended for adults at high risk (those with cardiorespiratory, hepatic, or renal disease). Children younger than 2 respond poorly to the vaccine.

Penicillin is the drug of choice in nonallergic patients. Penicillin not only causes lysis of the pneumococcal cells, but in low doses interferes with capsule production, rendering the organism susceptible to phagocytosis. In 1967 the first penicillin-resistant strains were reported; 10 years later multiply resistant strains were reported from South Africa. Multiply resistant strains of pneumococci are now distributed throughout the world, including the United States. The prevalence has been estimated as being approximately 2%. The mechanism of resistance to penicillin is due to altered transpeptidases, penicillin-binding proteins (PBPs) which do not bind penicillin so cell wall formation is not disturbed.

CHAPTER 11

Mycoplasmas

A 14-year-old boy presented with chills, fever, headache, cough, and chest pain 2 weeks after returning home from summer camp. There was a gradual onset of malaise, anorexia, fever to 39.4° C, and a cough that was at first nonproductive, but later productive of small quantities of mucoid sputum. He also developed a sore throat and "runny" nose, and complained of ear pain. On physical examination, rales were heard and a chest film revealed bilateral patchy infiltrates. A serum specimen gave a positive test for cold agglutinins and a *Mycoplasma pneumoniae* complement fixation test also was positive.

Mycoplasmas are the smallest free-living organisms that are able to replicate on cell-free media. They lack a cell wall, and consequently they are resistant to penicillin and other antimicrobials that inhibit cell wall synthesis. They are bounded by a single triple-layered cell membrane, consisting of two electron-dense membranes, high in lipids, separated by a clear zone. The cytoplasm contains DNA, typical ribosomes containing RNA, and other metabolic components. Mycoplasmas are pleomorphic and their morphology varies with the species, the stage in the growth cycle, and the environment. Spherical forms reproduce by binary fission or budding; filamentous forms extend and branch and eventually divide to produce new spherical bodies.

Mycoplasmas require lipids and lipid precursors for synthesis of the cell membrane, in addition to their other nutritional needs. Animal sera added to the medium provide lipoprotein and cholesterol, and glucose or arginine are utilized as an energy source. Growth of mycoplasmas is slower than that of most bacteria. The generation time is typically 1 to 3 hours (compared to about 20 minutes for *Escherichia coli*). An exception is *Ureaplasma*, a species that grows rapidly and utilizes urea as a substrate.

Colonies of mycoplasmas on agar media are barely visible to the unaided eye, and a dissecting microscope is employed to examine agar plates. Colonies of *Ureaplasma* (originally called T strains for "tiny") are still smaller.

Common human species of mycoplasmas include *Mycoplasma orale* and *M. salivarium*, normally found in the oropharynx, and *M. fermentans*, normally present in the genitourinary tract. Pathogenic species are *M. pneumoniae*, *M. hominis*, and *Ureaplasma urealyticum*.*

*Mycoplasmas have been known since 1898 as a cause of contagious bovine pleuropneumonia. Other species have been isolated from almost all domestic and laboratory animals and were originally referred to as "pleuropneumonia-like organisms," or PPLO.

MYCOPLASMA PNEUMONIAE

Mycoplasma pneumoniae is a spherical organism with a tapered, filamentous tip containing a dense central rodlike core. This specialized structure helps the organism attach to the respiratory mucosa. Colonies of *M. pneumoniae* growing on guinea pig blood agar are surrounded by zones of hemolysis. The hemolysin has been found to be hydrogen peroxide. The major antigenic determinants of *M. pneumoniae* are the proteins and glycolipids of the cell membrane.

Mycoplasma pneumoniae can attack all levels of the respiratory tract and can cause pharyngitis, tracheobronchitis, and pneumonia (Fig 11–1). The organism is spread from person to person by droplets, i.e., by inhalation of infectious aerosols. The virulence of the organism is considerable since only 1 to 100 colony forming units is capable of causing infection in 50% of volunteers. The pathogenicity of *M. pneumoniae* depends upon the attachment of the specific terminal structure to neuraminic acid receptor sites in the trachea and bronchi. The filamentous attachment moiety on the organism is a protein designated P1. The organisms attach to the ciliated respiratory epithelium between the cilia and the microvilli, the specialized attachment tip making contact with the sialoglycoprotein re-

ceptors. The organisms do not invade the mucosal cells, but damage them by producing large amounts of hydrogen peroxide, which appears to inhibit or overcome the catalase activity of these cells. Cell damage becomes apparent in 48 to 72 hours. The mycoplasmas interfere with ciliary action and cause cell death. This leads to an inflammatory reaction, with mononuclear cells infiltrating bronchial and peribronchial tissue and the walls of the alveoli. The incubation period for mycoplasmal pneumonia is 1 to 2 weeks, which is the time required for maximal infection. There is a gradual onset of symptoms: cough, fever, and malaise persisting for several weeks, followed by a slow convalescence.

Mycoplasmal pneumonia was originally termed "primary atypical pneumonia," meaning that no bacteria could be implicated as the cause and that patients failed to respond to penicillin. *Mycoplasma pneumoniae* was originally thought to be a virus, and was termed "Eaton agent" after its discoverer. *Mycoplasma pneumoniae* accounts for approximately 20% of all cases of pneumonia in teenagers and young adults. Most cases occur between the age of 5 and 20 years.

About 5% of patients with mycoplasmal pneumonia develop acute hemorrhagic bullous myringitis, a painful infection of the eardrum. Some patients may develop the Stevens-Johnson syndrome, which is characterized by vesicular

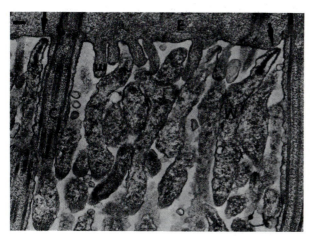

FIG 11–1.
M. Pneumoniae infection of a tracheal ring organ culture after 72 hours. Note the heavy parasitization of the mycoplasmas *(M)* with specialized tips *(arrows)* interacting with the epithelial cell *(E)* and in close apposition to the bases of the cilia *(C)* and microvilli *(m)*. The *bar marker* represents 0.1 μm. *(From Wilson MH, Collier AM: J Bacteriol 1976; 125:332–339. Used by permission.)*

and bullous lesions on mucocutaneous areas, hemolytic anemia, arthritis, and central nervous system manifestations.

During infection, a variety of humoral antibodies (IgM and IgG) are produced. Although these antibodies are cidal for *M. pneumoniae*, they are not protective and pneumonia can occur despite high serum titers. Local factors are important, and there is evidence to suggest that specific IgA in respiratory secretions prevents attachment of the organisms to respiratory epithelial cells. Cold agglutinins* appear in half of the cases of mycoplasmal pneumonia. Antibodies to mycoplasmal glycolipid may cause false-positive cardiolipin tests for syphilis. Circulating immune complexes have been detected in patients with mycoplasmal pneumonia. The immunoinflammatory reaction suggests that this disease is primarily a manifestation of the host's reaction to a rather benign infection, and that some of the pathogenicity is due to autoimmune mechanisms.

*Cold agglutinins are serum antibodies that cause red cells to clump at 4 to 6° C. Cold agglutinins are also present in some hemolytic anemias.

MYCOPLASMA HOMINIS

Mycoplasma hominis is found in the genitourinary tract. It has been related to recurrent abortion, endometritis, and salpingitis, and is isolated from the blood of about 10% of women with septic abortions or postpartum febrile episodes. It has also been recovered from the blood of febrile males following multiple trauma.

UREAPLASMA UREALYTICUM

This organism colonizes the urethra of more than 80% of sexually active persons. In males, it is the cause of at least half of the cases of nongonococcal, nonchlamydial urethritis. It has also been implicated in spontaneous abortion, low birth weight, prematurity, and other forms of fetal wastage.

CHAPTER 12

Bordetella pertussis

A 3-year-old child of recent Haitian immigrants was brought to the pediatric clinic because of severe and intractable coughing. The child had a "cold" 3 weeks previously which did not clear up; the cough became worse, paroxysmal, and was sometimes followed by vomiting. Physical examination revealed a tired-appearing child with a pale and somewhat edematous face. The only findings were several subconjunctival hemorrhages and an ulcerated lingual frenulum. A blood count showed a marked leukocytosis with a predominance of lymphocytes. The parents were unable to confirm that the child had received any immunizations. A diagnosis of pertussis was made which was confirmed when a culture of a nasopharyngeal swab grew out *Bordetella pertussis*.

Bordetella pertussis (less frequently *B. parapertussis* or *B. bronchiseptica*) causes whooping cough. The disease is spread by droplet infection and is one of the most contagious of all diseases; attack rates approach 100%. Fifty percent of all unvaccinated children have the disease by their second year. Seventy percent of the deaths associated with pertussis are in children under 1 year of age.

After an incubation period of about a week, the child develops an upper respiratory infection with a cough that persists for 1 to 2 weeks. The cough becomes worse, episodes of coughing become paroxysmal and more frequent at night. At the end of the paroxysm there is a deep inspiratory "whoop" and the older child often becomes cyanotic and anxious, and may vomit. A profound lymphocytosis is often present. The disease may persist for 1 to 4 weeks or longer. Unusual features of *B. pertussis* infection are the absence of fever, a lack of neutrophilia, and a high incidence of secondary bacterial pneumonias.

Bordetella organisms are small nonmotile gram-negative rods that are strictly aerobic. They are extremely susceptible to the fatty acids and peroxides present in peptone media and consequently an absorbent such as blood, charcoal, starch, or ion exchange resins must be added to the medium. A commonly used medium is Bordet-Gengou agar which contains potato extract, glycerol, and 25% blood. Growth occurs after 48 to 72 hours; the colonies glisten and resemble drops of mercury. *Bordetella* does not ferment carbohydrates; amino acids are utilized as energy sources. Three species are involved in human disease: *B pertussis*, *B. para-pertussis*, and *B. bronchiseptica*.

Fresh clinical isolates of *B. pertussis* have smooth colonies, and the organisms are encapsulated and virulent. These organisms are termed **phase I.** After continued transfer on laboratory media the colonies become rough, and the organisms lose their capsules and become avirulent. These organisms are designated as **phase IV.** (Phases II and III are intermediate stages.)

Bordetella pertussis has a complex structure, including a capsule of unknown composition and a large number of cell wall antigens. The organism attaches to the respiratory epithelium by means of pili or fimbriae. Fimbriated variants demonstrate strong adherence to epithelial cells in vitro and high infectivity in vivo. Nonfimbriated variants attach poorly to epithelial cells and have a low infectivity. The reservoir of *B. pertussis* is in humans.

A remarkable feature of the host-parasite relationship of *B. pertussis* is the strict viscerotropism of this organism which multiplies only in association with the ciliated epithelium of the tracheobronchial tree. The organism utilizes the amino acids abundant in the mucous layer of the respiratory tract, especially after inflammation and necrosis have occurred. The toxin produced by the organism causes a denuding of the bronchial epithelium and the infection may progress to a peribronchitis or bronchopneumonia.

Bordetella pertussis produces a large number of potentially virulent factors which may play a role in the pathogenesis of pertussis. These include pertussis toxin (PT), filamentous hemagglutinin (FHA), adenylate cyclase (AC), tracheal cytotoxin (TCT), hemolysin, endotoxin, dermonecrotic or heat-labile toxin, and fimbriae. PT is a unique exotoxin that functions as an NAD-dependent adenosine diphosphate (ADP)–ribosyltransferase. Like diphtheria and cholera toxins, *Escherichia coli* LT and pseudomonas toxin A, it affects target cell function by transferring ADP-ribose to the guanosine diphosphate (GDP)–binding proteins involved in intracellular

mediator systems. PT consists of an active A subunit enclosed by five subunits making up the B portion. The B portion is required for binding to specific cell receptors while the A portion catalyzes the ADP ribosylations of proteins. The toxin enters the bloodstream and is responsible for some or all of the systemic manifestations of the disease, including the promotion of lymphocytosis, sensitization to histamine, and hypoglycemia.

The lymphocytosis-promoting factor increases stem cell production of lymphocyte precursors causing the lymphocytosis associated with whooping cough. This component is thought to be the protective antigen; antibodies to this antigen neutralize the infectivity of the organism. This factor also has an adjuvant effect in that it enhances the immune response to other antigens. The histamine-sensitizing factor is believed to mediate the increased sensitivity to biochemical and environmental stimuli that occurs during the paroxysmal stage of the disease. Islet activation factor causes increased insulin secretion in response to normal insulinogenic stimuli such as glucose or adrenergic outflow. In some instances this can cause symptomatic hypoglycemia.

An essential step in the pathogenesis of pertussis is adherence of the organism to host cells. Attachment and adherence to cilia of respiratory epithelial cells is mediated by FHA. AC induces a profound bactericidal defect in neutrophils and macrophages associated with a suppression of superoxide production; chemotaxis is also affected. Blood monocytes are unaffected and exhibit enhanced migration to the site of inflammation. AC catalyzes the uncontrolled formation of cyclic adenosine monophosphate (AMP), disrupting normal cellular function. Activation of AC requires an activator protein which resembles calmodulin, a calcium-dependent protein regulator widely distributed in eukaryotic cells. TCT is highly specific for ciliated cells, resulting in destruction of the clearance mechanism of the respiratory tract. The dermonecrotic toxin causes necrotic lesions when injected simultaneously. Its role in the pathogenesis of pertussis is unclear, as is the role of the hemolysin and endotoxin.

Pertussis may be prevented by active immunization with a killed suspension of the organism. The vaccine is usually combined with diphtheria and tetanus toxoids (diphtheria-pertussis-tetanus, DPT).

In the 1930s whooping cough affected over 250,000 persons per year in the United States, with as many as 12,000 deaths (4.5% mortality). Following the introduction of the pertussis vaccine and the immunization of more than 90% of school-children, the annual number of cases dropped to 1,000 to 2,000 with 5 to 20 deaths. The vaccine has a fairly high frequency of side effects, some of which are potentially serious, but which rarely result in permanent neurologic sequelae or death. Despite these side effects, the benefit-risk ratio clearly favors the benefits by a large margin. When pertussis vaccination was discontinued in England, outbreaks occurred. Vaccine-induced protection is not lifelong and cases of pertussis in adults occur often in medical personnel. Vaccination is not used in adults.

A new acellular pertussis vaccine is under development that may be safer and as effective as the current vaccine. Erythromycin eradicates the organism from the respiratory tract and if given prophylactically may prevent the disease in nonimmunized children and adults.

CHAPTER 13

Legionella

A 31-year-old black man employed in the garment district of Manhattan was admitted with dyspnea, chest pain, chills, and fever of several days' duration. He was well until 1 week prior to admission when he noted a persistent headache. Several days before admission he experienced shaking chills, fever, a cough productive of blood-tinged sputum, right pleuritic pain, and dyspnea. He smoked one pack of cigarettes per day. Physical examination revealed a coherent man in mild respiratory distress. His temperature was 38.8° C; pulse, 110; respiratory rate, 26; and blood pressure, 130/90 mm Hg. Chest examination revealed rales in the right midaxillary line and at the base of the right lung. The white blood cell count was 13,900/mm^3, with 81% neutrophils and 11% band forms.

The chest film showed an infiltrate in the hilum and middle lobe of the right lung. Gram stain of the sputum showed a few neutrophils and mixed oral flora; acid-fast stain was negative. A test for cold agglutinins was negative.

The patient was treated with penicillin. After 36 hours he was still febrile and a repeat radiograph showed progression of the infiltrates to involve the entire right lung. He developed diarrhea. Therapy was changed to gentamicin and cefuroxime. On the fifth hospital day the patient became hypothermic, hypotensive, and required intubation. Erythromycin and clindamycin were added to his regimen. On the eighth hospital day a radiograph showed a right pleural effusion which was not tapped. The patient died on the eighth hospital day.

In 1976 a large outbreak of pneumonia occurred in Philadelphia among participants at an American Legion convention. There were 221 cases with 34 deaths. After considerable effort, a previously unknown bacterium was recovered from a number of the cases, and all of the infected patients showed an antibody response to this organism during their convalescence. The bacterium was named *Legionella pneumophila*.

The organism is a fastidious gram-negative rod that stains so faintly with the Gram stain in clinical material that it may be missed. Legionellae are sometimes coccobacillary; occasionally long filamentous forms are seen. Although the organism is nonmotile, polar flagella and pili have been seen in organisms grown in culture, but not in clinical specimens. On electron microscopy, the organism has a double layer of triple-unit membranes typical of gram-negative bacilli. The organism is strictly aerobic and does not grow on the usual bacteriologic media such as blood agar. Special media such as charcoal-yeast extract agar with iron, cysteine, and α-ketoglutarate are required. The organism prefers 90% humidity, and a temperature of 35° C. Colonies appear in 2 to 7 days. The organism does not ferment carbohydrates other than starch; amino acids are utilized as energy sources. *Legionella* species produce extracellular enzymes including phosphatases, lipase, DNAse, a protease, and a celphalosporinase. The organism has a weakly active endotoxin, a cytotoxin, and a hemolytic exotoxin. The role of these substances in the pathogenesis of legionellosis is unknown.

Eight serogroups of *L. pneumophila* are now recognized, as well as 25 other species of *Legionella,* 14 of which have been shown to cause human cases of pneumonia (Table 13–1).

Legionella organisms are part of the natural aquatic environment and are capable of surviving extreme ranges of environmental conditions. They can survive over a year in tap water. The organisms have been found in water from heat exchange apparatuses, evaporative condensers, and cooling towers utilized in air conditioning equipment, as well as in domestic supplies of potable tap water and shower water.

Aerosol transmission of contaminated water is probably the most important means of transmitting the infection. The pathway of infection is probably retrograde; organisms reach the alveoli and in turn infect the respiratory bronchioles, large bronchioles, and the interstitium of the lung whence, they spread to the pleura, lymphatics, the thoracic duct, and the blood.

Infection with *Legionella* species results in a wide spectrum of consequences ranging from asymptomatic seroconversion to a self-limited, mild febrile illness characterized by headache, chills, and myalgia (Pontiac fever), to a severe, potentially fatal progressive pneumonia.

Community-acquired *Legionella* pneumonia has an incubation period of 2 to 10 days. The onset is abrupt; early symptoms are chills and fever, myalgia, headache, and a nonproductive cough. The fever continues to rise steadily, often reaching 40.5° C. One third of the patients exhibit changes related to the central nervous system such as lethargy, confusion, delirium, or stupor, and 50% have diarrhea. The cough often becomes productive of purulent or blood-streaked sputum. The illness becomes progressively worse during the first week unless adequately treated. At least two thirds of the patients are smokers or have some significant underlying disease, frequently a cardiopulmonary disorder, diabetes, ethanol abuse, or malignancy. Nosocomial cases are usually immunocompromised; a high proportion of affected patients are recipients of renal transplants. Surgery may also be a predisposing factor.

Infection with *Legionella* is believed to be fairly common but the disease is rare. The attack rate is thought to be about 2%. It is estimated that there are seven subclinical cases for each clinical case. Legionnaire's disease may account for 4% to 6% of all undiagnosed pneumonias.

TABLE 13–1.

Legionella Species Shown to Cause Pneumonia

L. pneumophila
L. micdadei
L. bozemanii
L. dumoffii
L. longbeachae
L. jordanis
L. gormanii
L. feeleii
L. hackeliae
L. maceachernii
L. wadsworthii
L. cincinnatiensis

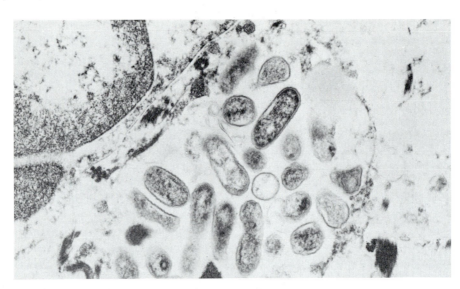

FIG 13–1.
Lung specimen showing numerous intracytoplasmic *Legionella* within alveolar macrophages. The nucleus is in the *upper left corner. (From Weisenburger DD:* Arch Pathol Lab Med *1981; 105:130. Used by permission.)*

Asymptomatic seroconversion has been demonstrated in 12% of some populations, and in 40% in some hospital employee groups.

The pathogenesis of legionnaires' disease is unclear. It is recognized that the cellular immune system is most important; organisms multiply intracellularly in blood monocytes and have been found inside of macrophages (Fig 13–1). Erythromycin and rifampin inhibit intracellular growth but do not kill the organism. Beta-lactam antibiotics are not effective but fluoroquinolones are also inhibitory when they enter the alveolar macrophages. Complement, specific antibodies, and polymorphonuclear neutrophils have little effect on resistance or immunity.

The specific diagnosis may be made by direct immunofluorescent staining of respiratory secretions, optimally obtained by transtracheal aspiration, and *L. pneumophila* can be cultured from sputum on charcoal-yeast extract agar. The organism can also be detected in sputum by DNA probe. Detection of urinary *Legionella* antigen is also useful. About one fourth of the cases show elevated antibody titers within 1 week of onset of pneumonia.

CHAPTER 14

Mycobacteria

A 22-year-old female, a Vietnamese refugee, presented with a persistent cough, fever, and 15-lb weight loss over the past 2 months. She had previously been in good health but had spent some time in crowded conditions in refugee camps where there was often not enough food. She did not smoke and denies hemoptysis or chest pain. Recently she had been waking up at 2 or 3 A.M. covered with sweat. An uncle with whom she lived had been treated for tuberculosis. Physical examination was unrevealing, but a chest film showed an infiltrate in the left hilum. A skin test with intermediate-strength purified protein derivative (PPD) produced an area of redness and induration 17 mm in diameter. A smear of her sputum revealed many acid-fast bacilli.

Mycobacteria are thin, nonmotile, rod-shaped bacteria. The genus includes saprophytic species that occur in soil, water, and some foods; commensal species that are among the indigenous microflora of certain anatomic areas; and pathogenic species that cause disease in humans and animals. Mycobacteria have a number of characteristics that distinguish them from other bacteria. They have a thick cell wall and a very high lipid content—more than 60% of the dry weight of the cell (compared with 3.0% in gram-negative bacteria and 0.5% in gram-positive species). Most of the lipids are found in the cell wall and include some unusual, high-molecular-weight complexes such as mycolic acid, mycosides, wax D, trehalose 6,6'-dimycolate, and sulfonated glycolipids. Because of their high lipid content, mycobacteria are resistant to drying, alcohol, acids, alkali, many germicides, and most antibiotics. Mycobacteria are strict aerobes. Most pathogenic species multiply much more slowly than other bacteria. For example, *Mycobacterium tuberculosis* has a doubling time of 12 to 18 hours compared with 15 minutes for *Escherichia coli*, and *M. leprae* has a doubling time of about 12 days.

Mycobacteria and some *Nocardia* are the only organisms that are acid-fast. After intensive staining with certain dyes in the presence of phenol, they resist decolorization with acid or acid-alcohol and retain the dye, whereas other bacteria are readily decolorized by these agents. The property of acid-fastness is associated with the presence of certain lipids in the cell wall.

Pathogenic mycobacteria do not produce any toxins or tissue-destroying enzymes. The principal basis for their virulence is their ability to survive after ingestion by macrophages and to multiply intracellularly. This process damages tissue after cell-mediated immunity has become activated. Mycobacteria are readily phagocytosed by neutrophils and macrophages, even in the absence of opsonin. Attachment of the mycobacteria to the cell surface is facilitated by the affinity of the lipids in the mycobacterial cell wall for the lipids in the macrophage cell membrane.

The capacity of virulent mycobacteria to multiply within mononuclear phagocytes is a reflection of the adequacy of the intracellular nutritional environment, and the ability of the organisms to withstand the intracellular killing mechanisms of the phagocytic cell. Certain virulent mycobacteria (including *M. tuberculosis*) are able to resist intracellular killing by preventing fusion of the lysosomes within the phagocytic cell. This ability has been associated with surface sulfonated glycolipids, cell wall polyglutamic acid, and ammonia production. Resistance to intraphagosome killing of *M. tuberculosis* has been associated with the presence of a mycoside. It has been observed that virulent mycobacteria are good catalase producers, and this enzyme may render the phagocytic myeloperoxidase system ineffective.

Trehalose dimycolate has been termed **cord factor** because of its presence in virulent tubercle bacilli that grow in serpentine cords composed of parallel strings of bacilli. Cord factor can be extracted from the bacteria with solvents and has been shown to be lethal to mice; to inhibit the migration of polymorphonuclear leukocytes (negative chemotaxis); induce granuloma formation; and protect against experimental infection. The role of cord factor in the pathogenesis of tuberculosis is still unclear.

Waxes D are a group of substances composed of mycolic acid, polysaccharides, and peptides. When combined with proteins of the tubercle bacillus (tuberculoproteins), wax D can induce a cell-mediated immune response (delayed-type hypersensitivity) against the tuberculoprotein. Wax D has a marked adjuvant activity and can enhance antibody production against a protein antigen when injected together with the antigen in an emulsion. Tuberculoproteins such as old tuberculin (OT) and PPD are weak antigens that can induce antibodies but not cell-mediated immunity. They can be used to detect the presence of delayed-type hypersensitivity.

Mycobacterial diseases tend to develop slowly, follow a chronic course, and elicit a granulomatous response. The infectivity of *M. tuberculosis* is high, but the virulence for healthy humans is relatively low. Disease following infection with *M. tuberculosis* is the exception rather than the rule, except in patients with underlying defects of cellular immunity.

TUBERCULOSIS

Tuberculosis is a chronic disease caused by *M. tuberculosis*. Because this organism multiplies best in an environment with high oxygen tension, the predominant infection is most often found in the lung, but many other organs and tissues may be involved. Tissue damage occurs as a consequence of delayed-type hypersensitivity induced when infection is established. *Mycobacterium tuberculosis* is a slowly growing, strictly aerobic organism. It can be distinguished from other mycobacteria by its ability to produce niacin. Colonies are rough, buff-colored, and require 10 to 20 days to appear.

With the increase in urbanization in Europe associated with the Industrial Revolution, the incidence and mortality increased markedly and reached a high of 400 deaths per 100,000 population per year during the 18th and 19th centuries. Poverty, overcrowding, malnutrition, and poor hygiene play an important role in the incidence of tuberculosis, as does the stress of war or economic depression. In populations living in primitive and crowded conditions, tuberculosis causes a high infant and child mortality, with a second peak in young adults. In more developed societies the disease is more common in older people. In the United States in the early 1900s, the annual death rate due to tuberculosis was 200/100,000 population, but it has been steadily declining until 1985 when it began to rise again in urban areas primarily in young males and in individuals from developing nations. There has been a 200% increase in tuberculosis in some cities since 1990.

Tuberculosis is primarily a disease of man. Infection results from exposure of a previously uninfected person to virulent *M. tuberculosis*. Transmission most commonly occurs by inhalation of an aerosol of droplet nuclei coming from a person with cavitary tuberculosis. Coughing, sneezing, and talking produce droplets of saliva or mucus containing tubercle bacilli. Most of these droplets travel 3 to 4 ft and fall to the floor or on furniture, but some droplets evaporate leaving particles of 1 to 5 μm suspended in the air. These aerosols of infective particles remain for long periods of time and may be inhaled and deposited in the alveoli of a susceptible person, resulting in primary infection.

When one or more mycobacteria reach an alveolus, they are promptly ingested by alveolar macrophages. They continue to multiply intracellularly, and an inflammatory cellular exudate appears. After a few weeks, the multiplying tubercle bacilli spread to involve the hilar lymph nodes and then disseminate via the lymphatics and the bloodstream to seed all of the organs and tissues of the body. In the majority of cases, cellular immunity and delayed-type hypersensitivity begin to develop and become evident by 4 to 6 weeks after infection.

Delayed-type hypersensitivity can be demonstrated by skin testing with tuberculin. The metastatic foci become granulomatous lesions composed of macrophages, epithelioid and giant cells, and tubercle bacilli. With the development of cellular immunity, the macrophages become activated and increasingly lethal for the tubercle bacilli, and the bacterial multiplication

and dissemination cease. The organisms are destroyed by the body defenses, except in the apex of the lung where high oxygen tension and carbon dioxide favor growth. Tuberculoprotein is released into the tissue causing platelet thrombi and vascular occlusion, and the lesions undergo necrosis and caseation. The apical lesion becomes walled-off and calcified. In time, little or no evidence of infection remains. In young persons a residual calcified nodule in the lung and an enlarged hilar node (Ghon complex) may be seen on the radiograph.

Primary tuberculosis is essentially an asymptomatic, nondestructive disease that occurs in a nonimmune, nonallergic person. The consequences of primary infection are determined by the balance between the person's native resistance (age, race*) and the virulence of the infecting organism. In most cases the disease enters the quiescent stage, which may last for the entire lifetime of the person or may be reactivated many years later.

In a small number of persons the primary disease becomes progressive. Tubercle bacilli multiply in the pulmonary parenchyma with extensive exudate and caseous lesions which may extend to involve the pleura or the pericardium. Enlarged hilar nodes may obstruct a bronchus, resulting in bronchiectasis and a nonventilated fibrotic lobe or segment. This process continues until widespread disease and possibly death occurs.

The disease may be reactivated during adolescence, pregnancy, during the sixth and seventh decades of life, or whenever immunity decreases as a result of malnutrition, diabetes mellitus, or immunosuppression associated with steroid therapy or other diseases. Most reactivated cases show pulmonary involvement with cavitary apical lesions and subsequent tracheobronchial spread. In about 10% of cases, reactivated latent organisms may produce extrapulmonary disease involving the kidneys, pleura, bones, or meninges. All of these can lead to miliary disease which is invariably fatal if not treated.†

The major drugs used in the treatment of tuberculosis are isoniazid, rifampin, ethambutol, pyrazinamide, and streptomycin. With combinations of these drugs properly administered, tuberculosis is now virtually 100% curable. Tubercle bacilli resistant to some of these drugs sometimes are encountered. Unfortunately, drug resistance has become a serious problem in some parts of the U.S. In some cases the acquisition of drug resistance is associated with decreased virulence, but transmission of resistant bacilli is known to occur.

Prevention of tuberculosis has been approached in two ways. Many countries employ as a vaccine an attenuated strain of *M. bovis:* bacille Calmette-Guérin (BCG). BCG vaccination should be considered for infants that are tuberculin skin test–negative and that have repeated exposure to patients with sputum-positive pulmonary tuberculosis, and for groups in which an excessive rate of new infection can be demonstrated. BCG should not be given to persons with impaired immune responses or with preexisting fibrotic lung disease. The other major approach to prevention is the treatment of persons with subclinical tuberculous infection, i.e., without active disease, but whose tuberculin skin test is positive.

OTHER MYCOBACTERIAL INFECTIONS

Bovine tuberculosis is caused by an organism that is bacteriologically distinct from *M. tuberculosis*, but which produces a similar clinical picture. *Mycobacterium bovis* is most commonly spread by ingestion of milk from cows with mammary tuberculosis. The elimination of infected cows from dairy herds and the practice of pasteurization has virtually eliminated this disease in the United States.

Nontuberculous mycobacterial infections may resemble tuberculosis clinically, pathologically, and radiologically, but are caused by a group of mycobacteria that were originally classified as "atypical." The nontuberculous mycobacteria have been classified into four groups by Runyon,* each group containing several species. Some of the species are pathogenic.

Group I organisms are **photochromogens.** Colonies grown in the dark are buff-colored, but become yellow when exposed to light *(M. kansasii)*. Group II organisms are termed **scotochromogens** *(M. scrofulaceum)* and are pigmented when grown in the dark. Group III species are termed **nonphotochromogens** since the color of the colonies does not change when exposed to light *(M. avium, M. intracellulare)*. Groups I, II, and III are slow-growing, and require 7 to 14 days for colonies to appear. Group IV organisms are rapid growers and show colonial growth in 4 to 6 days *(M. chelonei)*.

The nontuberculous mycobacteria are generally resistant to the major antituberculous drugs and are significantly less virulent for guinea pigs than *M. tuberculosis*. All of them have environmental reservoirs such as soil, water, or organic debris, and infections are acquired from these sources by ingestion, inhalation of dust particles, or inoculation into the skin. Unlike tuberculosis, there is no person-to-person transmission. A tuberculosis-like disease is produced in immunocompromised persons— patients who have been immunosuppressed for organ transplantation or for the treatment of neoplastic disease. Serious pulmonary and disseminated infection with *M. avium-intracellulare* has been reported in patients with acquired immunodeficiency syndrome (AIDS).

Certain species of nontuberculous mycobacteria have strict temperature ranges for growth.

---

*Africans, American Indians, orientals, and Eskimos are more susceptible to tuberculosis infection than whites.

†At the Columbia University College of Physicians and Surgeons, unsuspected miliary tuberculosis has been known as "Hyde Park disease" ever since Eleanor Roosevelt succumbed to miliary tuberculosis while being evaluated for a fever of unknown origin.

*Runyon EH: *Med Clin North Am* 1959; 43:273–290.

Mycobacterium marinum and *M. ulcerans* grow at 32° C but cannot grow at 37° C. Disease produced by these species is limited to skin ulcers; e.g., "swimming pool granuloma."

Since the nontuberculous mycobacteria are all acid-fast bacilli, they cannot be distinguished from *M. tuberculosis* microscopically. Differentiation and speciation can only be done by culture biochemical testing or nucleic acid probes. Table 14–1 lists the various nontuberculous mycobacteria.

LEPROSY

Leprosy is a chronic infection that primarily affects the skin, peripheral nerves, and mucous membranes. The etiologic agent is *M. leprae*, an obligate intracellular parasite that has not been grown in artificial media or tissue culture. The organism can be grown in the mouse footpad, and produces disseminated disease in the nine-banded armadillo. *Mycobacterium leprae* occurs predominantly in modified mononuclear or epithelioid structures called lepra cells, which contain large numbers of bacilli in packets. A tuberculin-like substance, lepromin, is used in a skin test. It is prepared by grinding lepromatous nodules and autoclaving the material. Although the lepromin test is not diagnostic, it provides a useful measure of the patient's immune status. Leprosy tends to be a rural disease in contrast to tuberculosis, which has an urban distribution.

The exact mode of transmission of leprosy is not known, but respiratory spread is probable since the upper respiratory tract of patients with active lepromatous disease is heavily infected. These persons, when sneezing or coughing, produce aerosols that contain large numbers of ba-

TABLE 14–1.
Pathogenic Nontuberculous Mycobacteria

Species	Type of Infection	Reservoir
M. bovis	Pulmonary, cervical lymphadenitis	Humans, cattle
M. leprae	Leprosy	Humans, armadillos?
Photochromogens: Runyon group I		
M. kansasii	Pulmonary, skeletal, disseminated, sporotrichoid, genitourinary	Cattle, water
M. marinum	Swimming pool granuloma, sporotrichoid	Fish, water
M. simiae	Pulmonary	Monkeys
Scotochromogens: Runyon group II		
M. scrofulaceum	Pulmonary, cervical lymphadenitis	Soil, water
M. szulgai	Pulmonary	?
M. xenopi	Pulmonary	Hot water tanks
Nonphotochromogens: Runyon group III		
M. avium-intracellulare	Pulmonary, skeletal, disseminated, cervical lymphadenitis, genitourinary	Animals, soil, water
M. ulcerans	Chronic skin ulcer	?
M. malmoense	Pulmonary	?
M. haemophilum	Ulcers, abscesses (in renal transplant patients)	?
Rapid growers: Runyon group IV		
M. fortuitum	Pulmonary, sporotrichoid	Animals, soil, water
M. chelonae	Pulmonary, sporotrichoid, cervical lymphadenitis	Animals, soil, water

cilli. When these bacilli are inhaled by a susceptible person, the organisms presumably grow in the upper respiratory tract and disseminate via the bloodstream. The incubation period of leprosy is measured in years or decades. Although leprosy seems to be very contagious, the infectivity is very low because the majority of people are not susceptible.

The pathogenesis of leprosy appears to be related to the ability of *M. leprae* to survive and replicate in macrophages and nerve cells. The organism is benign and does not directly produce tissue damage. In normal people the invading bacilli are phagocytosed by macrophages and destroyed. It would seem that susceptible persons have a defective cell-mediated immune response specific for *M. leprae*. In such persons macrophages do not recognize the bacilli as

pathogens and multiplication and dissemination occur.

There are three clinical forms of leprosy: tuberculoid, borderline, and lepromatous. The initial form of the disease is determined by the degree of immune deficit that exists. Patients with the greatest resistance keep the infection localized and develop tuberculoid disease, while those persons with the least resistance develop the generalized lepromatous form. The majority of patients develop an unstable borderline form that tends to shift toward the lepromatous form unless there is adequate treatment.

In tuberculoid leprosy (Fig 14–1), the cell-mediated immune response appears to be intact and the lepromin test is positive. There is little circulating antibody and there are few leprosy bacilli in the tissue. Lesions are well defined,

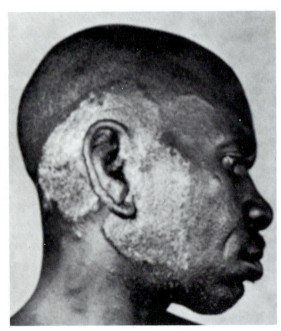

FIG 14–1.
Tuberculoid leprosy. An anesthetic plaque with well-defined edges and scaly surface extends over the cheek and into the scalp in a man from Zaire. *(From Binford CH, Connor DH (eds):* Pathology of Tropical and Extraordinary Diseases: An Atlas. *Washington, DC, Armed Forces Institute of Pathology, 1976.)*

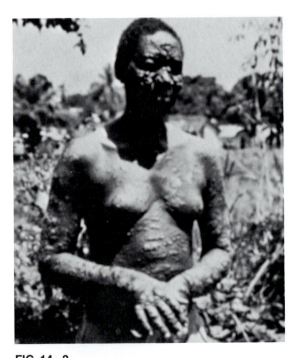

FIG 14–2.
Lepromatous Leprosy. Advanced lepromatous lesions over most of the body and gynecomastia in this adult Zairian man. *(From Binford CH, Connor DH (eds):* Pathology of Tropical and Extraordinary Diseases: An Atlas. *Washington, DC, Armed Forces Institute of Pathology, 1976.)*

hypopigmented, and localized. The organisms invade the nerves and colonize the Schwann cells, obliterating and destroying the peripheral nerves.

In lepromatous leprosy (Fig 14–2), the cell-mediated immune response is suppressed and the lepromin test is negative. There are high levels of circulating antibody, and the sera of these patients often contain immune complexes of antibacillary antibody and anti-immunoglobulin. These complexes precipitate at 4° C (cryoglobulins) and contribute to the pathogenesis of the disease. *Mycobacterium leprae* accumulate in large numbers because of the specific anergy to the organism. The bloodstream contains huge masses of bacilli. Skin lesions are extensive, diffuse, and symmetric and may contain 10^9 bacilli per gram of tissue. With treatment the lesions of lepromatous patients tend to become more tuberculoid.

The treatment of leprosy relies on sulfones such as dapsone, which blocks *p*-aminobenzoic acid metabolism in *M. leprae*. More definitive therapy is available with rifampin. Treatment must be continued for many years with dapsone.

CHAPTER 15

Fungal Agents of Pulmonary Infection

A 24-year-old male graduate student developed headache, chills, fever, weakness, severe substernal chest pain, and a cough productive of scanty amounts of sputum. Several weeks previously he had joined a group of amateur speleologists in exploring a small cave frequented by many bats. Physical examination revealed him to be in mild respiratory distress with a temperature of 40° C, and a palpable liver and spleen. The chest film showed a diffuse interstitial pneumonitis. Laboratory tests, including a Gram stain examination of sputum, were unremarkable. He was started on prednisone. His fever persisted for 10 days and then gradually returned to normal. At that time a histoplasmin skin test was strongly positive.

The above case serves to introduce a group of microorganisms somewhat different from the bacteria that have been described thus far. Fungi are eukaryotic cells with a distinct nucleus bounded by a nuclear membrane, and containing organelles including mitochondria and an endoplasmic reticulum. Most fungi are free-living and are widely distributed in soil and plant material throughout the world. A few species maintain a commensal existence as members of the indigenous microflora of man, particularly in the mouth, intestine, vagina, and skin.

Fungus (mycotic) infections may be acquired exogenously by the inhalation of spores or by the inoculation of spores or mycelial fragments into the tissues as a result of trauma. Endogenous infections follow some compromise in the host's defenses and are associated with fungal overgrowth or invasion of the tissues by a member of the indigenous fungal flora. Mycotic infections are not usually transferred from person to person. Fungi grow more slowly than bacteria and several days to weeks may be required for the appearance of colonies. Many fungi can grow on simple media and only require an organic source of carbon, e.g., glucose and a nitrogen source such as amino acid or ammonium or nitrate salts. Most fungi are strictly aerobic and can grow in a wide range of temperatures ranging from 18 to 37° C. The cell wall of fungi contains chitin (also found in the exoskeletons of Crustacea) and other carbohydrate polymers such as glucans and mannans. Sterols are present in the cytoplasmic membrane. Fungi are resistant to most of the antibiotics that affect bacteria.

The pathogenic fungi may exist in two forms: yeasts or molds. **Yeasts** are single spherical or oval cells slightly smaller than a red blood cell (3–5 mm in diameter). Yeasts reproduce by budding, an asexual process whereby small daughter cells are produced and pinched off. Colonies of yeasts are smooth and somewhat larger than bacterial colonies. **Molds** are multicellular filamentous forms, the basic element of which are hyphae. Molds reproduce by elongation and branching of the filamentous hyphal elements to form a tangled mass called a **mycelium.** Colonies of molds are often fuzzy or hairy. Table 15–1 lists some genera of yeasts, molds, and dimorphic fungi. The pathogenic fungi also reproduce by a variety of asexual spores. In some forms, the spores (conidia) are borne on specialized hyphal structures (conidiophores). Two forms of conidia can be distinguished: microconidia and macroconidia. Other asexual spores develop within the hyphae themselves and include **blastospores,** which bud from a hypha; **arthrospores,** produced by the segmentation of a hypha into rectangular, thick-walled cells; and **chlamydospores,** round thick-walled resting spores. Fungi can also reproduce sexually.

Under normal atmospheric conditions, some fungal species grow only in the yeast form, others only in the mold form. Many of the pathogenic fungi are dimorphic and grow in both yeast and mold phases. Dimorphic fungi appear as yeast in infected tissue and convert to the mold phase in culture. Growth at 37° C in a rich nutritive environment favors the yeast form, while growth in an increased carbon dioxide atmosphere at 18 to 25° C in a simple medium favors the development of the mycelial mold form. Some dimorphic species have been shown to contain two distinct forms of chitin synthetase. The interconversion of these two forms plays a role in the biosynthesis of cell wall and subsequent morphogenesis.

Fungus infections can be classified into four groups, each of which is associated with certain species of fungi (Table 15–2): **opportunistic infections,** secondary to a defect in host resistance;

TABLE 15–1.
Genera of Fungi Pathogenic for Man

Yeasts
  Candida
  Torulopsis
  Cryptococcus
  Rhodotorula
Molds
  Aspergillus
  Rhizopus
  Mucor
  Microsporum
  Trichophyton
  Epidermophyton
Diphasic fungi
  Histoplasma
  Blastomyces
  Coccidioides
  Paracoccidioides
  Sporothrix

TABLE 15–2.
Fungi Involved in Mycotic Infections

Systemic infections
  Histoplasma capsulatum
  Histoplasma duboisii
  Blastomyces dermatitidis
  Coccidioides immitis
  Paracoccidioides brasiliensis
  Cryptococcus neoformans
Opportunistic infections
  Candida albicans
  Candida spp.
  Aspergillus spp.
  Rhizopus spp.
  Mucor pusillus
Subcutaneous infections
  Sporothrix schenckii
  Fonseca spp.
  Cladosporium carrionii
  Phialophora verrucosa
Superficial infections
  Microsporum spp.
  Trichophyton spp.
  Epidermophyton floccosum

systemic infections involving the deeper tissue and organs, most commonly the respiratory tract; **subcutaneous infections,** limited to the deeper subcutaneous tissue and lymphatics; and **superficial infections,** involving only the skin, hair, and nails.

HISTOPLASMA

Histoplasmosis is an infection caused by *Histoplasma capsulatum,* a dimorphic fungus which despite its name does not have a capsule. The mycelial form of the organism is free-living in nature in the soil. The droppings of chickens, pigeons, and other birds provide an excellent culture medium for the organism, as does the excrement of bats. The soil in the area where birds and bats roost contains very high concentrations of *H. capsulatum.* Man (and animals) become infected by inhaling the spores (conidia) from the soil (Fig 15-1).

Individual cases occur in farmers who have cleaned out old chicken coops and inhaled infected dust, or persons exploring caves rich in bat guano. In one outbreak in Ohio, almost 300 people became infected following the raking and sweeping of a schoolyard containing trees that had served as a roost for blackbirds. The disease is worldwide in distribution, and endemic in certain areas of the United States, particularly the Mississippi, Ohio, and St. Lawrence river valleys. In these areas, almost all humans and wild and domestic animals are infected. More than 90% of the resident adults give a positive skin test to histoplasmin.

Histoplasma capsulatum is an intracellular parasite of reticuloendothelial cells where it exists in the yeast form (Fig 15–2). The pathogenesis of the disease parallels that of tuberculosis. After the spores are inhaled and reach the alveoli, the organism converts to the yeast forms which multiply by budding. Patchy areas of interstitial pneumonitis result. The regional lymph nodes become involved and the organisms enter the bloodstream. This primary form takes about 7 to 14 days and in the majority of persons is asymptomatic. A few patients may develop an influenza-like syndrome, particularly if the dose has been very heavy. At about 2 weeks following infection, humoral antibodies and cell-mediated immunity appear, the organisms are cleared from the blood by macrophages of the reticuloendothelial system, and the infected foci in the lungs become necrotic and granulomatous, and eventually calcify.

Primary histoplasmosis is a self-limited disease in most cases. In persons with underlying pulmonary disease such as the emphysema seen in heavy smokers, the infection may progress to a cavitary form with eventual fibrosis. In a few persons—infants, the elderly, and the immunosuppressed—the infections may disseminate to involve one or more organ systems, with fever, weight loss, and local lesions. Involvement of the adrenal glands can result in chronic adrenal failure (Addison's disease) and is a significant cause of death.

Cell-mediated immunity is the most important factor in limiting histoplasmosis. Humoral antibody is of no importance in limiting infection. Histoplasmosis is an important reactivation infection in patients with AIDS.

A variety of histoplasmosis found in Africa is caused by a related organism, *H. duboisii,* which primarily infects the skin and lymph nodes. Spread to bone is common, but lung lesions are uncommon. Current therapy for normal hosts is an azole: fluconazole or itraconazole.

BLASTOMYCES

Blastomyces dermatitidis, a dimorphic fungus, is the cause of North American blastomycosis. The organism resembles *Histoplasma* in that it exists in the mycelial form as a free-living soil saprophyte and converts to the yeast form in infected tissues. The geographic distribution of the disease is similar to that of histoplasmosis,

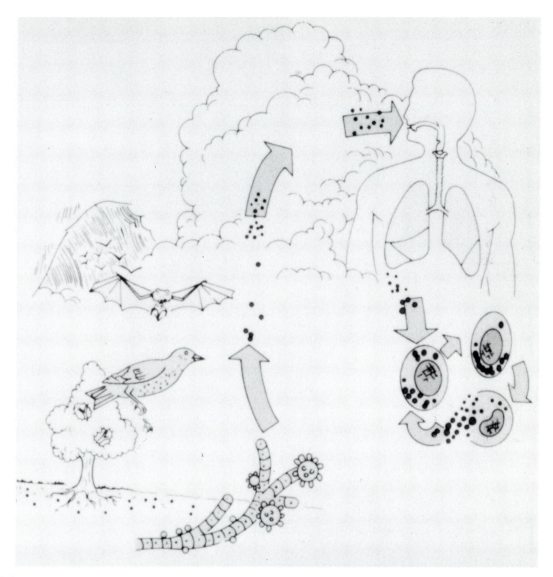

FIG 15–1.
Schematic illustration of the natural history of the saprobic and parasitic cycles of *Histoplasma capsulatum.*

namely, the Eastern and Central States, especially the Mississippi and Ohio river valleys. Bird droppings may be a source of human infection.

Infection results from the inhalation of spores (conidia), and the primary site is pulmonary. Primary blastomycosis is generally benign and self-limited. Symptoms may include fever, cough, and joint and muscle aches, or be limited to pleuritic chest pain. A few persons develop progressive pulmonary disease with cavitation and metastastic dissemination to skin, bone, and genitourinary sites. Granulomatous skin lesions are common on exposed areas and may progress

FIG 15–2.
Yeast cells of *Histoplasma capsulatum* phagocytized by bone marrow mononuclear cells (Giemsa-stained section).

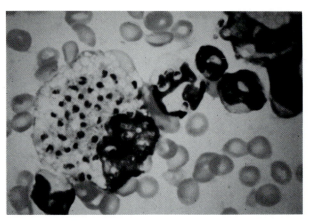

to extensive necrosis and scar formation which can be disfiguring. Chronic osteomyelitis results from bone involvement. The most common genitourinary site is the prostate.

The conversion from the mycelial to the yeast form is temperature-dependent, the yeast form growing at 37° C. It has been observed that the endogenous respiratory rate of the yeast form is several times higher than that of the mycelial form. At the temperature of the animal host, conversion from mold to yeast occurs, resulting in a greatly increased energy potential available to the invading organism. There has been speculation that the virulence of *B. dermatitidis* may be related to its high total lipid content. Phospholipids from the organism have been shown to elicit a granulomatous response in mice.

Cell-mediated immunity is more important than humoral antibody in recovery from *B. dermatitidis* infection. Current therapy is with an azole such as ketoconazole or itraconazole.

PARACOCCIDIOIDES

Paracoccidioides brasiliensis is the etiologic agent of South American blastomycosis. It is a dimorphic fungus that lives in the soil in the mycelial form and occurs in infected tissues in the yeast form. The disease is limited to tropical and subtropical areas of Central and South America.

The route of infection is believed to be via the inhalation of spores, leading to a primary pulmonary infection. The regional lymph nodes become involved and hematogenous dissemination to other organs occurs in about 70% of patients. Males are much more frequently infected than females, possibly because of the direct inhibitory effect of estrogens on the fungus. In persons with intact immune mechanisms, the disseminated lesions usually heal or become latent. Reactivation of latent lesions may occur many years later. In about one third of the patients, the pulmonary disease becomes progressive, characterized by chronic respiratory symptoms.

In rare instances—usually in patients younger than 20 years of age—the disseminated disease becomes severe. Extrapulmonary lesions consist of granulomatous cutaneous and mucocutaneous ulcers that slowly spread. Mucous membrane lesions occur most frequently on the lips, gums, tongue, and palate; they are painful and gradually deepen and enlarge with subsequent destruction of the underlying tissues. Cervical lymph nodes may enlarge and suppurate. Arteritis is common, and the liver and spleen may become involved. An acute form of the disease that may clinically simulate lymphoma occurs in children.

Paracoccidioides brasiliensis exhibits thermal

dimorphism. Conversion from the mycelial to the yeast phase occurs at temperatures higher than about 20° C. The yeast form grows well at 32° C, but growth slows and is reduced at 35 to 38° C, and ceases at 39° C. This may explain the predominance of cutaneous and mucocutaneous lesions.* Therapy with azole antibiotics appears to be curative.

COCCIDIOIDES

Coccidioides immitis, a dimorphic fungus, is the cause of coccidioidomycosis. The organism differs from other dimorphic fungi in that the tissue phase is a large round spherule rather than a yeast (Fig 15–3). In the soil the organism exists in the mycelial form. As the mycelia develop, they fragment into barrel-shaped arthrospores. These arthrospores are resistant to environmental conditions and are the infective form of the organism.

Coccidioidomycosis is sharply limited in the United States to the semiarid Southwest. Up to 90% of people resident in this endemic region have positive skin tests with coccidioidin, indicating previous infection. Infections have occurred in persons who have only spent a few hours in these areas.

The inhaled arthrospores reach the alveoli and convert to spherules (Fig 15–3). Phagocytosis of arthrospores and early spherules is impeded by some property of the outer cell wall; older spherules become too large (30–100 µm) to be ingested by phagocytic cells. Multiple endospores develop within the spherule and are released when the spherule ruptures. Each endospore subsequently develops into a new spherule.

The primary pulmonary infection lasts for a

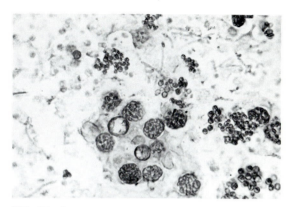

FIG 15–3.
C. immitis spherules in lung.

---

few weeks to a month or so. About half of the infected persons develop cough, fever, chest pain, and malaise (San Joaquin Valley fever). Twenty-five percent of white females and 5% of males have allergic manifestations such as rashes or arthralgia; the remaining 50% of infected persons are asymptomatic. The only evidence of their infection is a positive skin test to coccidioidin (a filtrate of the arthrospore phase culture).

A small number of infected people develop progressive pulmonary disease with chronic cough and cavitation. There is an association between diabetes mellitus and the development of progressive pulmonary disease. Less than 0.001% of infected persons develop disseminated disease. Compared with whites, Mexicans, blacks, Filipinos, and Orientals have an increased risk of dissemination. The most frequent sites of metastatic lesions are the bones and joints in which osteomyelitis and arthritis develop, and the meninges and subcutaneous tissues where nodules develop. The most serious form of infection is meningitis, which is extremely difficult to cure.

Disseminated coccidioidomycosis may develop as an opportunistic infection associated with pregnancy, Hodgkin's disease, or immunosuppressive therapy. Renal transplant recipients who have diabetes are particularly prone to this

---

*In this respect, *P. brasiliensis* resembles *Mycobacterium marinum* and *M. ulcerans* which can grow at 32° C but not at 37° C, and produce infections limited to skin ulcers.

complication. Therapy is with amphotericin, but fluconazole, an azole, also appears effective for the pulmonary and meningeal disease.

ASPERGILLUS

Aspergilli are rapidly growing molds that are widely distributed in nature and found in soil, vegetation, and organic debris. Infection is acquired by the inhalation of spores which reach the upper airway or the lungs. Outbreaks of aspergillosis have occurred in hospitals and are associated with colonized air conditioners or dust produced from insulating material during building construction. Although there are many species of aspergillus, the organism most commonly involved in human disease is *Aspergillus fumigatus* or *A. flavus*, but occasionally other species are implicated.

There are several clinical forms of aspergillosis. The lung is most often infected and may be involved in three distinct ways: **invasive pulmonary** disease in immunocompromised patients which takes multiple forms; pulmonary **aspergilloma** or fungus ball in which hyphae form a large mass within a residual cavity of healed tuberculosis or sarcoid disease; and **allergic bronchopulmonary disease** (farmer's lung), which is an allergic reaction to the inhaled spores. Another localized form of aspergillosis is external otitis. In debilitated patients, these superficial lesions can invade the inner ear, orbit, and paranasal sinuses. Disseminated disease is not seen in immunologically intact persons. Metastatic abscesses are common in the brain, heart, and liver.

The defense of humans against aspergillosis is first the alveolar macrophages which kill the spores, and second, polymorphonuclear leukocytes which kill phae. No specific immune functions are known. Macrophages kill conidia with nonoxidative killing systems which can be impaired by steroids. There is no evidence that antibodies are protective or that cellular immunity is involved. Predisposing factors are neutropenia and the use of cytotoxic drugs and corticosteroids in organ transplantation and the treatment of neoplastic disease. The diagnosis of fungal infections is based upon the recovery of the organism by culture. Therapy is with amphotericin B.

PART III

Cardiovascular Infections

CHAPTER 16

Overview of Cardiovascular Infections

Cardiovascular infections involve the lining of the heart or the valves (endocarditis), or both; the heart muscle itself (myocarditis); the sac that encloses the heart (pericarditis); and the blood vessels, primarily the veins (septic thrombophlebitis).

Bacteremia, the presence of bacteria in the normally sterile circulating blood, is a necessary precursor to cardiovascular infections. Bacteremia may be transient, intermittent, or continuous. In transient bacteremia, the organisms enter the bloodstream, remain there for a brief period (15–20 minutes), and are rapidly cleared by the reticuloendothelial system. Transient bacteremic episodes are usually asymptomatic and may be associated with physiologic functions such as menstruation and parturition, or with brushing the teeth. Transient episodes of bacteremia may also occur during medical or dental procedures that involve manipulation of anatomic sites that are normally inhabited by an indigenous bacterial flora (Table 16–1). Transient bacteremia may also occur in the early phase of certain infections (e.g., pneumonia, meningitis), and is frequently accompanied by shaking chills (rigor) and fever.

Intermittent bacteremia, characterized by recurrent episodes usually accompanied by chills and fever, often occurs with abdominal or pelvic abscesses (liver, kidney), biliary tract disease, or chronic meningococcemia.

Continuous bacteremia is almost always symptomatic with chills and fever and is present in bacterial endocarditis, septic thrombophlebitis, and in some multisystem diseases including typhoid fever, brucellosis, and leprosy. Continuous bacteremia of nosocomial origin may be the result of contaminated intravenous (IV) infusions. The organisms involved in bacteremia often reflect the involved anatomic site, e.g., a mouth organism such as viridans streptococcus may enter the bloodstream following dental manipulation, and a urethral species such as an enterococcus might cause bacteremia following a urologic procedure.

The consequences of bacteremia range from negligible, as in transient physiologic episodes, to potentially fatal shock, to colonization of the cardiac valves and endocardium leading to bacterial endocarditis.

BACTERIAL ENDOCARDITIS

Two factors must be present for the initiation of endocardial infection: bacteremia, and a modified endocardial surface that predisposes to colonization by the circulating bacteria (Fig

TABLE 16–1.

Clinical Procedures That Can Induce Transient Bacteremia

System	Procedure
Dental	Scaling of teeth
	Gingivectomy
Airway	Tracheal intubation
	Tonsillectomy
	Bronchoscopy
Gastrointestinal	Esophageal dilation
	Upper GI endoscopy
	Rectal examination
	Sigmoidoscopy
	Colonoscopy
	Barium enema
	Liver biopsy
Genitourinary	Bladder aspiration
	Catheterization
	Cystoscopy
	Urethral dilatation
	Biopsy of prostate
	Transurethral prostatectomy
	Placement of intrauterine contraceptive device (IUD)
Cardiovascular	IV catheterization
	Pacemaker placement
	Angiography
	Hemodialysis
	Cardiac catheterization
	IV drug abuse
Manipulation of septic foci	Incision and drainage of abscesses
	Burn surgery

16–1). The endothelium may be damaged by immune complex formation associated with acute rheumatic fever or certain connective tissue disorders (lupus, Marfan's syndrome). Endothelial alteration may also be the consequence of hemodynamic abnormalities such as high pressure gradients or regurgitant blood flow associated with congenital cardiac defects, or damaged by direct trauma resulting from intracardiac foreign bodies (e.g., catheters). Regardless of the cause, the altered, "roughened" endothelium

triggers the deposition of platelets and fibrin to form a thrombus.

For colonization of the platelet-fibrin thrombus to occur, circulating bacteria must be able to resist the bactericidal activity of serum complement; circumvent immunoglobulin-mediated clearance; perhaps trigger platelet aggregation; and adhere to the platelet-fibrin matrix. This adherence may be mediated by the ability of the organism to produce a glycocalyx of extracellular polysaccharide, or in the case of certain species (streptococci, staphylococci), by the interaction of lipoteichoic acid on the bacterial surface with fibronectin on the endothelial surface. Once the valve surface is colonized the colonies develop and by 24 hours they are encased in additional layers of fibrin and platelets forming a biofilm that protects the enlarging colonies from the action of phagocytic cells. This biofilm also functions to concentrate nutrients for bacterial growth. Local bacterial invasion can produce myocardial and valve ring abscesses leading to conduction defects, infarction, valve perforation, or pericarditis.

Enlarging bits of vegetation break off and are swept away in the bloodstream as microemboli. Although these emboli are not sterile they seldom cause metastatic infection because the organisms are usually of low virulence and they are exposed to phagocytic cells and to specific antibodies. The simultaneous presence of bacterial antigen and antibody leads to the formation of circulatory immune complexes. The deposition of these complexes is probably responsible for the petechiae, Roth's spots, Osler's nodes, Janeway's lesions, arthritis, and glomerulonephritis that often accompany bacterial endocarditis.*

Clinically, bacterial endocarditis is characterized by fever and heart murmur, chills, malaise,

---

*Petechiae are pinpoint intradermal hemorrhages; Roth's spots are retinal hemorrhages; Osler's nodes are tender, raised, discolorations on the pads of fingers and toes; Janeway's lesions are small painless areas of redness or hemorrhage on the palms or soles.

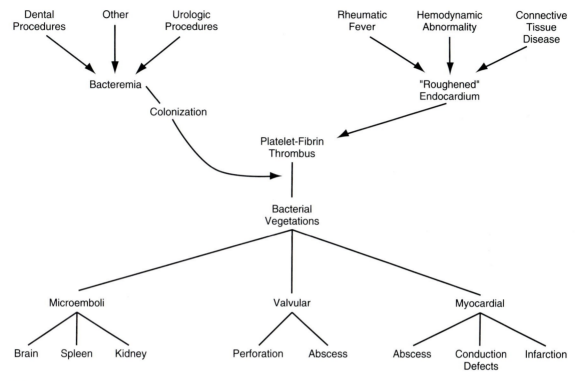

FIG 16–1.
Pathophysiology of endocarditis.

anorexia, weight loss, and evidence of peripheral embolization such as enlargement of the spleen. The mitral and aortic valves are most frequently involved, accounting for 60% to 80% of cases. Viridans group streptococci, stephylococci, and coagulase-negative staphylococci and *Staphylococcus aureus* are the next most frequent agents (10%–30%). Various gram-negative bacilli including *Cardiobacterium hominis, Actinobacillus actinomycetemcomitans, Haemophilus aphrophilus, H. paraphrophilus, H. parainfluenzae, Legionella* species, enterobacteria, and pseudomonads, occur in 1% to 5% of cases. Other bacteria, including the pneumococcus, group A streptococcus, corynebacteria, *Neisseria gonorrhoeae*, and so forth, are uncommon. Fungi causing endocarditis include *Candida albicans* and other species of *Candida, Aspergillus, Histoplasma, Blastomyces, Coccidioides, Cryptococcus*, and *Mucor*. Infective endocarditis may also be caused by *Coxiella burnetii*, the agent of Q fever.

Predisposing factors in endocarditis are the presence of prosthetic valves and IV drug abuse. The laboratory diagnosis of bacterial endocarditis is primarily dependent upon the recovery of the etiologic agent from blood cultures. Treatment requires prolonged therapy with an antimicrobial agent to which the organism has been shown to be susceptible in vitro. The most important complications of endocarditis are congestive heart failure due to valve damage and cerebra emboli.

MYOCARDITIS

Infectious myocarditis has been associated with almost every known bacterial, rickettsial, viral, and parasitic disease. In the past, myocarditis was found in patients with tuberculosis, diphtheria, and syphilis. Clinically, myocarditis is characterized by fatigue, dyspnea, cardiac enlargement, and arrhythmias and other electrocardiographic (ECG) abnormalities. Myocarditis may be caused by staphylococci, gonococci, pneumococci, or meningococci. Myocarditis may be seen in cases of leptospirosis, rickettsial diseases, and a wide variety of viral illnesses, including poliomyelitis, influenza, and the diseases caused by coxsackievirus.

PERICARDITIS

Organisms can reach the pericardium by extension of pleuropulmonary infections; via the bloodstream; or directly, during surgical or accidental trauma. Infectious pericarditis can be caused by a large number of viruses (coxsackievirus, echovirus, and mumps, influenza, Epstein-Barr, varicella-zoster, and herpes simplex viruses), bacteria (enterobacteria, staphylococci, streptococci, *Mycobacterium tuberculosis*, meningococci, *Haemophilus influenzae*, *Bacteroides*), fungi *(Histoplasma, Coccidioides, Blastomyces, Cryptococcus, Candida, Aspergillus)*, and parasites *(Toxoplasma)*. As a result of the inflammatory reaction, fluid or exudate fills the pericardial space. If the pressure within the pericardium increases, there may be interference with the contractions of the heart (tamponade) with limitation of cardiac output.

Clinically pericarditis presents with chest pain, a friction rub (detected by auscultation), cardiac enlargement, and ECG abnormalities. The diagnosis is usually made by clinical, ECG, and radiographic findings. On occasion, fluid is removed for culture by pericardiocentesis.

SUPPURATIVE THROMBOPHLEBITIS

Suppurative thrombophlebitis is an inflammation of the vein wall. This may occur as a complication of a skin infection, or of parturition, abortion, pelvic abscess, or gynecologic surgery. A thrombus may be a site for local entrapment and colonization by bacteria. The affected vein becomes enlarged, thickened, and the lumen becomes filled with pus and clots, and bacteremia and sepsis may be present. Superficial veins show signs of inflammation (warmth, redness, swelling, and tenderness). The most frequent causative agent is *S. aureus;* other organisms are aerobic gram-negative species *Klebsiella*, such as *Pseudomonas aeruginosa* (especially in burn patients), enterococci, and *Candida* species. Diagnosis is based upon the finding of gross pus within the veins; culture of the pus generally reveals the organism. Therapy often requires both antibiotics and surgical excision.

CHAPTER 17

Nonhemolytic Streptococci and Enterococci

A 27-year-old man was seen with a chief complaint of fever and generalized aches and pains for the past week. His history included tonsillitis, acute rheumatic fever with congestive heart failure, and recurring sore throat. Physical examination revealed a well-developed, well-nourished man, with a temperature of 38.8° C and a grade 2/4 apical systolic murmur radiating to the axilla. Laboratory results included a white blood cell count of 8,800/mm^3 and an erythrocyte sedimentation rate of 55 mm/hr.* Three blood cultures grew out an α-hemolytic streptococcus of the viridans group, subsequently identified as *Streptococcus mitis.*

The nonhemolytic streptococci affecting man include *S. pneumoniae* (pneumococcus), the viridans streptococci, and the Lancefield group D organisms, which contain enterococcal and non-enterococcal species (Table 17–1). They are all gram-positive cocci that appear in pairs, short

*The erythrocyte sedimentation rate (ESR or "sed rate") is a nonspecific indicator of inflammation. Normal values (Wintrobe) are 0–5 mm/hr for males, 0–15 mm/hr for females. Higher values suggest infection.

chains, or as single cells. They are facultative; pinhead colonies appear on blood agar in 24 to 48 hours at 35° C. Colonies may be surrounded by a green zone (alpha hemolysis) or there may be no visible alteration of the blood agar.

All of these organisms occur as major components of the indigenous flora inhabiting the mucous membranes of the mouth, pharynx, intestine, urethra, and vagina. They are normally harmless commensals, but they are capable of causing disease when they gain entrance to anatomic sites that are normally sterile.

VIRIDANS STREPTOCOCCI

Streptococcus mitis, S. sanguis, and *S. mutans* reside on the surfaces of the teeth and have been shown to cause endocarditis. *Streptococcus mitis* can also cause empyema, pericarditis, peritonitis, and septic thrombophlebitis. *Streptococcus salivarius* and *S. anginosus* also cause endocarditis. *Streptococcus mutans* is probably the most cariogenic species in the group. *Streptococcus anginosus,* also known as *S. milleri,* can also cause suppurative infections, including acute and chronic sinusitis, and abscesses of the brain, lung, liver, and appendix.

TABLE 17–1.

The Major Streptococci Affecting Humans

Hemolytic streptococci	
Lancefield group A *(S. pyogenes)*	
Lancefield group B *(S. agalactiae)*	
Lancefield group C	Usually β-hemolytic
Lancefield group F	
Lancefield group G	
Nonhemolytic streptococci	
Lancefield group D	
Nonenterococcal	
S. bovis	
S. equinus	Hemolysis varies with species of
Enterococcal	blood agar
Enterococcus faecalis	
E. faecium	
Viridans streptococci	
S. mitis	
S. salivarius	
S. mutans	
S. sanguis	Usually α-hemolytic
S. anginosus	
S. vestibularis	
Pneumococcus	
Str. pneumoniae	

NONENTEROCOCCAL GROUP D STREPTOCOCCI

The primary species is *S. bovis,* which is a normal intestinal inhabitant. *Streptococcus bovis* is a significant cause of septicemia and endocarditis, particularly in persons with neoplastic disease of the gastrointestinal tract. The high association of *S. bovis* bacteremia with carcinoma of the colon suggests that all patients with this organism in their blood need aggressive evaluation of their gastrointestinal tract.

ENTEROCOCCAL GROUP D SPECIES

Enterococci are found in the feces of most healthy adults reflecting the fact that the gastro-intestinal tract is the major site of human colonization. Enterococci can also be found in the biliary tract, attesting to their ability to grow in a high concentration of bile.

Enterococci are the third most common bacterial organism isolated from human infection (following *Escherichia coli* and staphylococci) and as such account for almost 10% of all bacteria recovered. Ninety percent of all enterococci isolated are *Enterococcus faecalis,* 8% are *E. faecium,* and other enterococcal species are rare.

The most frequent disease caused by enterococci are urinary tract infections. Enterococcal urinary tract infections are particularly common in elderly men, and are often asymptomatic. Enterococci account for about 15% of nosocomial urinary tract infections. Enterococci are the fifth most common cause of nosocomial infections.

Predisposing factors are prolonged hospitalization, instrumentation, or severe chronic illness. Enterococci are common causes of postoperative wound infections, especially following gastrointestinal surgery. Therapy with cephalosporin antibiotics tends to select out enterococci. Enterococci are frequently recovered together with other organisms (enterobacteria, anaerobes) from intraabdominal and pelvic abscesses, peritonitis, and cholecystitis. Foot infections in patients with diabetes are caused by enterococci in association with other bacteria.

Enterococcal bacteremia may follow instrumentation of the urinary tract, or intravenous drug abuse. Neonatal sepsis and meningitis can be caused by enterococci. Enterococci are the third most common cause of endocarditis, especially in men over 60 years of age. Fortunately, less than 3% of patients with enterococcal bacteremia develop endocarditis.

Enterococci have the ability to exchange genetic material, including resistance genes, with staphylococci and gram-negative species such as *E. coli.* Consequently they have become among the most resistant bacteria encountered in clinical practice. High-level resistance to gentamicin and other aminoglycosides is common and about 1% of isolates are resistant to ampicillin. Resistance to vancomycin is so far rare.

PART IV

Central Nervous System Infections

CHAPTER 18

Overview of Central Nervous System Infections

Infections of the central nervous system include meningitis (involving the pia and arachnoid coverings of the brain); encephalitis and brain abscess (involving the brain itself); and epidural and subdural infections (involving the dura mater of the brain and spinal cord) (Fig 18–1). This section will also consider infections of ventriculoatrial and ventricoloperitoneal shunts used to relieve hydrocephalus, and clostridial toxemic diseases (tetanus and botulism) the primary manifestations of which involve both the central and peripheral nervous systems.

MENINGITIS

The leptomeninges may be infected by bacteria, viruses, fungi, or amebas. Most bacterial and viral meningitides occur as acute clinical episodes with an abrupt onset and a relatively brief course. Meningitis due to fungi and some bacteria (*Mycobacterium tuberculosis, Treponema pallidum, Nocardia*) generally is more chronic in nature with a gradual onset and a more prolonged duration.

Meningitis may be characterized as **purulent,** in which the cerebrospinal fluid (CSF) contains many white blood cells and readily visualizable microorganisms (usually bacteria); or as **aseptic,** in which no microorganisms are seen in the CSF. Aseptic meningitis is usually due to a virus or to a leptospira. Bacterial meningitis is a life-threatening disease. The case fatality rate is 20% to 30% in neonates and adults, especially the elderly, and 3% to 5% in infants and children.

Bacteria reach the central nervous system from a distant focus via the bloodstream or by direct extension from an adjacent anatomic site, or by trauma to the skull. The pathogenesis of hematogenous infection begins with the attachment, colonization, and invasion of a distant site, often the nasopharynx but occasionally the skin, heart, or intestine. The organisms invade the blood, some bacterial species avoiding phagocytosis, while others survive in mononuclear phagocytes. The meninges are seeded by these bloodborne bacteria, probably via the choroid plexuses of the lateral ventricles and then to the extracerebral spinal space. Alternatively, bacteria from local foci such as the paranasal sinuses, ears, mastoid, or facial areas extend to infect the meninges. The bacteria spread rapidly throughout the subarachnoid space via the CSF

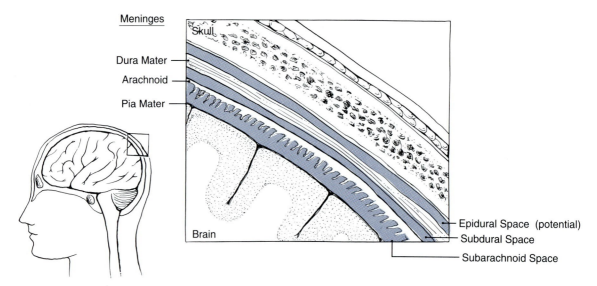

Meninges

Skull

Dura Mater

Arachnoid

Pia Mater

Brain

Epidural Space (potential)

Subdural Space

Subarachnoid Space

FIG 18–1.
Sites of infection of the meninges.

(which is completely exchanged every 3 to 4 hours, and does not normally contain phagocytic cells or high levels of antibodies). Meningeal pathogens are generally limited to the subarachnoid space; the cerebrum tends to resist bacterial invasion.

Bacterial products such as cell wall teichoic acid fragments from pneumococci, or lipooligosaccharide from *Haemophilus influenzae* trigger an inflammatory cascade of cytokines (tumor necrosis factor, interleukin-1, prostaglandin E_2) and the influx of polymorphonuclear neutrophils. The consequences of this inflammation include disruption of the blood-brain barrier with decreased glucose transport and more permeability to serum proteins; cerebral edema; intracranial hypertension; and alteration of the cerebral blood flow.

The bacterial etiology of meningitis varies with the age group: in neonates (birth to 2 months) the most frequent organisms are group B streptococci and *Escherichia coli;* other species less commonly encountered are enteric gram-negative bacilli (salmonella, *Klebsiella-Enterobacter, Citrobacter, Proteus*); *Listeria mono-*

cytogenes, and "water organisms" (*Flavobacterium, Pseudomonas*). Group B streptococcal and enterobacterial infections may be acquired from the maternal vagina or the hands of nursery personnel; *Listeria* infections are associated with dairy products and *Flavobacterium* or *Pseudomonas* infections can frequently be traced to contaminated humidification equipment.

The highest age-specific attack rates after the newborn period are between 3 and 8 months of age with the incidence remaining high up to 2 years. The three most important organisms are *H. influenzae, Neisseria meningitidis,* and *Streptococcus pneumoniae.* Together, these three organisms account for 70% of all cases of meningitis. *Streptococcus pneumoniae* is the most common etiologic agent when all age groups are considered. *Haemophilus influenzae* is the principal pathogen of the pediatric group aged 2 months to 6 years, with a peak incidence at 2 years. *Neisseria meningitidis* also occurs in the 1- to 4-year-old group with another peak in adolescence and young adults. *Streptococcus pneumoniae* occurs up to the eighth decade of life. Other organisms include other streptococci, *E.*

coli, Staphylococcus aureus, Pseudomonas aeruginosa, and leptospira.

Tuberculous meningitis is almost always due to *M. tuberculosis*. The highest incidence is in the first 5 years of life, but it can occur at any age. In children, tuberculous meningitis is usually a complication of primary infection; in adults it may develop during the course of chronic tuberculosis. If untreated, tuberculous meningitis is fatal in 1 or 2 months. It has been postulated that tuberculous meningitis occurs in two stages: tuberculous lesions form in the meninges or brain from hematogenous dissemination of organisms during primary infection. After a latent period of months or years meningitis develops when an adjacent caseous lesion discharges bacilli directly into the subarachnoid space. It has been suggested that the inflammatory reaction of the meninges is a delayed hypersensitivity reaction.

The pathogenesis of viral meningitis is somewhat different from bacterial meningitis in several ways: viral agents can reach the central nervous system via the olfactory tract (herpes simplex) or neural pathways (rabies) as well as hematogenously in blood monocytes; viruses are not restricted to the meninges but may also involve the brain (meningoencephalitis). The etiology of viral meningitis varies with the season, the geographic location, and the age and immune status of the patient. About 70% of cases are caused by enteroviruses, especially echoviruses and coxsackieviruses A and B. The majority of these cases are in children and occur in the late summer and early fall. Mumps virus meningitis is more frequent in winter months. Cases of herpes simplex and human immunodeficiency virus (HIV) meningitis occur sporadically. Meningoencephalitis caused by arboviruses (eastern equine encephalitis, western equine encephalitis, and St. Louis encephalitis viruses) is more common during the summer months. Adenovirus and cytomegalovirus meningitis are usually seen in immunocompromised persons. Other viral agents that may cause meningitis are lymphocytic choriomeningitis, varicella-zoster, and Epstein-Barr viruses.

Central nervous system infections caused by fungi usually present clinically as chronic meningitis. Meningitis caused by *Cryptococcus neoformans* is a common complication of immunocompromised patients. *Histoplasma capsulatum* and *Coccidiodes immitis* can also cause meningitis, as can *Borrelia burgdorferi*, several amebas, and *Toxoplasma gondii* (a parasite).

Acute meningitis typically presents with fever, headache, stiff neck, vomiting, photophobia, and lethargy, confusion, or coma. In infants, there may be jaundice, diarrhea, irritability, convulsions, and a bulging fontanel. The onset is usually abrupt and symptoms progress over a period of hours. The presence of petechiae or purpura suggest a meningococcal etiology, especially if accompanied by shock and intravascular coagulation. Chronic meningitis (tuberculous, fungal, syphilitic) usually has a gradual onset with headache, fever, and lethargy developing over a period of weeks.

The laboratory diagnosis of meningitis is primarily based upon examination of the CSF. In bacterial and fungal meningitis, CSF glucose is usually decreased below 50% of the blood glucose level, and CSF protein is increased above 50 mg/dL. In viral meningitis, glucose and protein are often normal. White blood cell counts may be greater than $1,000/mm^3$ with polymorphonuclear neutrophils predominating in bacterial meningitis, and lymphocytes in viral and fungal meningitis. A Gram stain of the CSF sediment often reveals the bacterial agent (gram-positive or gram-negative cocci, or gram-negative bacilli). Direct antigen detection by latex agglutination may be useful to rapidly define the common bacterial agents and is more sensitive for detecting cryptococcal infection than India ink preparations (Table 18–1).

Treatment of meningitis needs to be initiated promptly and consists of one or two antibiotics that are known to be effective against the majority of etiologic agents.

TABLE 18–1.

Characteristics of Various Types of Meningitis

Type	Etiologic Agents	Cerebrospinal Fluid			Ancillary Tests
		Sugar	Protein	Cells	
Bacterial	S. pneumoniae N. meningitidis H. influenzae Group B streptococci E. coli	Decreased	Elevated	Polys	Direct antigen defection by latex agglutination
Tuberculosis	M. tuberculosis	Decreased	Elevated	Polys and lymphocytes	——
Viral	Echo Coxsackie Mumps HSV HIV Adeno CMV LCM VZ EB	Normal or slightly decreased	Elevated	Predomin- ately lymphocytes	——
Fungal	C. neoformans C. immitis H. capsulatum	Normal or slightly decreased	Slightly elevated	Predom- inately lymphocytes	Detection of cryptococcal antigen

BRAIN ABSCESS

Although brain abscess can occur at any age, the peak incidence is during the second and third decades of life and again between 50 and 70 years of age. Abscesses may be single or multiple. The major sources of brain abscess are chronic pulmonary infections, sinusitis, and ear and odontogenic infections. Patients with cyanotic congenital heart disease or endocarditis may also be at risk for development of brain abscess because of the high incidence of cerebral embolization. Streptococci are the organisms most often involved in brain abscess; these are usually members of the viridans group, but anaerobic streptococci *(Peptostreptococcus)* are also frequently involved. Other anaerobes recovered are *Bacteroides* species. At least 50% of abscesses are polymicrobial, with two or more bacterial species. *Proteus* and other enterobacteria, *S. aureus, Haemophilus* species, *Actinomyces, Nocardia, Blastomyces,* and other fungi can also cause brain abscesses.

Diagnosis of brain abscess largely depends upon computed tomographic (CT) scan techniques and magnetic resonance imaging. Lumbar puncture should be avoided because of the risk of brain herniation; the CSF usually provides little useful information. Treatment is usually a combination of antimicrobial therapy and surgical removal when feasible.

PARAMENINGEAL INFECTIONS

These include subdural empyema, and cranial and spinal epidural abscesses. Subdural empyema, a severe, rapidly progressive, life-threatening infection, is a collection of pus in the space between the dura and the arachnoid. Epidural infections are localized between the dura and the overlying skull or vertebral column. Symptoms are headache or backache, fever, and focal neurologic signs. The sources of cranial infections are infections of the middle ear or sinuses, especially frontal; trauma; or neurosurgery. Streptococci and staphylococci are the most frequent causes. Diagnosis is by CT scan and treatment is a combination of antibiotics and surgical drainage.

Spinal epidural abscess can result from direct extension of vertebral osteomyelitis; perinephric, retropharyngeal, or psoas abscesses; or decubitus ulcers. Hematogenous seeding can also occur from furuncles, cellulitis, or infected acne. Symptoms include fever, localized tenderness, and nerve root pain. *Staphylococcus aureus* is the organism most commonly involved; occasionally gram-negative bacilli and anaerobes are involved. Diagnosis is by computer tomography, magnetic resonance imaging, and myelography; treatment is surgical drainage and antibiotics.

INFECTIONS OF CENTRAL NERVOUS SYSTEM SHUNTS

These devices are used to treat hydrocephalus by diverting CSF to the peritoneum or the jugular vein. Ten percent to 30% of patients with ventriculoatrial or ventriculoperitoneal shunts develop meningitis. Shunts may become infected at the time of surgery, hematogenously, or in a retrograde fashion from the contaminated distal end of the catheter. The clinical presentation ranges from low-grade fever to fulminant ventriculitis and sepsis. Coagulase-negative staphylococci are the leading cause of shunt infections and account for over half of them; other causative organisms are *Propionibacterium acnes*, gram-negative bacilli, and enterococci.

CHAPTER 19

Neisseria meningitidis

A 20-year-old naval trainee presented at sick call with a fever to 39.4° C, severe headache, and stiff neck. During the previous week he had a mild upper respiratory infection, but on this day he awoke with fever and severe headache. Physical examination revealed an acutely ill man with a blood pressure of 105/65 mm Hg, pulse rate of 120, and a temperature of 39.8° C. There were a few small petechiae on the volar surfaces of both forearms. Neurologic tests indicated meningeal involvement and a lumbar puncture was performed. The cerebrospinal fluid (CSF) was slightly turbid with a protein of 75 mg/dL and glucose of 20 mg/dL. The white blood cell count was 400/mm^3, 95% of which were polymorphonuclear neutrophils.* A Gram stain of the CSF revealed gram-negative diplococci, many of which were intracellular. Cultures of the CSF and of the blood both grew out *Neisseria meningitidis.*

*Normal CSF protein is 15–45 mg/dL; normal CSF glucose is about 50% of blood glucose, or 50–75 mg/dL. The spinal fluid is normally clear and should not contain any cells other than an occasional lymphocyte.

Neisseria are Gram-negative diplococci, most species of which are members of the indigenous flora of man and animals. Gram-negative bacteria differ from gram-positive species in several respects besides the final color they take in the Gram stain. There are significant differences in their resistance to antimicrobial agents and their susceptibility to disruption by physical and chemical forces. Many of these differences can be related to the structure of their cell envelope. Gram-negative bacteria have a two-layered cell wall; a thin layer of peptidoglycan, and an outer membrane of lipopolysaccharide and lipoprotein. (The cell envelope of gram-positive bacteria is typically a thick cell wall of peptidoglycan containing a small amount of teichoic acid.)

Neisseria are kidney-shaped cocci that characteristically occur in pairs with the flattened sides opposing. *Neisseria* are aerobic organisms that have a high level of cytochrome C oxidase (an enzyme that provides a ready means for the identification of this genus in the laboratory). Commensal species (*N. sicca, N. flava, N. lactamica,* etc.) inhabit the mucous membranes of the upper respiratory and genitourinary tracts and seldom cause disease.

The two pathogenic species of this genus are *N. meningitidis,* the meningococcus, and *N.*

gonorrhoeae, the gonococcus. Meningococci and gonococci have a number of characteristics that distinguish them from their nonpathogenic brethren besides their ability to produce disease. These two pathogens are more fastidious, i.e., they require enriched media such as heated blood (chocolate) agar supplemented with yeast extract; they grow only in the narrow temperature range of 35 to 37° C, and prefer a humid atmosphere enriched with 5% to 10% carbon dioxide. Most can grow on enriched agar containing colistin and vancomycin that inhibits the nonpathogenic *Neisseria* and many other members of the indigenous flora.

VIRULENCE FACTORS

Surface components and the products elaborated by meningococci that may play a role in the early steps of the disease process include IgA protease, the ability to obtain iron for growth, pili, lipopolysaccharide, peptidoglycan, outer membrane proteins I and II, and capsular polysaccharide.

The presence of IgA seems to be important in protecting mucosal surfaces from invasion by pathogenic bacteria. The ability of the meningococcus to produce an enzyme capable of hydrolyzing the immunoglobulin present on mucous membranes is thought to play a role in the pathogenesis of disease caused by this species, possibly by facilitating its adherence to epithelial cells and subsequent colonization.

In order to obtain the iron required for growth, bacterial pathogens must compete with the host's iron-binding and storage proteins. These proteins occur in serum (transferrin), in mucosal secretions (lactoferrin), and in tissues (ferritin). The meningococcus produces a low-molecular-weight chelating compound called a siderophore that acquires iron primarily from lactoferrin for the synthesis of membrane proteins. The gonococcus does not have a sidero-

phore, but is able to scavenge iron from transferrin by some unknown mechanism.

Meningococci isolated from clinical specimens have large numbers of pili emanating from their surface. The presence of pili is associated with a substantially enhanced ability to attach to human cells. Meningococci have lipopolysaccharide (endotoxin) in their outer membranes. The lipopolysaccharide appears to be a major site of binding of bactericidal antibody. Piliated meningococci attach to cells from the nasopharynx and oropharynx in high numbers, and to cells from other body sites in much lower numbers. This suggests that the surface of nasopharyngeal cells may have a specific pilus receptor.

Invasive strains have polysaccharide capsules covering the cell wall. The cell wall contains the lipopolysaccharide-endotoxin complex and outer membrane proteins. The polysaccharide capsules provide the means for serologic grouping. Presently, 12 known serogroups (A, B, C, D, H, I, K, X, Y, Z, W-135, and 29E) exist. Serogroups H, I, and K have been isolated in China, and a new serogroup provisionally designated as L has recently been described in Canada.* Although the capsule actually reduces the adherence of meningococci to epithelial cells, it also acts to interfere with phagocytosis, permitting the organisms to multiply extracellularly until anticapsular antibodies appear. The capsules are also implicated in the resistance of meningococci to killing by complement-mediated lysis. The capsule is clearly an important virulence factor.

The presence of large amounts of polysaccharide in the cell wall may also contribute to the virulence of meningococci. This lipopolysaccharide endotoxin is as potent as endotoxins from other gram-negative bacteria in the activation of the clotting cascade, with extensive fibrin deposition in small vessels (disseminated intravascular coagulation) and the production of altered vascular resistance leading to circulatory

*Meningococci may be grouped by the quellung reaction, in which the capsule swells when brought into contact with homologous antiserum.

collapse and death. However, meningococcal lipopolysaccharide is ten times more potent than the endotoxins of other gram-negative bacteria in eliciting the Shwartzman reaction.

Large increases in the virulence of *N. meningitidis* occur after the organism has been grown under iron-restricted conditions at a low pH. These environmental factors result in the expression of a new outer membrane protein.

Meningococci of groups B and C share an identical outer membrane protein designated type 2. Antibodies against this protein are bactericidal in the presence of complement.

PATHOGENESIS OF MENINGOCOCCAL INFECTION

The ability of certain strains of meningococci to adhere to the mucosa, colonize, invade, and produce disease in susceptible persons is a function of surface antigens such as the capsule, the outer membrane protein, and enzymes such as IgA protease. The lipopolysaccharide endotoxin of the cell wall may be involved in some of the manifestations of meningococcal disease.

Meningococcal disease must be preceded by nasopharyngeal colonization (Fig 19–1). The organisms are acquired by inhalation of aerosols of respiratory secretions from carriers. The nasopharynx is the site preferentially colonized by meningococci. This warm, moist area with a high carbon dioxide concentration provides ideal conditions for the multiplication of this organism. During nonepidemic periods, meningococci colonize the nasopharynx of up to 35% of the normal population. The carrier state persists for many weeks or months. Meningococci recovered from the nasopharynx or throat of healthy carriers are often nonencapsulated and therefore ungroupable.

About 7 to 10 days after colonization of the upper respiratory tract, bactericidal antibodies appear. These antibodies do not affect the meningococci that have colonized the pharynx, but

they prevent invasion, bloodstream multiplication, and dissemination.

Only a small percentage of the population develop disease, even when colonized by an encapsulated strain. In closed populations such as military training camps or boarding schools, carrier rates may approach 50% before and during an outbreak. The incidence of disease in such populations is usually less than 1%.

Susceptibility to meningococcal disease is directly related to the presence of specific antibody. The binding of IgG or IgM to the organism activates the complement cascade, which leads to lysis of the cell wall by C8 and C9.

Young adults infected with *N. meningitidis*, particularly group C, may be susceptible to dissemination of infection if they produce too much serum IgA antibody. This antibody attaches to the bacteria and blocks attachment of IgG and IgM antibodies that would induce complement-mediated lysis of the organism and protect against dissemination.

Three forms of meningococcal disease occur: (1) Acute meningitis characterized by the abrupt onset of fever, headache, stiff neck, confusion or stupor, and other evidence of meningeal involvement. Petechiae are seen in about 75% of persons with this disease and purpura may occur. (2) Fulminant meningococcemia (Waterhouse-Friderichsen syndrome) with or without meningitis may occur and is characterized by intravascular coagulation, circulatory collapse, and death within a few hours. (This syndrome may be an example of the generalized Shwartzman reaction.) (3) Chronic meningococcemia characterized by transient episodes of bacteremia, often accompanied by sterile arthritis and pustular dermatitis.

Group C meningococcal disease has been shown to have a significantly higher case fatality rate than group A disease because of the higher rate of fulminant meningococcemia associated with group C infection.

Allergic complications of meningococcal disease, such as vasculitis, arthritis, pericarditis,

A   **B**

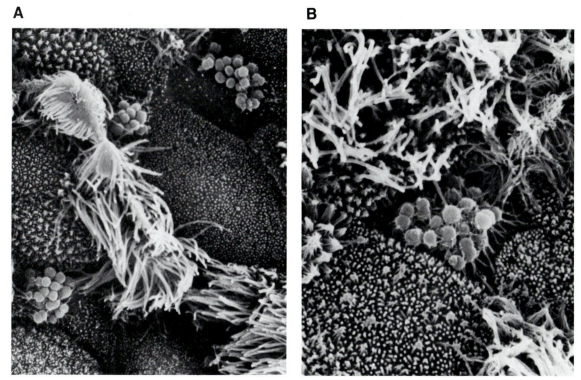

FIG 19–1.
Scanning electron micrographs showing interaction of *Neisseria meningitidis* with human nasopharyngeal mucosa. The meningococci attach by pili to the microvilli of nonciliated cells but not to ciliated cells **(A)**. Attachment stimulates folding of the epithelial cell membrane around the bacteria and subsequent internalization **(B)**. *(From Stephens DS, Hoffman LH, McGee ZA: J Infect Dis 1983; 148:369. Used by permission.)*

and episcleritis, occur in 5% to 10% of patients. These are more common following group C infection than group A disease. With the onset of the rash or arthritis, there is a fall in the circulating level of C3. Biopsies of skin and synovial membrane reveal the deposition of immune complexes containing capsular polysaccharide, IgG or IgM, and complement.

Group Y meningococci cause pneumonia four times more often than they cause meningococcemia or meningitis. One study has suggested that pneumonia may be the most common manifestation of meningococcal disease, with many cases being missed because of the responsiveness of such disease to penicillin.

Meningococci have been isolated with in-

creasing frequency from patients attending venereal disease clinics. The organism has been recovered from the urethra and rectum of patients who give a history of oral-genital contact. The meningococcus may cause a urethritis clinically indistinguishable from that produced by the gonococcus.

IMMUNITY TO MENINGOCOCCAL INFECTION

Passively acquired immunity to meningococcal infection is present during the first few months of life. With the disappearance of these maternal antibodies, the young infant is highly susceptible to disease. By 2 years of age most infants become colonized with *N. lactamica*, an organism closely related to the meningococcus, but of considerably less virulence. Colonization with *N. lactamica* results in the development of cross-reacting bactericidal antibody to meningococci of groups A, B, and C. Other sources of meningococcal A, B, and C antibodies are bacteria indigenous to the throat and intestine that have polysaccharide capsules similar to those of the meningococci. Such organisms include staphylococci, viridans streptococci, and certain strains of *Escherichia coli*.

In the past, groups A and C accounted for most of the cases of meningococcal disease in the United States; at the present time many cases are caused by group B. The capsular polysaccharides of groups A and C are highly immunogenic in man; they have been purified and combined in an effective vaccine. Specific bactericidal antibodies are produced that are protective. In the presence of complement these antibodies produce lysis of the organisms and act as a circulatory barrier to invasion and dissemination from the upper respiratory tract.

The group B capsular polysaccharide is not immunogenic in man, either because the *N*-acetylneuraminic acid capsular material is almost identical to the neuraminic acid residues on host cell membranes, or possibly because the capsular material is rapidly degraded by host enzymes before it can reach the cells involved in antibody production. Recently, two experimental group B vaccines show promise of success. In one of them the capsular material is combined with the outer membrane protein, and in the other, tetanus toxoid is combined with the polysaccharide.

Nasopharyngeal carriage (and the potential for meningococcal disease) can be temporarily eliminated by chemoprophylaxis with rifampin. This treatment is given to patients who have been exposed to cases of meningococcal meningitis. Penicillin, while effective in treating meningococcal disease, cannot be used for chemoprophylaxis because adequate levels of the drug cannot be achieved in the nasopharynx. Rifampin is used for prophylaxis. A group **A, C, X, Y,** 135**W** vaccine is available for military personnel and for travellers to areas where meningococcal disease is a problem.

CHAPTER 20

Viral Agents of Central Nervous System Infection

One week after arriving at college, an 18-year-old man had sudden onset of severe headache, a stiff neck, and photophobia. He had been in good health until the previous day when he had a sore throat and a slight fever. On physical examination, he was found to have a temperature of 37.7° C and an erythematous maculopapular rash over his trunk and arms. There was mild nuchal rigidity and a lumbar puncture was performed. His cerebrospinal fluid (CSF) was clear, with normal glucose and protein levels, but the white blood cell count was 200/mm^3, most of which were lymphocytes. No organisms were seen on Gram stain of the CSF sediment. A clinical diagnosis of viral meningitis was made and treatment consisted of an analgesic and bed rest. The following day he felt better, and by the end of the week all symptoms and the rash had disappeared. Culture of throat washings, obtained at the time of examination, grew an enterovirus, identified as coxsackievirus group B.

Many different viruses have the capacity to produce disease of the central nervous system manifested either as meningitis or encephalitis. These organisms include representatives of the enterovirus, arbovirus, arenavirus, rhabdovirus, paramyxovirus, and herpesvirus groups (Table 20–1).

ENTEROVIRUS

Enteroviruses are one subgroup of the picornaviruses, the other subgroup being the rhinoviruses. Enteroviruses differ from rhinoviruses in their ability to replicate at 37° C, and in their resistance to acid pH. All picornaviruses are very small, naked (unenveloped) agents with icosahedral symmetry, a single strand of positive-sense RNA, and four polypeptides. The enterovirus group includes the polioviruses, coxsackieviruses A and B, echoviruses, and agents characterized as enteroviruses.

Humans are the reservoir of the enteroviruses affecting man. The natural habitat of the enteroviruses is the gastrointestinal tract. They are excreted in large numbers in the stools of in-

TABLE 20–1.

Viral Agents of Central Nervous System Infection

Virus	Group	Characteristics	Reservoir	Transmission
Poliovirus Coxsackievirus A and B Echovirus Enterovirus	Enteroviruses	RNA Single strand(+) Naked	Man	Fecal-oral Respiratory secretions
Eastern equine* Western equine* St. Louis encephalitis* Japanese B encephalitis*	Arboviruses	RNA Single strand (+) Enveloped	Man	Mosquitoes
Lymphocytic choriomeningitis virus	Arenaviruses	RNA Single strand (−) Enveloped	Rodents	Rodent urine, feces, bites
Rabies	Rhabdoviruses	RNA Single strand (−) Enveloped	Wild and domestic animals	Bites, saliva
Mumps Measles	Paramyxoviruses	RNA Nucleocapsid Enveloped	Man	Direct contact Respiratory aerosols
Herpes simplex Varicella-zoster Cytomegalovirus	Herpesviruses	DNA Double strand Enveloped	Man	Direct contact

Encephalitis viruses.

fected persons and transmission is largely by the fecal-oral route, either directly by person to person or indirectly by ingestion of fecally contaminated food or water. Epidemics of enterovirus infection usually occur during the summer and fall. The highest rates of infection are in young infants and children of lower socioeconomic groups. This is probably the result of poor hygiene.

The incubation period is typically 3 to 5 days. After ingestion, viral replication takes place in the lymphoid tissues and epithelial cells in the pharynx and gastrointestinal tract. Virus can persist in the upper respiratory tract for up to 4 weeks and may be excreted in the stool for more than 4 months. During replication in the respiratory and gastrointestinal tracts the virus can enter the bloodstream. During this viremic phase other organs may be attacked. The localization in these target organs varies with the tropism of the particular virus. All of the enteroviruses can cause asymptomatic infection or meningitis. Some of the viruses can also cause paralytic disease, myocarditis, acute respiratory disease, or rash illness.

The initial tissue damage may be caused by the lytic effects of the virus, in which viral replication is accompanied by an inflammatory reaction and cell necrosis. Viral replication is terminated by the appearance of specific immunoglobulins (IgM and IgG). Examples of these primary lytic infections are viral meningitis, poliomyelitis, and acute respiratory disease. Other enteroviral syndromes are believed to represent immunomodulation by the virus, in which the host immune response results in antibodies that cross-react with certain host tissue determinants. Coxsackie B myocarditis may be one example of this autoimmune pathogenetic mechanism.

POLIOVIRUS

There are three serotypes of poliovirus (1, 2, and 3). Prior to the widespread use of oral polio vaccine, most cases of paralytic disease were caused by type 1. Following replication in lymphoid tissue a minor viremia occurs with infection of reticuloendothelial tissues. When the infection is confined to these tissues, the individual remains asymptomatic with the production of antibodies and lifelong immunity. If the reticuloendothelial tissues are unable to contain the infection, a major viremia occurs resulting in abortive poliomyelitis, aseptic meningitis, or paralytic poliomyelitis.

Polioviruses have a distinct tropism for the central nervous system, which may become infected hematogenously by passage through the blood-brain barrier, or via the axons or perineural sheaths of peripheral nerves. The virus replicates in the neurons of the gray matter of the anterior horn of the spinal cord and the motor nuclei of the pons and medulla. Motor and autonomic neurons are destroyed accompanied by a local inflammatory reaction.

The incubation period is 9 to 12 days. Ninety percent of cases are asymptomatic in young individuals. Abortive poliomyelitis is a 2- to 3-day febrile illness with no neurologic involvement. If aseptic meningitis occurs, recovery is usually complete within a few days. Paralytic poliomyelitis occurs in about 0.1% of poliovirus infections and is characterized by the abrupt onset of muscle pain followed by asymmetric flaccid paralysis with no significant sensory loss. In bulbar poliomyelitis the cranial nerves and the muscles of respiration are involved, which may result in respiratory failure. The mortality of paralytic disease is 2% to 3%.

Poliomyelitis can be prevented by immunization. There are two polio vaccines: inactivated polio vaccine (IPV, the Salk vaccine) which is administered subcutaneously, and live oral polio vaccine (OPV, the Sabin vaccine). Trivalent OPV induces both systemic and gut immunity, but has the potential of mutating to a virulent strain. IPV fails to elicit gut immunity and requires parenteral administration. Both vaccines are considered safe and effective.

COXSACKIE-, ECHO-, AND ENTEROVIRUSES

Most enteroviral disease in the United States is caused by the coxsackieviruses. More than half of these infections are asymptomatic. The most common syndrome caused by the coxsackie-, echo-, and enteroviruses is aseptic meningitis. Specific serotypes of these viruses can cause febrile rash illnesses; acute respiratory disease; paralytic disease; myopericarditis; herpangina; hand-foot-and-mouth disease; epidemic pleurodynia; generalized disease of the newborn; orchitis; and acute hemorrhagic conjunctivitis (Table 20–2). Febrile rash illness usually involves children less than 9 years of age. Outbreaks usually occur during the summer with fever and a rash resembling rubella.

Acute respiratory disease is indistinguishable from the common cold, and paralytic disease cannot be distinguished from poliomyelitis. Herpangina generally occurs in children aged 3 to 10 years and is characterized by fever and vesicles or ulcers on the tonsils and palate. Hand-foot-and-mouth disease usually affects children and is manifested by a vesicular eruption over the oral cavity and the extremities.

TABLE 20–2.

Clinical Syndromes Caused by Enteroviruses Other Than Poliovirus*

	Coxsackievirus A	Coxsackievirus B	Echovirus	Enterovirus
Aseptic meningitis	+	+	+	+
Febrile rash illness	+	+	+	+
Acute respiratory disease	+	+	+	+
Paralytic disease	+	+	+	–
Myopericarditis	+	+	+	–
Herpangina	+	(+)	(+)	–
Hand-foot-and-mouth disease	+	–	–	–
Epidemic pleurodynia	(+)	+	(+)	–
Generalized disease of newborn	(+)	+	+	–
Orchitis	–	+	+	–
Acute hemorrhagic conjunctivitis	(+)	–	–	+

*+ = caused by specific serotypes; (+) = uncommon or rare cause of syndrome; – = not known to cause syndrome.

Pleurodynia is a disease of the parietal pleural of the chest wall that affects older children and young adults. There is an abrupt onset of intense stabbing pain over the lower rib cage or upper abdomen. The pain is spasmodic and paroxysmal and accompanied by episodes of low-grade fever. The illness lasts for 4 to 6 days.

Generalized disease of the newborn usually occurs between the third and seventh day of life. It may be characterized by encephalitis and myocarditis, or hemorrhage and hepatitis. The mortality is about 50%.

Acute hemorrhagic conjunctivitis has occurred in widespread epidemics involving many thousands of cases. It is probably transmitted by direct contact of fingers carrying discharge material from infected eyes. Onset is sudden with pain, swollen eyelids, and subconjunctival hemorrhages. The incubation period is 12 to 48 hours.

ARBOVIRUSES

Arboviruses share a common means of transmission by bloodsucking insects: mosquitos, sand flies, and ticks. There are several hundred different viruses in this large group which includes a number of encephalitis viruses, yellow fever, dengue, and several hemorrhagic fevers. The reservoir of these viruses varies, but may include horses, cattle, sheep, other small mammals, birds, and arthropods. Transmission is via the bite of the arthropod.

Many of the encephalitis viruses are mosquito-borne, and consequently disease occurs in the summer and early fall. Infection may be asymptomatic or may vary from a flulike syndrome to severe encephalitis. Susceptibility to more severe disease is highest in infancy and old age. The incubation period varies from 5 to 15 days. Man is a dead-end host.

Following deposition of the virus under the skin by mosquito bite, the virus multiplies in the vascular endothelium and the reticuloendothelial system. The virus can reach the central nervous system during the viremia, and cross the blood-brain barrier, or the virus may reach the brain by neural pathways. Damage to brain tissue is largely the result of vascular involvement. Multiple small hemorrhages cause neuronal necrosis.

Clinically, there is headache, fever that may reach 40° C, chills, nausea, vomiting, myalgia, and lethargy or confusion that may progress to coma. Seizures are common in infants and children. Recovery usually takes place in 3 to 5 days but there may be neurologic sequelae ranging from mental retardation to paralysis, particularly in infants. The mortality is usually less than 1%, but may reach 20% in severe encephalitis.

ARENAVIRUSES

Arenaviruses are round to oval particles with a genome of single-stranded negative-sense RNA enclosed in a three-layer envelope covered with glycoprotein "spikes." Arenaviruses primarily attack rodents. The group includes the viruses of lymphocytic choriomeningitis (LCM), Lassa fever, and several hemorrhagic fevers. LCM is a disease of mice, hamsters, guinea pigs, and other animals. Man is incidentally infected. The reservoir is the infected rodent. Virus is excreted in the saliva, urine, and feces of infected animals. Man is probably infected by inhalation of aerosols or dust, by direct contact with the animal, or by animal bite.

Most infections occur in young adults, but are rarely fatal. The incubation period varies from 8 to 21 days. Clinically, there are 3 to 5 days of fever, headache, and myalgia, occasionally accompanied by lymphadenopathy and a maculopapular rash. The fever subsides, but after 2 to 4 symptomless days there is a second febrile episode with more severe headache, which may progress to aseptic meningitis. Some patients develop painful orchitis, or myopericarditis. During convalescence alopecia may occur and persist for several months. It is believed that the second febrile episode and its manifestations may be due to some form of immunomodulation. Lassa fever and other hemorrhagic viruses also can be contracted from blood or secretions of ill patients. Mortality is very high with these viruses, but ribavirin will treat Lassa fever.

RHABDOVIRUSES

Rhabdoviruses are bullet-shaped, helical, enveloped viruses with a single-strand negative-sense RNA genome. The most important member of this group is **rabies virus**, a neurotropic agent.

Rabies is an acute encephalitis of animals and humans. The reservoir is in wild and domestic canines (dogs, wolves, coyotes, foxes), cats, skunks, raccoons, and bats. Virus is often present in the saliva of rabid animals; the disease is transmitted by the bite of these animals. In the United States most human cases are associated with dog or cat bites.

The incubation period is highly variable, ranging from 10 days to 1 year; the average is 2 to 8 weeks. During the incubation period the virus remains localized near the site of the bite wound and replicates in skeletal muscle. The virus enters the peripheral nervous system at the neuromuscular junction, and spreads up the nerves to involve the spinal cord and the brain, especially the limbic system. Viral replication proceeds in the gray matter and then spreads along the efferent nerves to reach other organs and tissues. The primary pathologic finding is destruction of the nerve cells.

The disease begins with nonspecific symptoms of fever, headache, nausea, and vomiting that last 2 to 10 days. This is followed by the rapid development of neurologic manifestations including agitation, seizures, hallucinations, paralysis, and hyperactivity. About half of the patients demonstrate severe spasms of the pharynx and larynx when attempting to drink, resulting in choking and gagging. Symptoms progress to coma in about 4 to 10 days with death occurring a few days later.

Because of the long incubation period, rabies may be averted by immunization. Rabies immune globulin is infiltrated around the wound, and active immunization is initiated with human diploid cell rabies vaccine.

PARAMYXOVIRUSES

The paramyxoviruses include the mumps, measles, parainfluenza, and respiratory syncytial viruses. Parainfluenza and respiratory syncytial viruses are discussed in Chapter 4, Respiratory Viruses.

Mumps virus is a common cause of parotitis. The most frequent extrasalivary gland involvement is with the central nervous system, either as meningitis or encephalitis. Mumps meningitis is a relatively benign infection that may occur prior to, during, or following parotitis, or even in the absence of salivary gland involvement. The symptoms are essentially the same as other viral meningitides with headache, fever, vomiting, and nuchal rigidity. Symptoms usually resolve in 3 to 10 days with complete recovery. Mumps encephalitis is relatively rare, but more serious than viral meningitis. Early-onset encephalitis coinciding with the parotitis is due to neuronal destruction caused by viral replication. Late-onset encephalitis occurring 7 to 10 days after the salivary gland involvement is believed to be an autoimmune process resulting in demyelinating disease. Mumps is discussed in greater detail in Chapter 48.

Measles virus can cause acute encephalitic disease which may be mild or severe during convalescence from measles. The measles virus has also been implicated in subacute sclerosing panencephalitis (SSPE), a chronic degenerative disease occurring years after an attack of the measles. Patients with SSPE have very high titers of measles antibody in their serum and CSF. Measles is discussed in Chapter 52, Viral Exanthems.

HERPESVIRUSES

This group includes the herpes simplex, varicella-zoster, and cytomegaloviruses.

Herpes simplex virus (HSV-1) can cause an acute necrotizing, hemorrhagic encephalitis, usually involving the temporal lobes. All ages are susceptible. The virus reaches the central nervous system during primary or recurrent herpes infection via the neural route. Untreated patients rapidly deteriorate to coma and death within a few days. HSV-1 is a common cause of aseptic meningitis in adults and can cause encephalitis in neonates. The treatment of choice is acyclovir. Herpes is discussed in Chapter 27.

Cytomegalovirus (CMV) infection may be congenital or occur in immunocompromised persons. The nervous system manifestation is a meningoencephalitis associated with destructive demyelinating lesions and it is an important cause of retinitis in HIV-infected patients. Cytomegalovirus is discussed in Chapter 57, Viral Opportunists.

CHAPTER 21

Cryptococcus neoformans

A 52-year-old Wall Street broker complained of several weeks of headache, irritability, and inability to concentrate. He had previously enjoyed good health. Physical examination and routine laboratory tests were all normal, and within a few days he began to feel better. Three months later his symptoms recurred and persisted for several weeks. A lumbar puncture was performed and the cerebrospinal fluid (CSF) had a slightly increased protein level with five lymphocytes per cubic millimeter. India ink and Gram stains failed to reveal any microorganisms. A careful neurologic examination was unrevealing and he again felt better. He remained symptom-free for 2 months when he developed severe headaches, nausea, and dizziness. A repeat lumbar puncture showed an elevated opening pressure; the CSF had increased protein and decreased glucose levels, and the white blood cell count was $300/mm^3$, most of which were lymphocytes. India ink examination was negative, but a latex test for cryptococcal antigen was positive, and culture of the CSF grew out a yeast identified as *Cryptococcus neoformans*. Subsequent investigation revealed that the window air conditioner in his office was heavily contaminated with pigeon droppings. He was treated with amphotericin B and 5-fluorocytosine, and he eventually recovered.

Cryptococcus neoformans is a yeastlike fungus. The cell is round to oval, about 5 μm in diameter, and has a prominent capsule. Reproduction is by budding; buds form, enlarge, and pinch off to become individual cells. The organism grows readily on blood agar at 35 to 37° C, forming smooth colonies in 2 to 5 days. *Cryptococcus neoformans* gives a positive test for urease. There are four serotypes, A, B, C, and D, based on the antigenic specificity of the capsular polysaccharide. Most clinical isolates are serotypes A and D.

The reservoir of serotypes A and D is in the excreta of birds, especially pigeons, in soil contaminated by bird feces, and on fruit. The reservoir of serotypes B and C is not known. Infection occurs by inhalation of the organisms with dust or dried soil. Person-to-person transmission does not occur. There is increased susceptibility to cryptococcal infection in immunodeficiency

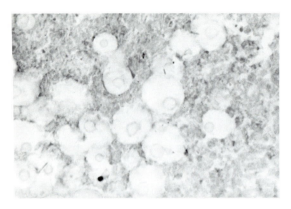

FIG 21–1.
C. neoformans in brain.

states, especially acquired immunodeficiency syndrome (AIDS); in Hodgkin's disease and other lymphoreticular disorders; in sarcoidosis; and during corticosteroid therapy. A small number of patients have no obvious deficit in host resistance.

Following inhalation, organisms are usually phagocytosed by neutrophils and macrophages, and killed. Occasionally the disease progresses in the lungs and spreads to the central nervous system. The primary determinant of virulence is the capsule which inhibits phagocytosis. Noncapsular variants are avirulent. The capsule is composed of a polysaccharide of mannose units together with minor amounts of glucuronoxylo-

and galactoxylomannans. The polysaccharide may be immunosuppressive, and may also affect leukocyte migration.

Phagocytosis of encapsulated organisms is enhanced by opsonization with anticapsular IgG antibodies. The complement system is activated by the alternative pathway and C3 fragments are deposited on the surface of the yeast. Sensitized T cells function to activate the phagocytes and enhance intracellular killing by the myeloperoxidase-halide system.

The predisposition of the organism to localize in the central nervous system may be related to the absence of IgG and complement in the CSF. There is minimal tissue reaction in the brain, but accumulations of the capsular polysaccharide develop within the cortical gray matter, and on the leptomeninges (Fig 21–1). Lesions may also occur in bone and kidneys, particularly in renal transplant recipients.

Clinically, cryptococcal meningitis has an insidious onset with headache, vertigo, behavioral changes, and low-grade fever over a period of weeks or months. Diagnosis is based upon the demonstration of the organism in the CSF, by India ink staining (Fig 21–2), detection of antigen by latex agglutination, or by culture. Since cryptococcal antibodies are present in a large proportion of the healthy population, they are not useful diagnostically. However, a decreasing

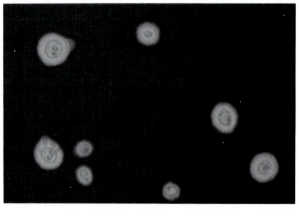

FIG 21–2.
Encapulated budding yeast cells of *Cryptococcus neoformans* highlighted with India ink. (From Murray P, Kobayashi G, Thompson J, et al (eds): *Medical Microbiology.* St. Louis, Mosby–Year Book, 1990, p 339. Used by permission.)

antigen level and a rising antibody titer are favorable prognostic indicators.

Immunity involves both humoral and cell-mediated responses. Treatment is based upon amphotericin B, usually combined with 5-fluoro-cytosine. Maintenance therapy in AIDS patients is fluconazole. Mortality is about 30% in treated patients, except in AIDS, where the mortality is much higher.

CHAPTER 22

Neurotoxic Clostridia

Clostridia are gram-positive, spore-forming, anaerobic bacilli. Some species occur in soil as saprophytes, others exist as commensals in the lower intestinal tract of man and animals. The spores of clostridia are resistant to drying, cold, boiling, and most disinfectants, and can survive in soil, food, tissues, etc. for long periods of time. When environmental conditions become suitable, the spores germinate into vegetative cells which reproduce by binary fission like non-spore-forming bacteria.

The ability of the pathogenic clostridia to invade healthy tissue varies considerably. At one extreme, the organisms remain at the site of inoculation (tetanus) or never even enter the body (botulism), but elaborate potent neurotoxins that produce the disease. At the other end of the spectrum (clostridial myonecrosis), the clostridia elaborate toxic enzymes that enable the organisms to progressively invade healthy tissue.

The clostridial neurotoxins (botulinus toxin and tetanus toxin) are two of the most poisonous substances known to man. On a weight basis, these toxins are about 2 million times more poisonous than potassium cyanide and more than 1,300 times more deadly than cobra venom. The lethal dose of these toxins for humans has been estimated to be less than 0.1 mcg.

BOTULISM

Botulism is an intoxication that results from the action of a toxin produced by *Clostridium botulinum*. There are eight types of *C. botulinum*, each type producing an immunologically distinct form of neurotoxin. The majority of cases of botulism are caused by types A, B, and E. *Clostridium botulinum* spores are found in the soil. Vegetables, meat, fish, or other foods are contaminated with soil containing the spores which are capable of surviving many hours of boiling. Improper processing of such contaminated foods—usually home canning procedures—can produce conditions of anaerobiosis that favor germination of the spores, vegetative growth, and toxin production.

Classic botulism results from the ingestion of toxin-containing food. Two other forms of botulism occur. In infant botulism, babies between

3 and 26 weeks of age ingest *C. botulinum* spores which germinate and produce toxin within the intestine. Honey, sometimes added to the nutritional formula, has been found to contain *C. botulinum* spores, and has been implicated in this form of the disease. Wound botulism, the rarest form of the disease, results from infection of a wound with *C. botulinum* with subsequent toxin production within the wound and absorption into the system.

Botulinum toxins are synthesized during the death and lysis of the vegetative cells. The association between toxin production and lysogenization by bacteriophages has been demonstrated. Toxin-producing strains can be cured of their lysogenic bacteriophages and rendered nontoxic; nontoxic strains can be infected with bacteriophages and rendered toxic. Type A and B toxins are synthesized as protoxins that require a protease for transformation to full toxicativity. Type E toxin is synthesized in a fully active form.

Botulinum neurotoxin is the most potent biologic toxin known, with a median lethal dose of 5 to 50 ng/kg body weight. Its primary action is in the cholinergic nerve terminals of the peripheral nervous system, where it blocks the release of the neurotransmitter acetylcholine. Botulinum toxin is composed of two components: a neurotoxin and a hemagglutinating factor. The neurotoxin binds to a receptor on the external surface of presynaptic nerve terminals, moves to a new site within the nerve terminal, and binds to an internal receptor site where it blocks the exocytosis of acetylcholine-containing vesicles. During the binding step to the external receptor, the toxin is vulnerable to the action of type-specific antitoxin. After binding, the toxin is unaffected by antitoxin.

The blockade of acetylcholine release is most prominent in cranial nerves, autonomic nerves, and at the neuromuscular junction, which accounts for the most common clinical manifestations of diplopia and dysphagia. The cause of death is respiratory paralysis due to blockade of transmitter release from the phrenic nerve to the muscles of the diaphragm. Symptoms of weakness, lassitude, and dizziness appear 12 to 36 hours after ingestion of the contaminated food, followed by the symmetric involvement of cranial nerves and a descending pattern of weakness or paralysis. Antitoxin is administered to patients, but the mainstay of therapy is respiratory support.

TETANUS

Tetanus is an infectious complication of wounds, caused by the toxin of *Clostridium tetani*. This organism is found in the soil and in the feces of various animals and some humans. The disease occurs when wounds become contaminated with soil containing spores of *C. tetani*; the spores germinate and the vegetative cells produce tetanus toxin which is absorbed into the system, eventually reaching the central nervous system.

Mere contamination of a wound is not sufficient to produce tetanus. The oxidation-reduction (redox) potential (E_h) of the wound must be lowered from the +120 mV of normal tissues to less than +10 mV in order for tetanus spores to germinate. Lowering of the E_h is associated with tissue necrosis following trauma (puncture wounds, compound fractures) or the injection of necrotizing substances.

Tetanus neonatorum occurs when the umbilical cord is cut or tied with objects contaminated with tetanus spores. Tetanus has also been associated with subcutaneous self-administration of narcotic drugs such as heroin.

Infections with *C. tetani* remain localized at the site of inoculation. After the spores germinate in necrotic tissue, vegetative growth and toxin synthesis begins. Toxin can reach the central nervous system by two routes: humorally through the lymph and blood, and neurally by way of the tissue spaces of the peripheral nerves. The tetanus neurotoxin—tetanospasmin—is only slightly less toxic than type A bot-

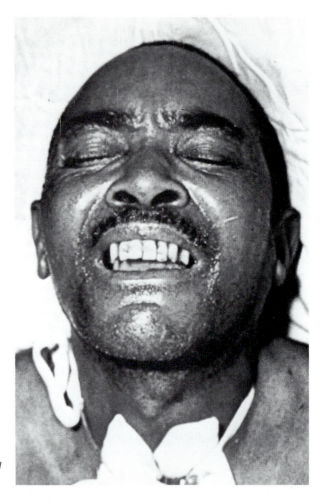

FIG 22–1.
Risus sardonicus in tetanus, due to spasms in the masseter muscles. *(From Lambert HP, Farrar WE: Infectious Diseases Illustrated. London, Gower Medical Publishing, 1982. Used by permission.)*

ulinum toxin. Tetanospasmin contains about 100 million mouse lethal doses per milligram. It is a simple protein composed of two polypeptide chains held together by a disulfide and a peptide bond. One of these polypeptide chains is responsible for binding to tissue receptor sites. Tetanus toxin shows particular affinity for a ganglioside rich in sialic acid. The specific neurotoxic action of tetanospasmin is primarily the inhibition of the release of glycine and γ-aminobutyric acid, which are major inhibitory transmitters in the anterior horn cells of the spinal cord. The uncontrolled propagation of im-

pulses through the motor neurons of the central nervous system results in the spasmodic contraction of the muscles characteristic of tetanus (Figs 22–1 and 22–2).

The incubation period of tetanus is 7 to 8 days. Early symptoms are developing rigidity and spasm of the masseter muscles, i.e., lockjaw. Other muscle groups become progressively involved with developing rigidity of the neck, chest, abdominal wall, back, and limbs. Tonic convulsions are frequent and patients suffer extreme pain from muscle spasms. Symptoms may last for several weeks and the mortality in gener-

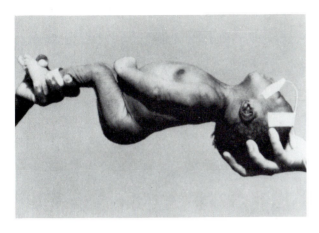

FIG 22–2.
An infant with tetanus and opisthotonus resulting from persistent spasms in the back muscles. *(From Lambert HP, Farrar WE:* Infectious Diseases Illustrated. *London, Gower Medical Publishing, 1982. Used by permission.)*

alized tetanus may be 50% or more.

Tetanus may be prevented by active immunization with tetanus toxoid, a component of the pediatric DPT (diphtheria-pertussis-tetanus) vaccine. Booster injections of tetanus toxoid given up to 20 years after the initial immunization series results in an antibody response of antitoxin well above the protective level in about 5 days .

Previously unvaccinated patients with contaminated wounds that are not amenable to surgical excision should be treated with tetanus antitoxin, followed by active immunization with tetanus toxoid. Clinical tetanus does not induce immunity because so little toxin is released. It is important to actively immunize patients recovering from tetanus.

PART V

Skin and Subcutaneous Infections

CHAPTER 23

Overview of Skin and Subcutaneous Infections

The skin, an important barrier to the invasion of deeper tissues by microorganisms, is itself subject to infection. The indigenous microflora of the skin is largely gram-positive and consists of coagulase-negative staphylococci, *Propionibacterium acnes*, aerobic corynebacteria (diphtheroids), mycobacteria, and yeasts. The primary limiting factor for skin bacteria is the availability of water; moist skin always has higher numbers of bacteria (including transient gram-negative species) than dry skin. Sweat contains sodium chloride, lactic acid, urea, amino acids, ammonia, protein, carbohydrate, and iron, all of which affect bacterial growth. The skin also contains free fatty acids and lipids which inhibit many bacterial species.

Various types of skin lesions can be distinguished: **macules** (small—less than 10 mm—flat discolored spots); **papules** (small, solid, elevated lesions); **nodules** (small, palpable solid lesions); **vesicles** (small elevated lesions containing serous fluid); **bullae** (larger vesicles); **pustules** (small elevated lesions containing pus); and **ulcers** (circumscribed lesions characterized by loss of epidermis and part of the dermis).

Superficial skin infections are those that are limited to the epidermis. They include erythrasma, and the dermatophytoses. Erythrasma is characterized by scaly, reddish patches, caused by *Corynebactium minutissimum*. Lesions generally occur in the genitocrural area, and are more common in obese diabetic men.

Pyodermas are purulent infections of the skin. They include **impetigo**, a vesicular infection of the skin usually caused by group A streptococci, sometimes in combination with *Staphylycoccus aureus*; **folliculitis**, infection of the hair follicles; and **furuncles** and carbuncles, single or multiple skin abscesses. These infections are almost always caused by *S. aureus*. *Staphylococcus aureus* can also cause bullous impetigo and the scalded skin syndrome.

Vesicular lesions may represent herpesvirus infection. Papular lesions occur with yaws, a treponemal infection; or warts, a viral disease. Granulomatous lesions are seen with leprosy and swimming pool granuloma.

Infections in which the typical skin lesion is an ulcer are cutaneous diphtheria, cutaneous anthrax, and Buruli ulcer. **Cellulitis** is an infection of the subcutaneous tissues. Erysipelas is cellulitis caused by group A streptococcus. Another form of cellulitis with similar lesions is erysipeloid, caused by *Erysipelothrix insidiosa*. Anaerobic cellulitis may be due to one of several *Bacteroides* or clostridial species. Gangrenous cellulitis, also termed **ecthyma,** may be caused by group A streptococci, *Pseudomonas aeruginosa, or other organisms.*

Mycetoma is a chronic, progressive, destructive infection that involves skin, subcutaneous tissue, and sometimes muscle and bone as well. Mycetoma may be caused by actinomycetes, *Nocardia*, or several species of fungi.

The pathogenesis of skin infections varies with the organism, but in most cases the agent is introduced into the skin by trauma, or the material containing the microbe comes into contact with abraded skin. Some of the more virulent organisms, (e.g., group A streptococci) may be able to initiate disease in intact skin.

The diagnosis of skin infections can often be made by microscopic examination and culture of the skin lesion on appropriate media.

CHAPTER 24

Staphylococci

A 23-year-old woman consulted a physician because of recurrent skin abscesses. She had been in good health until 8 months prior to her visit when she noted an area of tenderness, erythema, and induration on her left forearm. The lesion subsequently drained pus spontaneously. She has had 15 or 20 such lesions during the ensuing months. On physical examination the only positive findings were "boils" on her legs. Blood count, urinalysis, glucose tolerance test, and serum protein electrophoresis were all normal. One of the lesions on her leg became fluctuant and was incised and drained creamy pus. A Gram stain of the pus revealed many gram-positive cocci in clusters (Fig 24–1), and a culture grew out *Staphylococcus aureus.*

Staphylococci are gram-positive cocci that appear in packets or grapelike clusters when viewed microscopically. They are facultative anaerobes, but grow best under aerobic conditions. Staphylococci are able to grow in relatively simple laboratory media, utilizing glucose or other carbohydrates as energy sources and amino acids as sources of nitrogen. Colonies on agar are 1 to 3 mm in diameter after 18 to 24 hours incubation at 35°C, and are opaque with yellow or white pigmentation. Staphylococci produce catalase which distinguishes them from streptococci.

Staphylococcus aureus is the most virulent species and is unique in its production of coagulase.* The remaining 11 species that involve humans are all coagulase-negative. The most important coagulase-negative species are S. *epidermidis* and S. *saprophyticus.*

Some strains of staphylococci are free-living in nature, but most human pathogenic strains are constituents of the normal indigenous flora of the skin and the mucous membranes of the nose, pharynx, urethra, and vagina. Staphylococci are quite resistant to drying, heat, and high salt concentrations, which contributes to their survival on environmental surfaces and on skin. Many strains produce lipase which facilitates colonization of the skin despite the presence of fatty acids, which are inhibitory to many other bacterial species. Staphylococci generally act as opportunists, requiring some defect in

*Coagulase production can be demonstrated in the laboratory in several ways: A small portion of a coagulase-positive staphylococcal colony will clump within a few seconds when mixed on a glass slide with a drop of plasma. Alternatively, a small volume of plasma in a test tube will clot within 1 hour after the addition of coagulase-positive staphylococci.

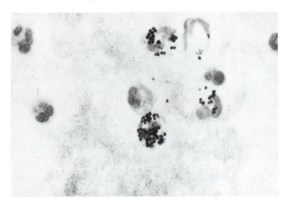

FIG 24–1.
Staphylococci in pus.

host resistance, commonly trauma or foreign bodies, to establish infection. The source of the organism is usually endogenous, but exogenous strains may be introduced during a surgical procedure.

STAPHLYOCOCCUS AUREUS

Up to 40% of adults are carriers of *S. aureus*, most frequently in the anterior nares but also on the skin of the perineal region and the mucous membranes of the pharynx. The organism may also be present in the stool. The fingers and hands are readily contaminated from the nares, and hospital personnel often spread infection by neglecting handwashing.

Staphylococcus aureus strains are susceptible to a number of lytic bacteriophages. Strains may be fingerprinted for epidemiologic investigations by testing them with an internationally accepted standard battery of 24 phages to determine which ones can lyse the organism. With this technique, staphylococcal strains can be grouped (I, II, III, and miscellaneous) and typed (e.g., 80/81/52).

Staphylococcus aureus has a number of structural and soluble factors that may play a role in pathogenesis. The cell wall is composed of a large rigid polymer called **peptidoglycan**

which enables the organism to withstand severe environmental osmotic variations. This polymer of cross-linked amino sugars and amino acids can be hydrolyzed by lysozyme, an enzyme present in tears, saliva, polymorphonuclear leukocytes, and macrophages. The cell wall also contains **ribitol teichoic** acid, a phosphate-containing polymer. The ribitol teichoic acid is linked to the peptidoglycan and the teichoic acid–peptidoglycan complex makes up 40% to 60% of the cell wall and is the site of action of the penicillins and cephalosporins used to treat staphylococcal infections. The teichoic acid–peptidoglycan complex induces teichoic acid antibodies present in low titers in a large percentage of the population. These antibodies may have opsonic activity and increase significantly during staphylococcal bacteremia or endocarditis. The other cell wall constituent is **protein A**, a surface protein covalently linked to the teichoic acid–peptidoglycan complex.

The protein A surface layer reacts with serum IgG molecules by combining with the Fc portion, leaving the Fab sites free and exposed. The interaction of protein A with the Fc portion is responsible for producing a variety of reactions, including the inhibition of phagocytosis, the activation of complement, induction of T and B lymphocyte proliferation, and hypersensitivity reactions such as anaphylaxis and the Arthus phenomenon.

Some strains of *S. aureus* have a slime layer or capsule external to the cell wall. This material is composed of galactose and galacturonic acid. It is antigenic and antiphagocytic, interfering with the interaction between the underlying teichoic acid–peptidoglycan complex and complement, thus protecting encapsulated strains from complement-mediated phagocytosis. The capsule increases the ability of the organism to spread through tissue, which enhances the virulence of these strains.

Protein A, peptidoglycan, and teichoic acid all play a role in the activation of the classic and alternative complement pathways. The peptidoglycan–teichoic acid complex is another potent promoter of chemotaxis by complement activation. The deposition of C3b on the surface of some encapsulated strains is not sufficient for promoting optimal phagocytosis; such strains also require specific IgG (nonencapsulated strains require nonimmune IgG and complement for phagocytosis). The peptidoglycan exposed at the cell surface promotes opsonization. Encapsulated strains are more virulent than nonencapsulated strains, presumably because the capsule masks the peptidoglycan.

Staphylococcus aureus has surface-associated proteins that have a strong affinity for fibronectin, a glycoprotein present on tissue cells and in plasma. Fibronectin mediates the adherence of staphylococci to endothelial cells. Extracellular soluble substances produced by *S. aureus* include coagulase, which can result in the deposition of fibrin on the surface of staphylococci, thereby altering their ingestion by phagocytic cells, and decomplementation antigen. Decomplementation antigen is an extremely stable, nondialyzable macromolecule, provisionally identified as a water-soluble teichoic acid, which reacts with IgG to form immune complexes that activate the classic complement pathway. This antigen could protect staphylococci from complement attack by inducing abortive complement-consuming reactions up to and including C5.

A group of **hemolysins**—alpha, beta, gamma, and delta—are collectively called exotoxins. Alpha hemolysin, produced by 80% of virulent *S. aureus* strains, interacts with the lipoprotein of cell membranes to cause cellular disruption. Alpha hemolysin affects the heart, peripheral circulation, and central nervous system, and is dermonecrotic. Beta, gamma, and delta hemolysins are also membrane-damaging toxins. Beta toxin is sphingomyelinase; delta toxin may be a lecithinase; the exact mode of action of gamma toxin is not yet known.

Leukocidins are substances that kill white blood cells. There are two components, F and S, which act synergistically on leukocyte membranes, producing an altered permeability to cations, particularly potassium.

Exfoliative toxins cause a separation of the stratum granulosum layer of the epidermis associated with the scalded skin syndrome. Two forms of the epidermolytic toxins, A and B, have been identified. Most strains producing these toxins are in phage group II. The production of the toxin is genetically regulated by plasmids.

Seven antigenically distinct types of **enterotoxins** are produced by strains of *S. aureus* involved in food poisoning. Some of these enterotoxins act directly on the bowel, causing hypermotility; others affect the vomiting center of the brain. As little as 25 µg of enterotoxin b will produce vomiting and diarrhea in humans.

Toxic shock syndrome toxin (TSST-1) is a potent pyrogen that induces T lymphocyte proliferation, requiring the release of interleukin-1 from macrophages. TSST-1 enhances endotoxin shock and hypersensitivity skin reactions, and suppresses immunoglobulin production. TSST-1 is a potent inducer of tumor necrosis factor.

Lipase production increases staphylococcal survival on the skin. Strains producing large amounts of lipase, hemolysin, and nuclease can colonize the skin and cause furunculosis. Lipase production correlates with enhanced mortality in bacteremia. Strains producing low amounts of lipase, hemolysin, and nuclease cannot colonize the skin but can colonize the mucous membranes of the anterior nares and vagina. Catalase production may protect ingested staphylococci from the lethal action of myeloperoxidase.

The virulence of *S. aureus* is not associated with any single factor but rather seems to correlate with several factors, such as soluble toxins and surface structures that interfere with phagocytosis. The ability to survive and multiply in a host is essential for pathogenicity; protection is related in part to promotion of phagocytosis, and in part to antitoxic immunity. For example, mice immunized with alpha toxoid were protected against lethal doses of alpha toxin but succumbed to the intraperitoneal injection of *S. au-*

reus. Other mice, immunized with a heat-killed whole vaccine, resisted intraperitoneal challenge but were killed by alpha hemolysin.

Staphylococcus aureus produces two distinct types of disease: invasive and toxigenic.

INVASIVE STAPHYLOCOCCAL DISEASE

Invasive disease is characterized by abscess formation which may occur in any organ. Skin is especially prone to infection, and superficial skin abscesses (furuncles) are common following infection of a hair follicle. This infection provokes an acute inflammatory response, characterized by the accumulation of tremendous quantities of leukocytes. The lesion becomes walled off owing to the deposition of fibrin, and central necrosis occurs. Furuncles may coalesce to form larger and deeper abscesses (carbuncles) where the skin is thick and inelastic, e.g., on the nape of the neck.

Staphylococci are the most frequent cause of wound infections. Virulent strains may produce impetigo, conjunctivitis, umbilical stump infections, pneumonia, or septicemia in the newborn. These strains may originate from another baby in the nursery or from a carrier among the nursing personnel. The infection may be transmitted to other babies by nurses who handle the infants and neglect handwashing. Infants may also carry infection to their mothers who can develop breast abscesses by nursing infected babies. Deep abscesses may form in persons debilitated by disease, malnutrition, extensive surgery, or who are immunocompromised.

The most serious consequence of staphylococcal infection is bloodstream invasion, with the high risk of metastatic abscess formation or involvement of the cardiac valves. Endocarditis is present in up to 14% of patients with bacteremia. Staphylococcal endocarditis may occur following open heart surgery (e.g., valve replacement with a prosthesis), or in persons who inject nonsterile materials into their veins (e.g., heroin addicts). Staphylococcal pneumonia or lung abscess may occur as a complication of severe viral pneumonitis, such as influenza, or in hospitalized patients at high risk (postsurgical or neonates). Acute osteomyelitis is most often seen in children under 12 years old and results from the localization of *S. aureus* in the metaphysis of a long bone. The infection may spread to involve a contiguous joint. Staphylococcal bacteremia frequently leads to bacteriuria; rarely pyelonephritis may result from the seeding of the kidney via the bloodstream.

Host factors predisposing to invasive staphylococcal infections are foreign bodies such as prostheses, implants, sutures, etc. For example, it was necessary to inject 5 million *S. aureus* cells into the skin of human volunteers in order to produce a lesion. However, a suture containing only 100 staphylococci that was tied into the skin of human volunteers promptly produced an abscess. Other predisposing factors are underlying disease (diabetes or uremia) or immunosuppression with adrenocortical steroids. These conditions are associated with reduced migration, ingestion, and killing by phagocytic cells.

TOXIGENIC DISEASES

Toxigenic staphylococcal disease includes food poisoning (enterotoxemia), scalded skin syndrome, and toxic shock syndrome. **Staphylococcal enterotoxemia** accounts for a significant number of foodborne illnesses. The organisms are usually introduced into the food by a food handler with an insignificant infection, such as paronychia, due to a strain of *S. aureus* that produces one or more enterotoxins. The foods involved are those that do not undergo a final heat treatment (ham salad, cream pie, etc.). The staphylococci multiply and produce enterotoxin if these foods are permitted to stand for several hours at warm temperatures. The victim eating the food ingests the preformed toxin. Within 1 to 6 hours there is abrupt onset of nausea, vomiting, and headache, sometimes accompanied by diarrhea. The symptoms usually subside after 24 hours.

Scalded skin syndrome refers to several exfoliative types of dermatologic disease produced by staphylococcal exfoliative toxins. The disease occurs in children under 5 years of age, and rarely in immunocompromised adults. The disease begins with the appearance of a diffuse scarlatiniform rash or bullae (large fluid-filled blisters). The bullae break down and the epidermis separates and peels off in large sheets. Eventually the exposed areas become dry and crusty and desquamate in thick flakes.

Toxic shock syndrome is a recently recognized disease that most often affects women during their menses, although males are occasionally affected. It is characterized by fever, hypotension leading to vascular collapse, a scarlet fever–like rash that eventually desquamates, and involvement of multiple organ systems (kidney, liver, gastrointestinal). Cultures of blood, spinal fluid, throat, etc. are negative. The disease has been associated with the use of vaginal tampons that encourage overgrowth of certain strains of *S. aureus* by alteration of the Mg^{++} concentration in the vaginal fluid. These strains are nonhemolytic and produce little or no hemolysin, lipase, or nuclease. Toxic shock syndrome is caused by *S. aureus* strains that express TSST-1, enterotoxin b, or enterotoxin c. TSST-1 is associated with menstrual cases and with about half of nonmenstrual cases; the other two toxins cause the remainder of the nonmenstrual cases.

Toxic shock syndrome clinically resembles streptococcal scarlet fever and Kawasaki syndrome.* TSST-1 shares many biologic properties with the exotoxin (erythrogenic toxin) of *Streptococcus pyogenes*. It induces fever, enhances delayed-type hypersensitivity skin reactions,

*Kawasaki syndrome (mucocutaneous lymph node syndrome) is a disease of unknown etiology that occurs in children under 5 years old. It is characterized by fever, cervical lymph node enlargement, changes in the oral mucosa, and an erythematous rash that desquamates.

produces a rash, deregulates IgG synthesis by inducing immunosuppression to T lymphocyte–dependent antigens, and (in rabbits) enhances host susceptibility to endotoxin shock. However, toxic shock syndrome has a clinical profile that is very different from endotoxin shock. TSST-1 is a potent inducer of interleukin-1 by monocytes, and this may play a central role in this disease. A significant proportion of *S. aureus* strains recovered from patients with nonmenstrual toxic shock syndrome do not produce TSST-1, and the production of the toxin may not be essential to the pathogenesis of the disease. The pathogenesis of toxic shock syndrome is complex and probably multifactorial.

COAGULASE-NEGATIVE STAPHYLOCOCCI

Coagulase-negative staphylococci were previously considered to be harmless commensals and environmental contaminants. Some of these organisms are now recognized as significant pathogens involved in a number of disease processes. *Staphylococcus epidermidis* is a major cause of infections of central venous and other vascular catheters, prosthetic heart valves, peritoneal dialysis catheters, central nervous system shunts, and orthopedic prostheses. Complications of these infections include bacteremia, endocarditis, mediastinitis, meningitis, and progressive joint destruction. The mortality rate of septicemia due to coagulase-negative staphylococci approaches 30%.

Coagulase-negative staphylococci, particularly *S. saprophyticus*, are responsible for 12% of urinary tract infections in young children, and 10% of urinary tract infections in young women. *S. hemolyticus* has a great affinity for plastic materials and is resistant to many antibiotics.

The cell wall of *S. epidermidis* (and other coagulase-negative species) lacks protein A, and the teichoic acid is based upon glycerol. However some of these organisms produce a wide variety of potential virulence factors including hemolysins, cytotoxins, DNAse, lipase, and fibrinolysin. Most strains of *S. epidermidis* can activate the alternative pathway of complement and be ingested and killed by neutrophils in the absence of specific antibody.

Coagulase-negative staphylococci colonize in-dwelling medical devices by hydrophobic binding. These prosthetic implants are rapidly coated with a film of fibronectin, collagen, fibrin, and other host proteins, which further bind staphylococci. Staphylococci from the skin are introduced during the implantation of the catheter or prosthesis, or transiently enter the bloodstream from an endogenous source and colonize the implant. Once attached, the staphylococci produce a viscous, extracellular polysaccharide glycocalyx or slime, forming a biofilm on the surface of the prosthesis that completely covers the bacteria. This biofilm provides a protected microenvironment that acts as a barrier to phagocytic cells, antibodies, and antibiotics while concentrating nutrients for the replicating bacteria.

ANTIMICROBIAL RESISTANCE IN STAPHYLOCOCCI

In the 1940s most staphylococci were susceptible to penicillin. Today, almost all strains recovered from patients are penicillin-resistant. In most cases, resistance is due to staphylococcal β-lactamases which destroy penicillin by hydrolyzing the β-lactam ring of penicillin. The major mechanisms of resistance to β-lactam antibiotics are enzyme-mediated, in which the antibiotic is inactivated, and intrinsic, which may be due to alterations in the penicillin-binding proteins of the organism.

There are at least four different staphylococcal β-lactamases, which probably accounts for the varying resistance to the cephalosporins. The production of β-lactamases is controlled by plasmids.

Drugs such as oxacillin, nafcillin, and cephalosporins such as cefazolin are minimally hydrolyzed by staphylococcal β-lactamases. Shortly after the availability of methicillin, strains of staphylococci resistant to this drug appeared. The mechanism of resistance to methicillin, which is chromosomally mediated, is due to the production of a unique penicillin-binding protein (PBP) termed PBP2a. Susceptible strains of *S. aureus* produce four or five PBPs most of which are essential for cell growth and survival, and function as trans-, endo-, and carboxypeptidases. PBP2a has a reduced affinity for all β-lactam drugs. Multiresistant strains of *S. aureus* have appeared that are methicillin-resistant, but which are also resistant to aminoglycosides, tetracyclines, chloramphenicol, and fluoroquinolones.

The most resistant coagulase-negative species are *S. hemolyticus* and *S. epidermidis*. Most strains produce β-lactamases and are also resistant to erythromycin. *Staphylococcus saprophyticus* frequently appears to be susceptible to penicillin and resistant to methicillin when tested in the laboratory, but treatment failure with penicillin is common.

CHAPTER 25

Bacterial Agents of Skin and Subcutaneous Infections

GROUP A STREPTOCOCCUS

Group A streptococci (S. pyogenes) can cause several types of skin infections ranging from impetigo, a superficial pyoderma, to severe cellulitis. If the infecting streptococcus is one of the nephritogenic types (2, 49, 55, 57, 60, 61), acute glomerulonephritis may occur several weeks later.

Impetigo is a crusty, vesicular eruption that often appears on the face around the nose or mouth. The early lesions are vesicopustules that rupture leaving a moist eroded base. The exudate eventually dries, leaving thick crusts. In about 10% of the cases, *Staphylococcus aureus* is also present in the lesion, particularly if there are bullous lesions. Impetigo most commonly occurs in the late summer or early fall in young children. It is highly communicable; transmission is probably by direct contact. Spread within families is common, especially if hygiene is poor. Healing generally occurs within a few days.

Erysipelas is a superficial cellulitis characterized by a raised area of erythema, edema, heat, and tenderness that may occur on the face or the lower extremities. The organisms enter the skin through abrasions or breaks in the skin, from the respiratory tract of the patient or other persons. The infection involves the regional lymphatics and may extend into the deeper tissues. Recurrences are common. Rarely, streptococci may cause a rapidly progressive form of gangrene, usually at the site of trauma. The infection rapidly extends along fascial planes, and bacteremia, metastatic abscesses, and death may result unless treatment is prompt and effective. Streptococci of groups B, C, and G also cause disease of this type in diabetics.

ERYSIPELOTHRIX INSIDIOSA (E. RHUSIOPATHIAE)

This organism is a facultative, gram-positive non-spore-forming rod that is the cause of swine erysipelas, and erysipeloid in humans, a cellulitis that is an occupational disease in persons handling fish, shellfish, poultry, or meat. The organisms are introduced through abrasions, usually on the hands, and a painful erythematous elevated lesion develops which spreads peripherally. Occasionally septicemia, endocarditis, or septic arthritis may result.

BACILLUS ANTHRACIS

Bacillus anthracis is an aerobic gram-positive spore-forming rod that is the cause of anthrax in animals and man. Spores enter the skin through abrasions or wounds and after 2 to 5 days a papule appears at the site which develops into a painless ulcer with a black eschar surrounded by erythema and edema of the adjacent tissues (Fig 25–1). If untreated, the infection may spread to the regional lymph nodes; septicemia and meningitis may develop. A vaccine is available. A pulmonary form of the infection (woolsorters' disease) occurs in persons handling hides, woolen rugs, etc. Inhaled spores cause a rapidly progressive pneumonitis with respiratory distress, shock, and death within a few days.

PASTEURELLA MULTOCIDA

Pasteurella multocida is an aerobic gram-negative bacillus that is a constituent of the indigenous oral flora of cats, dogs, and some humans. The organism is a frequent cause of infection of bite wounds and on occasion may be recovered from the sputum of patients.

BACTEROIDES AND FUSOBACTERIA

Bacteroides comprises a number of species of obligately anaerobic gram-negative rods that are often very pleomorphic. *Bacteroides* organisms are normally found as indigenous members of the microflora of mucous membranes of the upper respiratory and lower gastrointestinal tracts.

The species most commonly recovered from infections is *B. fragilis* (Fig 25–2). This organism has characteristics unique among *Bacteroides:* a cell wall lipopolysaccharide (LPS) devoid of endotoxin activity, and a polysaccharide capsule. *Bacteroides fragilis* has been involved in suppurative lesions at all anatomic locations,

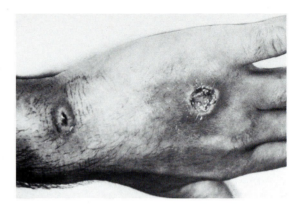

FIG 25–1.
Cutaneous anthrax.

sometimes in pure culture. The organism is recovered from more than 65% of intraabdominal infections and 25% of pleuropulmonary and female genital tract infections. Seventy percent to 80% of clinical isolates of *B. fragilis* are encapsulated, while only 0.5% of fecal strains have a capsule. The capsule has been shown to interfere with phagocytosis. Only encapsulated strains are capable of producing abscesses in experimental animals and the purified polysaccharide itself can induce abscess formation. The cell wall lipopolysaccharide of *B. fragilis* is atypical and has essentially no endotoxic activity. Unlike the lipopolysaccharides of other gram-negative species, the *B. fragilis* LPS does not contain 2-

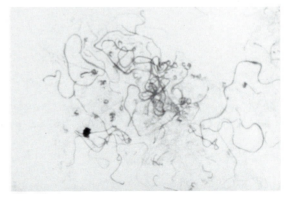

FIG 25–2.
Bacteroides fragilis.

ketodeoxyoctanoate (KDO). The LPS does act on complement to activate the C5a chemotactic factor. Virulent strains of *B. fragilis* produce more neuraminidase than strains recovered from stool specimens, and some strains produce fibrinolysin, lipase, proteases, nucleases, and heparinase. The heparinase may be responsible for the thrombophlebitis often associated with *B. fragilis* infections. *Bacteroides fragilis* is usually resistant to penicillin by virtue of chromosomally mediated β-lactamase production.

The second most frequent species is *Bacteroides melaninogenicus*. This species usually occurs in mixed anaerobic infections, and is seldom isolated from an abscess or other clinical material in pure culture. It is an important contributor to synergistic mixtures of bacteria by virtue of several virulence factors, the most important of which is collagenase. This enzyme is bound to a particulate fraction of the bacterial cell wall and is probably responsible for establishing localized infections. Other potential pathogenic factors produced by *B. melaninogenicus* include fibrinolysin, ribonuclease, and deoxyribonuclease. The organism contains endotoxic lipopolysaccharide, but the role of this component in infection is not known. In contrast to *B. fragilis*, isolates of *B. melaninogenicus* are usually penicillin-sensitive.

Normal human serum contains low titers of IgM antibodies against O antigens of *B. fragilis* and *B. melaninogenicus*, but their protective function is not known. A rise in IgM and IgG antibodies has been observed in patients after *B. fragilis* infections.

Fusobacteria are thin, gram-negative anaerobic rods that usually have pointed ends. They differ from *Bacteroides* primarily by production of butyric acid as a major end product of carbohydrate fermentation. The normal habitat of fusobacteria is the mouth, and many of the diseases caused by these organisms are associated with the respiratory tract. Fusobacteria have been recovered from pleuropulmonary infections, bacteremia, and soft tissue infections such as wounds and abscesses. They are often isolated from mixed infections with facultative bacteria, *B. fragilis*, *B. melaninogenicus*, or anaerobic cocci. Fusobacteria are components of synergistic fusospirochetal infections, an example of which is necrotizing ulcerative gingivitis (Vincent's angina, trench mouth). These synergistic infections usually involve necrotic tissue. Purulent lesions occur when fusobacteria occur with bacterial species, or alone, as in brain abscess or periapical dental abscess. Some commonly recovered species are *Fusobacterium necrophorum* and *F. nucleatum*.

The only known virulence factor of fusobacteria is its lipopolysaccharide which resembles the LPS of other gram-negative organisms. The LPS contains heptose and KDO, and has been shown to be very potent. Fusobacterial endotoxins have been implicated in human periodontal disease and fatal cases of septic shock. Some strains of *F. necrophorum* produce lipase, but the significance of this enzyme in the pathogenesis of lesions is not known.

Human sera have been shown to contain antibodies to fusobacterial antigens, particularly the LPS, but the capacity of such antibodies to protect against tissue invasion by fusobacteria is not known.

ACTINOMYCES

Actinomycetes are gram-positive, anaerobic, branching rods that commonly occur together with other organisms in the oral cavity, tonsillar crypts, and colon. They tend to grow more slowly than most bacteria and require 3 to 5 days for colonies to appear. Actinomycetes grow as branching filaments which fragment to resemble pleomorphic bacteria. The species involved in human disease are *Actinomyces israelii* and *A. bovis*.

Actinomycosis is a chronic, suppurative, and granulomatous disease in which abscesses with thick yellow-green pus form in the tissues.

These abscesses often expand to form tortuous sinus tracts which eventually burrow to the skin surface and drain pus. The pus contains yellow grains or granules, erroneously called "sulfur granules," composed of masses of the branching organisms held together by a polysaccharide-protein complex secreted by the organisms. The complex is cemented together by calcium phosphate deposited as a result of the phosphatase activity of the organisms.

The clinical forms of actinomycosis are cervicofacial which usually follow injection of the organism into traumatized oral tissues; thoracic actinomycosis with pleural effusions and draining sinuses in the chest wall which follows aspiration of the organism; and the abdominal form presenting as masses that may mimic appendicitis or carcinoma.

Although actinomycetes are not considered part of the normal vaginal flora, pelvic infections such as tubo-ovarian abscesses occur in women using intrauterine contraceptive devices and pessaries.

Various antibodies appear during the course of clinical actinomycosis which may play a role in the histopathologic manifestations of this disease. The continuous presence of antigenic material could form local immune complexes that initiate a hypersensitivity reaction, but little is actually known at the present time.

NOCARDIA

Nocardia are gram-positive filamentous bacteria that show branching. They resemble actinomycetes except that *Nocardia* are strict aerobes. The species most commonly involved in human infections—*N. asteroides* and *N. brasiliensis*—are weakly acid-fast. *Nocardia* are commonly present in soil. Growth on artificial media appears in about 2 to 3 days. The colonies are dry and by 7 to 10 days become wrinkled with yellow or red pigment.

Nocardia produce chronic suppurative in-

fections. Three clinical forms of nocardiosis are seen: pulmonary, central nervous system, and subcutaneous tissue infections. Pulmonary infection is most commonly due to *N. asteroides*. The organisms are inhaled with dust or soil. Approximately half of the patients who develop pulmonary nocardiosis have some underlying disease. About 30% of the patients have been treated with steroids or similar immunosuppressive therapy, but the disease also occurs as an opportunistic infection in patients with neoplastic diseases, especially lymphoma, leukemia, and Hodgkin's disease. The initial lesion is an acute inflammation with suppuration that develops into multiple large, confluent abscesses scattered throughout the lung. The organisms find their way into the bloodstream and establish metastatic abscesses most frequently in the brain, and to a lesser extent in the spleen, skin, peritoneum, and kidney. Cell-mediated immunity is the most important defense mechanism.

Subcutaneous infection is usually secondary to some minor trauma, such as a splinter or a thorn. The most common species in this type of infection is *N. brasiliensis*. Subcutaneous infections are slowly progressive and destructive of muscle and bone. Eventually, sinuses develop which drain pus containing sulfur granules (Fig 25–3).

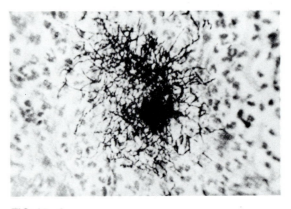

FIG 25–3.
Nocardia in pus.

MYCOBACTERIA

Mycobacterium marinum is a photochromogenic acid-fast rod that is found in water and marine organisms. The optimal growth temperature of this organism is 32°C; no growth takes place at 37°C. Human infection (swimming pool granuloma) follows minor trauma to skin in swimming pools. After an incubation period of 2 to 8 weeks, papules appear at the site of injury, and enlarge, becoming bluish-purple. Eventually the papules break down and become ulcers. The infection is limited to the cooler, superficial tissues; dissemination is rare. A similar organism, *M. ulcerans*, is the agent of Buruli ulcer, a chronic, painless infection prevalent in Africa, Australia, and Mexico.

Leprosy, caused by *M. leprae*, is discussed in Chapter 14, Mycobacteria.

CHAPTER 26

Fungal Agents of Skin and Subcutaneous Infections

A 35-year-old pine tree nurseryman presented with multiple painless, ulcerating nodules on the volar surface of his right forearm. These lesions had been present over the past 6 months. The initial lesion was a painless papule at the site of a scratch from a pine tree seedling. He was otherwise in good health and feeling well. Prior to being seen at the hospital, he had consulted a local physician who treated him with 10 days of penicillin with no response. A Gram stain of the lesion did not demonstrate any microbial forms, but a culture of the lesion grew a fungus identified as *Sporothrix schenckii*, a pathogen present on plant material. He was treated with potassium iodide with subsequent complete healing of the lesions.

The fungi causing subcutaneous infections have certain features in common: they are all dimorphic; in nature they exist on wood or vegetation; infection is usually via the traumatic introduction of spores into the tissues; they are of low pathogenicity so that infection tends to remain localized; and dissemination is rare and only in the compromised host.

SPOROTHRIX

Sporothrix schenckii is a dimorphic saprophytic organism that grows as a mold in nature and as elongated yeastlike cells in tissue. The organisms live on vegetation such as the thorns of carnations and roses, in sphagnum moss, and on pine trees. Man becomes infected when the fungus is introduced into the tissue by trauma caused by wood splinters or thorns. The organisms may also enter the tissues if abraded skin is exposed to soil or infected plant material.

Sporotrichosis is an occupational disease occurring in farmers, horticulturists, gardeners, and laborers. It is worldwide in distribution, but the growth of the fungus is favored by a warm, moist climate. The primary lesion usually occurs on the hands, fingers, or arms. It appears 2 to 12 weeks after the inoculation of spores and characteristically as a painless papule. The papule evolves into a reddish-purple nodule which eventually ulcerates leaving an open sore. After about a week the infection begins to spread along the lymphatics, and a chain of red, indurated nodules appear, some of which may break down, suppurate, and ulcerate (Figs 26–1 and 26–2). If the disease is untreated, additional ulcers develop and become chronic. Progressive or disseminated infection is rare and may involve the lungs, eyes, bones, or the brain and meninges. Sporotrichosis may be effectively treated with potassium iodide, administered orally.

Other subcutaneous fungi are *Petriellidium*, which can cause mycetoma, a subcutaneous infection of the foot; and *Cladosporium* and *Phialophora*, which cause chromoblastomycosis, a tropical disease of barefoot laborers.

DERMATOPHYTES

Most human cutaneous fungal infections are caused by a group of organisms known as dermatophytes. These organisms are able to infect only the superficial cornified layers of skin, hair, and nails.

The three genera involved are *Epidermophyton*, *Microsporum*, and *Trichophyton*. These organisms exist as molds, i.e., in the mycelial form both in nature and in the tissues. Dermatophytes may be grouped according to their habi-

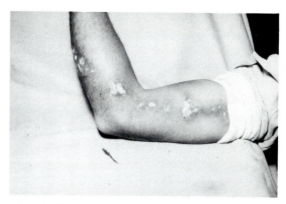

FIG 26–2.
Sporotrichosis.

tat as zoophilic (animal), anthropophilic (man), or geophilic (soil). Only a few geophilic species infect man and such infections are usually transient. Humans are infected by zoophilic species by direct contact with infected animals (cats, dogs, horses, cattle). These infections are usually highly inflammatory, well circumscribed, and often heal spontaneously.

The outcome of a dermatophyte infection is a function of the growth rate and morphology of the infecting species, the degree of inflammation, and the rate of desquamation of the skin. A loss of virulence of a dermatophyte is associated with a decrease in growth rate. In order to infect, the fungus must grow inward at the same

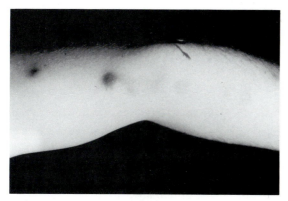

FIG 26–1.
Sporotrichosis.

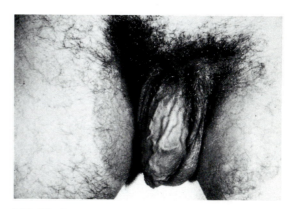

FIG 26–3.
Tinea cruris.

rate or faster than the keratinized layers are shed. The immunologic state of the host is important in determining the type of infection. Patients that do not develop delayed-type hypersensitivity to the organism have lesions that are chronic, scaling, and noninflammatory. If hypersensitivity is present, an inflammatory lesion (kerion) may occur with large vesicles, edema, and pustulation. Such lesions may resolve without treatment because the intense inflammatory response sterilizes the fungus. It is conjectured that the pathogenicity of anthropophilic species is increased by their ability to induce a specific anergy, i.e., suppress the cell-mediated immunity of the host. Chronic dermatophytosis is associated with modification of cell-mediated immunity.

Dermatophytes are not fastidious in their nutritional requirements. They are able to grow in keratin-bearing structures and are able to utilize the keratin because of their production of keratinolytic enzymes. They require a moist atmosphere and are sensitive to oxygen and carbon dioxide tension. Carbon dioxide causes arthrospore formation and enhances infectivity. Infectivity is enhanced if an area of superficial abrasion comes in contact with the spores. The spores reach the stratum corneum where humidity is higher than in intact skin. If the infection site is occluded by clothing or shoes that prevent water evaporation, abrasion is unnecessary.*

The ability of dermatophytes to penetrate and grow in cornified tissues may be due to the production of proteolytic enzymes such as keratinases. The organisms cannot invade beyond the stratum corneum and survive. There are factors in serum and in live epidermal cells that destroy the invading fungus.

The antigenic component that contributes to the local inflammatory response and induces the development of delayed-type hypersensitivity is the galactomannan glycopeptides.

Secondary allergic reactions, known as **dermatophytids,** may occur at a site distant from the primary fungal infection, often on fingers and palms. These eruptions may be papular, vesicular, or bullous, and are often accompanied by intense itching. They are thought to be due to a massive liberation of the sensitizing galactomannan glycopeptide antigen.

The various superficial infections are called ringworm or **tinea** according to the body site: tinea capitis (ringworm of the scalp), tinea barbae (beard), tinea corporis (body), tinea cruris (groin, "jock itch") (Fig 26–3), tinea pedis (athlete's foot), etc.

---

*The commonest dermatophyte infection in the United States is tinea pedis (athlete's foot), probably because occlusive shoes are worn. Tinea pedis is uncommon in countries where people go barefoot or wear open sandals.

CHAPTER 27

Viral Agents of Skin Infections

There are three major groups of viruses that produce skin disease: herpesviruses, poxviruses, and papillomaviruses.

Herpesviruses are responsible for a variety of human diseases including cold sores, a venereal disease, chickenpox, shingles, mononucleosis, congenital and perinatal infections, and certain neoplastic diseases. Herpesviruses are large, enveloped, double-stranded DNA viruses. The dense core is covered by an icosahedral capsid which in turn is surrounded by an amorphous protein coat called the tegument. The tegument is enclosed within a bilayered envelope composed of lipids and glycoproteins.

A characteristic common to herpesviruses is their ability to produce latent infections after the initial overt episode. During latency the viral genome is present in the cell but infectious virus cannot be recovered. Alterations in the immunity of the host can result in reactivation of the virus and recurrent infection.

Three subfamilies of herpesvirus have been described: alpha-herpesviruses, which replicate rapidly, killing the infected cell and becoming latent in ganglia; beta-herpesviruses, which are slower-acting, killing the infected cells and becoming latent in various tissues; and gamma-herpesviruses, which have an affinity for lymphocytes and lymphoblastic cells, producing persistent or latent infections. Herpes simplex

(HSV) and varicella-zoster (VZV) viruses are in the alpha group; cytomegalovirus (CMV) is in the beta group; and Epstein-Barr virus (EBV) is in the gamma group. Additionally, a herpesvirus, HV6, has been recovered from patients with B cell lymphomas. HV6 has also been found to be a relatively frequent cause of high fever in normal young children. Many of these children have a rash and illness consistent with a diagnosis of roseola.

Herpesviruses produce disease by destruction of tissue, by provoking immunopathologic responses, and in some instances by inducing neoplasia.

HERPES SIMPLEX VIRUSES

Two antigenic and epidemiologic types of HSV exist: HSV-1 and HSV-2. Both can cause primary and recurrent infections. The reservoir of both types is man, and transmission is by direct contact. The incubation period is 2 to 12 days. Transmission is by contact with HSV-1 in the saliva of carriers. Approximately 5% of asymptomatic persons excrete the virus in their saliva.

Oral-facial infections are usually due to HSV-1. Most primary infections occur in children under the age of 5 years and are usually asymptomatic. In the 10% that develop symptoms, vesicular lesions occur on the lips, tongue, gingiva, palate, and pharynx, and become painful ulcers. The infection lasts for about 10 days, accompanied by fever and irritability. Recurrent episodes may take place any time during the life of the victim as a result of reactivation of the latent infection. Reactivation can be precipitated by trauma, fever, menstruation, exposure to sunlight, or emotional stress. Recurrent infections usually take the form of vesicles on the face and lips (fever blisters, cold sores) which crust and heal within a few days. In immunosuppressed persons the infection may extend into deeper mucosal and cutaneous tissues, with bleeding, necrosis, and severe pain.

Genital infections occur principally in adults and are transmitted by sexual contact. Over 70% are caused by HSV-2. In women primary infection is characterized by itching and the development of painful vesicles that ulcerate; the principal sites are the cervix and vulva (Fig 27–1), but the infection may extend to involve the perineal area and the buttocks. The local symptoms are often accompanied by fever and headache. In men, lesions occur on the penis, and in the anus and rectum of homosexuals. The proximal illness lasts approximately 3 weeks. Recurrent infection due to reactivation is usually less severe, of

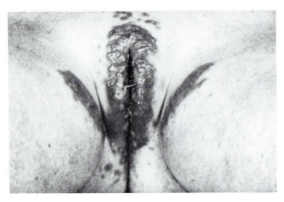

FIG 27–1.
Herpes vulvovaginitis.

shorter duration (about 2 weeks), and with fewer lesions. Reactivation may be precipitated by menses or sexual intercourse. Approximately 1% of patients develop an episode of aseptic meningitis, which is usually self-limited, but can result in sacral plexus involvement preventing urinary and bowel control.

Herpetic whitlow is HSV infection of the finger, and is an occupational hazard of physicians, dentists, nurses, and other medical and laboratory personnel. Transmission is usually the result of inoculation through abrasions or small cuts. Painful lesions develop, but recurrences are infrequent.

Burn wounds may become infected with HSV and disseminate to another organ(s).

Eye infections are usually caused by HSV-1. The primary infection is typically unilateral follicular conjunctivitis, but the cornea may also be involved. If the infection is limited to the conjunctiva, healing takes place in 2 to 3 weeks. Recurrent infections may result in corneal damage and eventual scarring. Herpetic infection is the most frequent cause of corneal blindness in industrialized countries.

Herpes encephalitis typically presents with the abrupt onset of fever and focal temporal or parietal lobe symptoms. Most adults do not have clinical evidence of a mucocutaneous infection since the disease is due to reactivation of the virus and passage of the virus from the ganglion back to the brain. Untreated, the mortality is 70% (see Chapter 20).

Most neonatal herpes infections are caused by HSV-2 and are the result of contact with infected genital secretions at the time of delivery. Symptoms develop a few days to several weeks post partum and are manifested by neurologic abnormalities and conjunctivitis. Vesicles may not be present. Congenital infection is less common and is characterized by jaundice, hepatosplenomegaly, seizures, chorioretinitis, and skin vesicles. Infection with HSV-1 may also occur postnatally through contact with the saliva of infected nursing staff or family members. The mortality of untreated neonatal infection is 85%.

The pathogenesis of HSV infection is initiated with the entry of virus through mucous membrane or abraded skin; normal intact skin is not penetrated. The virus binds to the surface of epithelial cells; HSV-1 and HSV-2 appear to attach to different receptors. Following attachment the viral envelope fuses with the cell membrane liberating the nucleocapsid into the cytoplasm. The nucleocapsid is disassembled, releasing the DNA-containing viral core which is transported to the cell nucleus. Within the nucleus the viral genome is replicated, structural proteins are synthesized, and nucleocapsids are assembled. The envelope is formed as the nucleocapsids bud through the nuclear membrane into the perinuclear space. Infected cells eventually lyse, releasing virus.

The initial cellular response is an infiltrate of polymorphonuclear neutrophils, followed by mononuclear cells. The viruses infect local sensory nerve endings and are transported in or on axons or supporting cells to the local sensory and autonomic ganglia. The trigeminal ganglion is infected from oral-facial infections; genital infections reach the sacral ganglion. Viral replication occurs in the ganglia and adjacent neural tissues during active disease. When reactivation occurs the virus migrates to other mucosal and skin surfaces via the peripheral sensory nerves. The mechanisms of latency and reactivation are unknown.

Humoral and cellular immune responses are both important in herpetic infections. Humoral neutralizing antibodies to HSV are able to neutralize the virus, but recurrences occur in the presence of high titers of neutralizing antibody. This is probably explained by the cell-to-cell spread of virus, although viremic episodes have occurred in patients with neutralizing antibody. Natural killer cells, macrophages, certain T cells and their lymphokines all play a role in the host's defense against HSV infection.

The laboratory diagnosis of HSV infection may be made by recovering virus by culture or demonstrating viral antigen by ELISA (Enzyme-Linked Immuno Sorbent Assay) in vesicle fluid or material from the ulcer. Serology is not very helpful since antibodies to HSV are present in a large proportion of the population.

Acyclovir is used in the treatment of primary genital herpes in immunocompetent patients, and for suppression of recurrent mucocutaneous infection in the immunocompromised patient. Acylovir is used to treat neonatal herpes and HSV encephalitis.

VARICELLA-ZOSTER VIRUS

Infection with VZV produces two distinct syndromes: varicella (chickenpox) and zoster (shingles). The reservoir of the virus is man.

Chickenpox represents a primary infection by the VZV. It is highly contagious, and transmitted from person to person by direct contact with vesicle fluid or by respiratory aerosols. Ninety percent of the population have had the disease by the age of 10 years. The incubation period is 2 to 3 weeks. In the immunocompetent child, chickenpox is a relatively mild disease with the sudden onset of slight fever, a few generalized constitutionalized symptoms, and an eruption that is initially maculopapular, but which rapidly becomes vesicular. The vesicles appear initially on the scalp, face, and trunk and then spread to involve the extremities. Lesions are intensely pruritic, last for 3 to 4 days, and then scab over. Lesions occur in successive crops for several days.

In adults, the fever and symptoms may be severe, and one-third develop viral pneumonia. Recovery is usual, but the most common cause of death is the pulmonary manifestations.

Neonates that develop chickenpox within the first 5 to 10 days of life or whose mother has developed the disease within a week before or

48 hours after delivery are at risk of severe, generalized disease with a mortality of 15% to 20%. Children with acute leukemia, even if in remission, are at risk of disseminated fatal disease. An epidemiologic association has been reported between chickenpox and Reye's syndrome, especially if aspirin has been used as an antipyretic. This syndrome is characterized by vomiting, seizures, and alteration of consciousness, and pathologically by severe fatty infiltrates of the liver, kidneys, and other organs.

Herpes zoster occurs mainly in older people and represents a local manifestation of reactivated VZV. Vesicles appear on skin areas supplied by one or more sensory nerves of dorsal root ganglia; most frequently in thoracic dermatomes. The skin lesions are accompanied by paresthesias and sensations of burning or aching. Herpes zoster is more severe in the immunocompromised host and may persist for many months.

The pathogenesis of chickenpox and herpes zoster is identical. The initial site of viral replication is not known, but a viremia develops. With viral replication in the skin, degenerative changes are seen in the epithelial cells with ballooning and the appearance of multinucleated giant cells with eosinophilic nuclear inclusions. As circulating antibodies appear, the viremia disappears and the skin lesions begin to decrease.

The diagnosis of chickenpox and herpes zoster is clinical but can be readily confirmed by a Tzanck smear in which scrapings from the base of fresh vesicles stained with Giemsa show the multinucleated giant cells with eosinophilic nuclear inclusion bodies. These cells may also be seen in the sputum of patients with varicella pneumonia. The VZV can be recovered in tissue culture and by direct fluorescent antibody methods.

No treatment is needed for uncomplicated chickenpox in immunocompetent children. Immunocompromised persons exposed to chickenpox should be given immunoprophylaxis with zoster immune globulin (ZIG) which must be administered within 72 hours of exposure to be effective. Acyclovir and vidarabine have been used to treat herpes zoster in immunocompromised patients.

CYTOMEGALOVIRUS

Infection with CMV is very common, but associated disease is infrequent. The reservoir of human strains of CMV is man. Infection is usually asymptomatic and the development of disease is dependent upon the age and immune status of the host. Like other herpesviruses, CMV causes a primary infection followed by latency that usually persists for life. Symptomatic primary infections, while uncommon, are more serious and have a higher fatality rate than reactivation disease. Most significant disease occurs in the immature neonate and the immunocompromised, particularly organ transplant recipients and patients with acquired immunodeficiency syndrome (AIDS).

During primary or reactivation infections, virus is secreted in urine, saliva, breast milk, cervical secretions, and semen. Viremia may be present in asymptomatic persons, and the virus may be transmitted by blood transfusions.

Infection of the neonate may be acquired in utero. Only about 10% of infected infants are symptomatic at birth, showing lethargy, jaundice, convulsions, thrombocytopenia, purpura, hepatosplenomegaly, microcephaly, intracerebral calcifications, chorioretinitis, and pulmonary infiltrates. An additional 60% of infants born to infected mothers acquire the disease by breast milk during the perinatal period. More than 90% of the surviving infected infants develop complications later in life that include mental retardation, hearing loss, chorioretinitis, and learning disabilities. Up to 80% of children become infected with CMV by puberty as a result of horizontal transmission from infected peers, parents, or other adults. The majority of these infections are asymptomatic and are followed by lifelong latency.

In immunocompetent adults, primary CMV infection occurs as heterophil-negative infectious mononucleosis syndrome.* This syndrome is characterized by fever, headache, malaise, and generalized lymphadenopathy. The infection is transmitted by intimate or sexual contact. Post-transfusion mononucleosis appears 3 to 8 weeks after receiving blood from an infected person; the virus is probably transmitted by infected lymphocytes. Uncommon complications of CMV-induced mononucleosis include interstitial pneumonitis, Guillain-Barré syndrome (a rapidly progressive ascending form of muscular weakness and sensory loss), meningoencephalitis, myocarditis, hemolytic anemia, and hepatitis. CMV infection is common in recipients of organ transplants, patients with malignancies, and those with AIDS. These infections may be expressed as interstitial pneumonia, hepatitis, retinitis, or gastrointestinal or central nervous system disease. CMV DNA has been found within the tumor cells of Kaposi's sarcoma in Central Africa and in homosexual men with AIDS.

CMV infects lymphocytes and epithelial cells. Characteristic intranuclear and intracytoplasmic inclusions are seen in infected epithelial cells. The virus replicates in the salivary glands, the respiratory tract, and the kidney. Neonates that die with CMV usually have disseminated intravascular coagulopathy suggesting that the virus may induce a vasculitis. Immune complexes circulate in infants with congenital infection during the first year of life. Deposition of these immune complexes in renal glomeruli may occur. Congenitally infected infants also show impaired cell-mediated immunity that is highly specific for CMV.

The diagnosis of CMV infection is readily

*More than 90% of cases of infectious mononucleosis are caused by the Epstein-Barr virus. These persons usually develop heterophil antibodies, i. e., agglutinins for sheep red blood cells.

made by culturing the urine and blood for the virus. Gancyclovir has recently been introduced for the treatment of CMV retinitis, pneumonitis, and other serious infections. CMV disease in seronegative transplant patients may be reduced by administration of immune globulin.

EPSTEIN-BARR VIRUS

Epstein-Barr virus infection is very common. The reservoir is in man, and a large percentage of infections are acquired in early childhood and are asymptomatic. The virus is excreted in the saliva of many healthy adults and convalescent carriers and young children become infected by saliva on the hands of adults. Although the virus may be transmitted to the fetus in utero, primary EBV infection is rare during pregnancy because of the small number of susceptible women. Young adults in their second decade who have escaped primary infection in childhood may become infected by the exchange of saliva in kissing and develop the acute viral syndrome of **infectious mononucleosis**. The incubation period is 4 to 6 weeks. This syndrome is characterized by sore throat, fever, and lymphadenopathy. The onset is abrupt and there may be chills, sweats, anorexia, and malaise. About one half of the cases have an enlarged spleen. The disease lasts 3 to 4 weeks and complications are uncommon. Pharyngeal excretion of the virus may persist for a year, and 15% to 20% of healthy adults with EBV antibodies are pharyngeal carriers.

The pharyngeal epithelial cells are the initial site of viral replication which is followed by infection of B lymphocytes. The virus enters the lymphocytes via the CD3 receptors and EBV antigens appear in the nuclei of infected cells. Approximately 20% of B lymphocytes carry EBV antigen during an episode of infectious mononucleosis. There is a polyclonal increase of B lymphocytes during the first week. During the second week T cell–mediated suppression occurs characterized by a reversal of the normal helper-suppressor ratio.

The diagnosis of infectious mononucleosis may be made by a white blood cell count containing more than 50% mononuclear cells and more than 10% atypical lymphocytes (Downey cells); the transient appearance of heterophil antibodies, and specific EBV antibodies. Heterophil antibodies are demonstrated as agglutinins for sheep, beef, and horse red blood cells. The first EBV antibody to appear is the viral capsid IgM, followed by early and nuclear antigens that persist for life.

EBV is believed to be the cause of Burkitt's lymphoma, a malignant childhood B cell lymphoblastic tumor predominantly found in Central Africa. EBV has also been associated with nasopharyngeal carcinoma, and certain lymphomas.

POXVIRUSES

The poxviruses are large DNA viruses that affect insects, birds, and mammals. The poxviruses infecting man include the agents of molluscum contagiosum, ecthyma contagiosum, vaccinia, and variola (smallpox).

Molluscum contagiosum is a benign disease characterized by small white-to-yellow papules present on the genital areas of adults and the exposed skin areas of children. It is transmitted by close contact, including sexual intercourse. The reservoir is man, and the incubation period varies from 7 days to 6 months. Lesions usually resolve spontaneously, except in AIDS patients in whom they may persist and become more numerous and severe.

Ecthyma contagiosum (orf) is a cutaneous disease of sheep and goats, and an occupational hazard of farm workers, shepherds, and veterinarians. There is typically a single maculopapular lesion on the hands, arms, or face that progresses to an umbilicated weeping nodule.

The lesion usually resolves spontaneously in 30 days.

Vaccinia is a "laboratory virus," probably derived from cowpox, and does not exist in nature. It is serologically related to smallpox, and was used to immunize against that disease. When the skin of a nonimmune person is scarified through a drop of fluid containing vaccinia virus, a papule appears after 4 days which evolves into a vesicle and pustule over the next 5 days. By the 20th day, a scab appears and drops off, leaving a small permanent scar and immunity against smallpox.

Variola (smallpox) was a severe viral disease that had a death rate as high as 50% with one form. As a result of tremendous efforts in surveillence and vaccination, global eradication was confirmed in 1979.

PAPILLOMAVIRUSES

The human papillomaviruses (HPV) are small, unenveloped viruses with an icosahedral capsid enclosing a genome of circular, double-stranded DNA. Over 50 genotypes have been identified in human papillomas. The reservoir is man. Transmission is the result of direct, close contact. The incubation period is 3 to 4 months.

Papillomas are epithelial tumors of skin and mucous membranes and include common, flat, and plantar warts, venereal warts (condylomata acuminata), and laryngeal papillomas. Common and flat warts occur frequently among children and are associated with HPV types 1, 2, 4, and 41. Genital warts are sexually transmitted and are caused by HPV types 6, 10, 11, 40–44, and 51. Laryngeal papillomas are associated with HPV types 6 and 11; laryngeal papillomas are transmitted during the birth process. Laryngeal papillomas and genital warts occasionally become malignant; women with a history of genital warts due to types 16 and 18 are more likely to develop cervical carcinoma than women without that history.

PART VI

Infections of Muscle, Bone, and Joints

CHAPTER 28

Overview of Muscle, Bone, and Joint Infections

MUSCLE

Muscle pain (myalgia) is often associated with systemic viral or bacterial infection. Infection of skeletal muscle (myositis) is uncommon and may be associated with trichinosis, cysticercosis, or toxoplasmosis. Bacterial myositis (pyomyositis) may follow penetrating wounds, and abscesses of adjacent skin, subcutaneous tissue, or bone. On occasion, pyomyositis may occur via the bloodstream from a distant site.

The organism most frequently involved in pyomyositis is *Staphylococcus aureus*. There is a gradual onset of localized pain, tenderness, induration, and fever. Abscess of the psoas muscle may be due to gram-negative bacilli, sometimes mixed with *S. aureus*, or *Mycobacterium tuberculosis*.

A much more severe infection is myonecrosis (gas gangrene), which is rapidly progressive and often fatal. Myonecrosis usually follows contamination of a wound with soil and is commonly caused by *Clostridium perfringens*, but other histotoxic clostridia, streptococci, *Bacteroides*, or mixtures of bacteria may be recovered.

BONE—OSTEOMYELITIS

Osteomyelitis can be divided into groups on the basis of the pathogenic mechanism: (a) hematogenous; (b) contiguous (soft tissue and postoperative infections); and (c) traumatic contamination. Acute hematogenous osteomyelitis most often involves rapidly growing bone, particularly the metaphysis of long bones. Nutrient arteries that supply the blood to bones make sharp loops near the epiphyseal growth plate. Blood in the large sinusoidal veins flows slowly and is connected with the medullary network of vessels. There are no phagocytic cells in this area since vessels in the metaphysis are capillaries. The loops of capillaries are 15 to 60 μm in diameter and blood flow is slow. Capillary loops adjacent to the epiphyseal growth plate are nonanastomosing branches of the nutrient artery; hence, any obstruction such as microthrombi produces small areas of avascular necrosis. Thus, if bacteria lodge in the area they proliferate and cause extensive damage.

The anatomy of the bones and joints explains why osteomyelitis is different at different ages. In the child below 1 year of age capillaries perforate the epiphyseal growth plate and infection, which begins in the metaphyseal sinusoid areas, spreads to the epiphysis and causes a septic arthritis. The epiphyseal growth plate can be destroyed in these children.

Between 1 year of age and puberty, infection will be contained in the metaphyseal sinusoidal veins since vessels no longer perforate the epiphysis. Infection spreads laterally, perforating the cortex, and lifts the loose periosteal layer producing a subperiosteal collection. The epiphysis is saved at this age. Spread into a joint at this age occurs only if the attachment of the joint capsule is below the epiphyseal plate, as in the hip and shoulder. In the adult, after reabsorption of the growth cartilage, there may be anastomoses between metaphyseal and epiphyseal blood vessels so that bone infection can enter the subarticular space. Since the periosteum is firmly attached in the adult, it is rare to see subperiosteal abscess formation.

Bacteria in bone cause accumulation of leukocytes and a fall in pH, damage to collagen, edema, and ultimately destruction of bone trabeculae with loss of matrix and calcium. Infection will spread to nearby osseous structures via haversian and Volkmann's canals, with a septic thrombophlebitis of the diaphyseal vessels, impairment of venous return, and death of osteocytes. Segments of bone in the area of infection separate from the rest of the bone. The dead pieces of bone are called sequestra.

There is central necrosis with large numbers of polymorphonuclear cells and fibrin material surrounded by an area of granulation tissue with lymphocytes and plasma cells, and there is an outer layer of fibrous tissue with new bone formation of a disordered type that contains few osteoclasts.

Irrespective of the primary pathologic changes, once infection of bone becomes established and self-sustaining, osteomyelitis becomes chronic. With the availability of effective therapy, the incidence of chronic osteomyelitis has

diminished. A higher frequency of chronic osteomyelitis occurs when the blood supply is poor, especially in diabetes mellitus and artherosclerotic peripheral vascular disease.

The pathologic picture is one of dead, devitalized bone with draining sinuses and open wounds. Systemic signs usually are absent, although some patients will present with acute exacerbations appearing much like primary episodes. Evaluation reveals the tissue changes of chronic disease. Physical findings, except for sinuses, may be absent. Radiographic findings are often dramatic, showing new bone formation and sequestra.

Acute hematogenous osteomyelitis occurs primarily in children between infancy and puberty. Ten percent of the total cases of hematogenous osteomyelitis occur before 1 year of age, 70% by 10 years, and 90% by 15 years. In recent years, a shift in age to patients in the fourth to sixth decades has been attributed to a rise in vertebral osteomyelitis in elderly adults. Hematogenous osteomyelitis also is encountered in persons who inject illicit drugs.

Most reported series of osteomyelitis of hematogenous origin note a very high incidence (up to 40%) of notable, but physically minor, trauma immediately prior to the onset of presenting symptoms.

The distal femur, proximal and distal tibia and fibula, foot, and proximal humerus are involved in approximately 80% of cases of osteomyelitis. Osteomyelitis of the femoral neck, proximal humerus, and distal fibula may allow bacteria to penetrate at the point of joint attachment into the adjacent hip, shoulder, and ankle joints, causing secondary septic arthritis.

Signs and symptoms of hematogenous osteomyelitis vary from minimal to severe, depending on the site of involvement, age of the patient, and the degree of chronicity. Most patients have fever, chills, malaise, and even nausea, vomiting, and headache. In infants, irritability or poor feeding are common. Temperature may be in the range of 39 to 39.5° C with tachycardia and dehydration notable in younger patients. Limping, regional pain in bone, swelling, warmth, erythema, and guarding of the affected region or limb are found in most cases of acute osteomyelitis. Pain may be severe enough to cause pseudoparalysis of the affected limb in infants and small children.

In vertebral osteomyelitis the lumbar region is the most frequent site followed by the thoracic and then the cervical area. Collection of soft pus between the dura and vertebral periosteum may cause neurologic compromise, or extend or perforate to form extraspinal abscesses. Hematogenous vertebral osteomyelitis occurs in the body of the vertebrae which has a very extensive blood supply. Anastomotic venous channels between adjacent vertebrae cause the illness to spread to adjacent vertebrae. The pathologic process is similar to that seen in long bones.

Patients with vertebral osteomyelitis may have nondescript complaints of headache, fever, and chills. The only physical findings may be rigidity of involved areas of spine, and paravertebral spasm presenting much like chronic low back pain. Physical findings without fever are common.

CONTIGUOUS (DIRECT EXTENSION) OSTEOMYELITIS

This form mostly affects patients 50 years old or older. A soft tissue infection or infected surgical site extends directly to contiguous bone. The surgery most often implicated is open reduction of fractures using nails, plates, and similar prosthetic devices. The fractures most often requiring internal fixations are femoral head and tibial fractures, these bones being the ones most often affected by osteomyelitis, although skull flap infections after craniotomy are not uncommon. Examples of soft tissue infections that can involve bone include lung abscess spreading to the ribs or spine, infected teeth resulting in mandibular infections, as well as sinus and ear infections leading to involvement of the skull

and mastoids, and the bones of the feet secondary to ulcers.

Pain and erythema developing in the immediate postoperative period or after control of the original infection should arouse suspicion of osteomyelitis. Low-grade, steady pain with development of ulcerations or sinus drainage is the usual presenting complaint of osteomyelitis that follows a contiguous infection.

TRAUMATIC CONTAMINATION OSTEOMYELITIS

This most commonly follows compound fractures, percutaneous surgical procedures, and trauma where skin and environmental organisms are driven into bone or tissue close to bone. Males in the trauma years, ages 15 to 30, constitute most of the patients. The physical findings are similar to the preceding categories of osteomyelitis.

Osteomyelitis of the foot following puncture wounds in children or adults is a special problem in this category. *Pseudomonas aeruginosa* is the most important organism. Symptoms are entirely local and the diagnosis is easily missed if unsuspected and a radiograph is not obtained.

INFECTING ORGANISMS

These vary depending on the age of the patient. Staphylococci predominate, with other isolates less common. Despite the increased incidence in recent years of gram-negative sepsis in both adults and children, a corresponding increase in osteomyelitis due to gram-negative bacteria has not been seen. A specific bacterial etiology can be obtained in 50% to 70% of cases. Overall, the prognosis for hematogenous osteomyelitis is good. With proper therapy started early, cure rates of 90%, without disability, can be expected.

Haemophilus influenzae and group B streptococci are important causes of osteomyelitis in children aged 6 months to 5 years. *Staphylococ-*

cus aureus and gram-negative enteric bacteria must also be considered since they are acquired in neonatal intensive care units. Hematogenous osteomyelitis in adults is most often due to *S. aureus*, but gram-negative bacteria such as *Escherichia coli* and pseudomonads are very important.

Up to 90% of nonhematogenous osteomyelitis will yield anaerobes on culture. This represents 80% to 90% of all osteomyelitis in adults. The skull, mastoid, mandible, maxilla, and peripheral extremities are the sites most likely to yield these organisms. In these patients there frequently is vascular insufficiency. The loss of a normal blood supply allows organisms of low virulence such as anaerobic bacteria to grow in the devitalized tissue and bone. Diabetes and atherosclerotic vascular insufficiency are the underlying diseases found in most of these patients. The presence of foul odor or pus is of great diagnostic value. Microorganisms commonly recovered include *Bacteroides* and *Fusobacterium* species and anaerobic cocci (Table 28–1). A clear-cut pathologic role is difficult to define because pure cultures are obtained only in a few cases. Usually these organisms are mixed with nonaerobic species.

DIAGNOSIS

Looking for changes of bone lysis in early osteomyelitis by means of radiographs is unsatisfactory since it takes at least 10 to 14 days to develop damage that can be seen on the x-ray film. Only about 1 μm of bone is resorbed each day and it takes about a 12- to 14-μm loss to be visible. Radiographically demonstrable changes may never develop with antibiotic therapy. Soft tissue changes on radiograph juxtaposed to bone in the correct clinical setting can be a valuable early clue and should not be ignored.

To assist in early diagnosis, use has been made of bone scintigraphy with technetium and labeled polypyrophosphate compounds. These materials accumulate in areas of rapid bone turnover, and may define an area of involvement as early as 24 to 48 hours after the onset of symptoms. Bone scans are not pathognomonic, and demonstrate only focal areas of increased osteoclastic or osteoblastic activity which may be

TABLE 28–1.

Osteomyelitis: Commonly Isolated Organisms Hematogenous Osteomyelitis (Monomicrobial Infection)

Infants (<1 yr)	Children (1–16 yr)	Adults (> 16yr)
Group B streptococcus	*Staphylococcus aureus*	*S. aureus*
S. aureus	*Streptococcus pyogenes*	*Staphylococcus epidermis*
Escherichia coli	*Haemophilus influenzae*	Gram-negative bacilli
	Salmonella spp.	*Pseudomonas aeruginosa*
		Serratia marcescens
		E. coli

Contiguous Focus Osteomyelitis (Polymicrobial Infection)
S. aureus
S. epidermidis
Str. pyogenes
Enterococcus Spp.
Gram-negative bacilli (*E. coli, Klebsiella, Psuedomonas, Serratia*)
Anaerobes (*Bacteroides* spp.)

due to any inflammatory process such as osteomyelitis, neoplasm, trauma, and infarctions, as occur in sickle cell disease. Positive bone scans must be interpreted with regard to the clinical setting; a negative bone scan does not exclude the diagnosis of osteomyelitis. Gallium citrate scans also outline areas of inflammation but are not specific for bone; their value in osteomyelitis is unknown. Other radiologic techniques that may be particularly helpful are computed tomography and magnetic resonance imaging.

In hematogenous osteomyelitis blood cultures are positive in only 50% of patients. Thus biopsy of bone is necessary. In contiguous infection osteomyelitis or traumatic osteomyelitis, skin surface or draining sinus cultures often do not reflect the organism(s) in the bone. Biopsy should be done after scans are complete to avoid false-positives caused by trauma to the bone during therapy.

In acute osteomyelitis, an elevated erythrocyte sedimentation rate (ESR) and an elevated white blood cell count with a predominance of immature forms may be present. These parameters are useful in diagnosis and for following the effectiveness of therapy.

THERAPY

Antibiotic therapy of osteomyelitis is dependent upon the specific etiologic agent. It requires long periods of administration of antibiotics, i.e., 4 to 6 weeks. Even with such therapy recurrences are common and some forms of osteomyelitis probably are never cured.

Surgical intervention is often required to establish a diagnosis and to remove foreign material. Otherwise, surgery is limited therapeutically to a small number of cases where drainage of a subperiosteal collection or debridement of necrotic bone is necessary. Failure to respond to appropriate treatment, coupled with continued pain, swelling, fever, and an elevated white blood cell count and ESR are all clues to the need for surgery. In the case of vertebral osteomyelitis, neurologic compromise requires immediate surgical intervention to relieve cord compression. Surgery should also be used to drain a septic hip when it accompanies osteomyelitis.

JOINT—INFECTIOUS ARTHRITIS

Bacterial arthritis is a common and serious problem. Bacterial involvement of a joint most frequently results in a suppurative arthritis of a single joint, but some bacteria characteristically involve several joints. Some forms of arthritis are "postinfectious," whereas others are due to viruses, fungi, and even parasites. There are a limited number of ways in which changes in the joint can be manifested, and it often is difficult to differentiate infectious arthritis and arthritis due to other causes.

Infectious arthritis can be of hematogenous origin; due to inoculation when a joint is entered, such as intraarticular injection of a steroid, arthroscopy, or prosthetic joint surgery; or secondary to a contiguous focus of infection in soft tissue or bone. In infants less than 1 year of age the infection usually is secondary to osteomyelitis since the capillaries perforate the epiphyseal growth plate. Trauma may allow bacteria in the blood to penetrate joints more readily.

Within 24 to 48 hours of bacteria reaching a joint, there is polymorphonuclear cell infiltration and vascular congestion. Host defenses may eradicate the bacteria, or bacteria continue to multiply and fluid accumulates in the joint. Polymorphonuclear leukocytes damage the articular cartilage by proteolysis. Subsequently, proliferating synovial cells invade the cartilage-bone matrix. Bacterial toxins and cell wall components also produce an inflammatory response.

A number of factors predispose to septic arthritis. In children, other infections (25%) and trauma (30%) are important while in adults preexisting osteoarthritis or rheumatoid arthritis occurs in a third of patients. Corticosteroid injections have been administered to patients who have developed infectious arthritis.

Noninfectious but infection-related arthritis follows infections such as meningococcal disease, and appears to be due to circulating immune complexes and complement aggregating in the joint. The arthritis that follows *Salmonella, Shigella,* and *Yersinia* infection of the intestine occurs most often in persons with the histocompatibility antigen HLA-B27. The role this particular histocompatibility antigen plays is unknown.

CLINICAL FEATURES

Patients who have septic arthritis characteristically have pain on motion in the joint, limitation of joint motion, swelling of the joint, and fever. Small children may be unable to move a joint and appear at times to be paralyzed. The joints can be markedly tender or show minimal tenderness. The exception is the hip in which it is difficult to demonstrate an effusion.

Inflammation of the tendon sheaths is primarily seen with *Neisseria gonorrhoeae.* Gonococcal arthritis is the most common form of arthritis in young females. The arthritis can exist in two forms. In the most common form the patient has systemic symptoms with fever, chills, skin lesions, and polyarticular complaints which begin as tenosynovitis of the wrists or ankles, or both. The patient usually has skin lesions—erythematous, petechial papules that evolve into vesicles and may become pustular. The lesions characteristically are on the hands or other peripheral areas and are transient.

Bacterial arthritis is most often monoarticular in children and adults. The sole exception is gonococcal arthritis which is primarily polyarticular. The knee is the most common single joint affected in both children and adults. Children have the hip, elbow, and ankle affected in about the same percentage. Hand joints are involved infrequently except with gonococcal arthritis or after bites (Table 28–2).

TABLE 28–2.

Frequency of Joint Involvement in Bacterial Infectious Arthritis

Joint(s)	Children (%)	Adults (%)
Knee	40	50
Hip	20	25
Ankle	15	7
Elbow	15	10
Wrist	5	7
Shoulder	5	15
Interphalangeal and metacarpal	1	1
Sternoclavicular	1	8
Sacroiliac	0	2

INFECTING ORGANISMS

The frequency with which certain agents cause bacterial arthritis is dependent upon the age of the patient. In the newborn, group B streptococci and staphylococci are the most common bacteria although gram-negative bacilli such as *E. coli* may also be involved. The infant between 2 months and 2 years of age most often is infected with *H. influenzae* type b, which is the cause of many serious infections in this age group. After 2 years of age, *S. aureus* causes most bacterial arthritis as it does in the elderly. In adults aged 15 to 65 years, *Neisseria gonorrhoeae* is the most common agent. Throughout life, group A streptococci account for about 10% of cases, with group B streptococci more common in neonates and the older diabetes patient. *Streptococcus pneumoniae* was common in the preantibiotic era, but is fairly rare today.

Most patients who develop gram-negative arthritis have underlying chronic illness or chronic arthritis in the infected joint. Heroin addicts have been found to have *P. aeruginosa* and *Serratia marcescens* arthritis. Arthritis in these patients often occurs in the sternoclavicular or sacroiliac joints. *Salmonella* arthritis occurs predominantly in persons with hematologic disorders, such as sickle cell anemia, in whom hemolysis is common. *Pasteurella multocida* occurs after dog or cat bites. Anaerobic organisms such as *Fusobacterium*, *Bacteroides*, and *Clostridium* are infrequent.

Mycobacteria characteristically produce a monoarticular arthritis often involving the knees. The infections are indolent and may involve tendon sheaths. *Mycobacterium kansasii* and *M. intracellulare* tend to involve the wrists and the hands. *Sporothrix schenckii* is the most common fungus to infect joints such as the knee, wrist, and elbow. Monoarticular arthritis also occurs with *Coccidioides immitis* and other fungi such as *Blastomyces dermatitidis* (Table 28–3).

DIAGNOSIS

Examination of joint fluid is crucial to the diagnosis. The joint fluid is characteristically turbid or purulent and the leukocyte count is greater than 100,000/mm^3 in half of the patients, with more than 90% of the cells being polymorphonuclear leukocytes. The joint fluid protein is usually elevated and without its normal viscosity. The joint fluid glucose is usually low, less than 40 mg/dL.

Gram stains of joint fluid will show the organisms in most cases in which *S. aureus* is involved, but in less than 30% when other organisms are the cause. There are many problems since the Gram stain of the mucinous fluid often gives false-positive results. Similarly, it is difficult to see gram-negative bacteria. Blood cultures are useful adjuncts to diagnosis since they are positive in about half of the cases. Joint fluid cultures are positive in at least 90% of patients with infectious arthritis.

Radiographic studies will generally show distension of the joint capsule and adjacent soft tissue swelling. There may be rarefaction of subchondral bone if the illness has been present for several weeks. Subsequently, there is erosion of articular bone with narrowing of the joint space. Technetium 99m pyrophosphate scans have been used to detect early infections of the hip, shoulder, and spine, but the findings may not be specific.

The ESR is useful in the evaluation of septic arthritis. It is uniformly elevated in bacterial arthritis except in sickle cell patients. Most chil-

TABLE 28–3.

Etiologic Agents in Bacterial (Suppurative) Arthritis

Organism	Children (%) 2 year	Children (%) 2–10 yr	Adults (%)
Staphylococcus aureus	7	25	70
Haemophilus influenzae type b	40	5	<1
Streptococcus spp.*	15	15	15
Gram-negative bacilli	10	6	10
Anaerobes	0	1	<1
Neisseria	4	11	†

*Includes SS. pneumoniae, groups A and B streptococci, viridans streptococci, microaerophilic and anaerobic streptococci.
†Fifty percent of adults aged 18 to 40 years.

dren have a marked leukocytosis, whereas some adults do not have elevated white blood cell counts. Anemia, if present, is related to the underlying disease. Patients with gonococcal arthritis often have a normal or mildly elevated ESR and may not have any leukocytosis. Synovial fluid cell counts can be below 40,000/mm³. Synovial cultures are positive, but blood cultures are negative.

Although all patients who present with acute monoarticular arthritis should be considered as having a bacterial infection, other diseases, such as acute rheumatoid arthritis, gout, and chondrocalcinosis (pseudogout) will produce a similar clinical picture and show high polymorphonuclear cell counts in synovial fluid. The other diagnostic parameters of joint fluid—glucose, protein, mucin clot, viscosity—often are abnormal in noninfectious causes of arthritis. Joint fluid must be examined for crystals to determine whether the joint findings are due to gout or pseudogout.

THERAPY

Antibiotics are administered parenterally and are able to enter the joint space in concentrations adequate to kill bacteria. The agents used are based on the organisms isolated. However, β-lactam antibiotics or fluoroquinolines are the preferred drugs. Aspiration of the fluid repeatedly is needed to prevent synovial damage caused by white blood cells. Surgery is rarely necessary, except with hip infections in which the mechanical difficulties of closed needle aspiration make it wise to utilize surgical drainage initially.

This aspiration allows decompression of the joint and also removes destructive enzymes. If after 4 days there is no significant improvement in joint fluid findings, the joint can be opened.

CHAPTER 29

Histotoxic Clostridia

A 23-year-old woman was brought to the emergency room in a semiconscious state. Three days prior to admission she had attempted to terminate a 12-week pregnancy by inserting and manipulating a wire coat hanger into her uterus. On physical examination she was sweating profusely despite a normal temperature, respirations were shallow and rapid, and she was hypotensive. Pelvic examination revealed a tender uterus and a thin, brownish, foul-smelling exudate coming from the cervix. Gram stain of the exudate showed many large gram-positive rods and a few white blood cells. A urine specimen obtained by catheter was colored red, and a blood specimen likewise showed the serum to be red.* The abdominal film revealed gas in the uterus. The patient was started on pressor agents and antibiotics, a unit of blood was transfused, and she was taken to the operating room where an emergency hysterectomy was performed. The patient developed renal failure and irreversible shock and died 8 hours later. Cultures of blood and the uterine exudate obtained on admission both grew out *Clostridium perfringens*.

*The red color of the urine and serum was due to free hemoglobin.

Clostridia are anaerobic gram-positive rods. They are widely distributed in nature, and universally present in soil and the intestinal tracts of man and other animals. Anaerobic bacteria probably evolved about 2 billion years ago when the primordial atmosphere was devoid of oxygen. Even after atmospheric oxygen and aerobic life appeared, anaerobes have continued to survive in ecologic niches in which a suitably low oxidation-reduction (redox) potential* exists.

Anaerobes lack the cytochromes required for electron transport to oxygen. They are able to reduce oxygen to hydrogen peroxide and to superoxide, but they lack enzymes such as catalase, peroxidase, and superoxide dismutase that can break down these products. Consequently, oxygen is toxic to anaerobes. Clostridia vary in their sensitivity to oxygen; some species such as *C. histolyticum* are aerotolerant, while others like *C. novyi* are strictly anaerobic and fail to grow in an atmosphere that contains more than 0.05% oxygen.

A number of clostridial species produce exotoxins. Two species that produce neurotoxins, *C.*

*The oxidation-reduction potential of a system is expressed on an E_h scale somewhat analagous to the pH scale of acidity and alkalinity. The most oxidized condition is pure oxygen at +810 mV, while the most reduced condition is pure hydrogen at −420 mV. Some representative E_h values are: venous blood, +250 mV; abscesses and infection sites, −250 mV and lower; intestinal tract, −300 mV.

tetani and *C. botulinum*, have been described in Chapter 22. The remaining toxigenic species form tissue-damaging toxins and enzymes and include *C. perfringens*, *C. novyi*, *C. septicum*, *C. histolyticum*, *C. ramosum*, *C. difficile*, *C. sordellii*, and several other species. These organisms can cause a variety of infections that include bacteremia, and intraabdominal, biliary tract, female genital, pulmonary, and soft tissue infections. In addition, *C. perfringens* is a significant agent in food-borne gastroenteritis (see Chapter 31), and *C. difficile* is the etiologic agent of antibiotic-associated pseudomembranous colitis (see Chapter 33).

Transient **clostridial bacteremia**, most commonly due to *C. perfringens*, may be seen in older persons with intestinal obstruction, perforated ulcer, carcinoma of the colon, or, in some cases, unrelated to any obvious clinical condition. These episodes are generally totally benign and self-limited, and often resolve without antibiotic therapy. Paradoxically, *C. perfringens* causes a devastating **septicotoxemia** in cases of uterine myonecrosis; the septicemia is associated with profound intravascular hemolysis, hemoglobinemia, hemoglobinuria, renal shutdown, and shock, and is often fatal. Bacteremia due to *C. septicum* is a special situation. It rarely occurs in the absence of underlying gastrointestinal malignancy, leukemia, or lymphoma.

Intraabdominal infections due to clostridia are often secondary to intestinal surgery or penetrating wounds of the abdomen when intestinal contents have been released into the peritoneal cavity. Such infections are usually polymicrobial and could involve several species of clostridia together with other members of the intestinal flora. Clostridia are also present in some gallbladders and are occasionally the source of biliary tract infections.

Clostridial cellulitis follows the introduction of spores into a severe wound grossly contaminated with soil or fecal material. The spores germinate and vegetative growth occurs in the necrotic, devitalized, or poorly profused tissues.

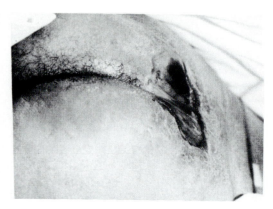

FIG 29–1.
Clostridial cellulitis.

Multiple organisms are often involved and there may be marked crepitance.* The infection spreads along fascial planes, but there is no invasion of healthy muscle or systemic symptoms (Fig 29–1).

Clostridial myonecrosis (gas gangrene) is a rapidly progressive and highly lethal infection of previously healthy muscle by one or more of the histotoxic clostridia. More than 80% of cases of gas gangrene are caused by *C. perfringens*. The infection follows contamination of traumatic or surgical wounds. Lacerated, crushed, or dead tissues have redox potentials as low as -150 to -250 mV and provide excellent growth conditions for clostridia. Lactic acid, a product of anaerobic glycolysis, accumulates and the pH falls, which also favors the growth of anaerobes.

The hallmark of gas gangrene is liquefaction of the muscle fibers caused primarily by the clostridial lecithinase which destroys cell membranes. The incubation period is 1 to 4 days, and the initial symptom is pain around the wound. The skin around the wound develops a bronze color and hemorrhagic bullae may be present (Fig 29–2). There is often a serosanguinous exudate with an unpleasant sweet odor. Gram stain of this material usually shows large, gram-positive rods

---

*Bubbles of gas in the tissues that result from the fermentation of tissue carbohydrates. The overlying skin has a crackling quality when palpated.

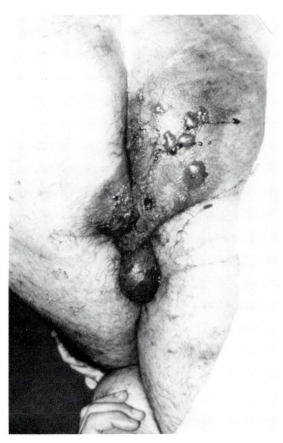

FIG 29–2.
Clostridial myonecrosis.

with few or no leukocytes. On exploration, the muscle fibers are pale and friable. Gas may be present in the tissues. Systemic symptoms include sweating, tachycardia, and extreme anxiety. The mortality is about 25%.

Clostridial myonecrosis of the uterus (postabortal septicotoxemia) is almost exclusively due to *C. perfringens.* The infection rarely involves the nongravid uterus and frequently follows amateur attempts to mechanically induce abortion by the introduction of nonsterile objects into the uterus. *Clostridium perfringens* from the vaginal flora or from an exogenous source is inoculated

at the same time that necrotic tissue is produced and the result is rapid invasion and destruction of the myometrium. The process is accompanied by bacteremia, intravascular hemolysis, hemoglobinemia, hemoglobinuria, and renal shutdown.

Most histotoxic clostridial infections are endogenous. Clostridia are poorly invasive in healthy tissue. The pathogenesis of these infections is primarily due to the toxins and enzymes produced by these bacteria. The histotoxic clostridia produce a variety of toxic materials, many of which contribute to tissue injury. These substances include several hemolysins, lecithinase, collagenase, proteinase, deoxyribonuclease, and lipase. The phospholipase (lecithinase, alpha toxin) of *C. perfringens* is probably the major factor responsible for the pathologic events in myonecrosis. In addition to its hemolytic properties, phospholipase has been shown to cause hypotension and increase vascular permeability. The toxin requires calcium ions for activation.

One of the major defense mechanisms against clostridial or any anaerobic infection is the normal redox potential of healthy tissues (E_h of +120 mV). Factors that lower (reduce) this potential predispose to anaerobic infection. Such reduction may be associated with poor perfusion secondary to cold, trauma such as a crush injury, intramuscular injection of vasoconstrictor agents, diabetes, or rapidly growing malignant tumors.

The diagnosis of histotoxic clostridial infection is primarily clinical. Gram stains of exudate show the large gram-positive rods, and few leukocytes. Recovery of clostridia requires anaerobic culture technique.

The most important aspect of therapy is surgical debridement with excision of all involved tissues, supplemented by antibiotics. Most clostridia are susceptible to penicillin, cephalosporins, clindamycin, chloramphenicol, and tetracycline.

PART VII

Gastrointestinal Infections

CHAPTER 30

Overview of Gastrointestinal Infections

Diarrheal diseases are extremely common in all parts of the world. Diarrheal disease is the largest single cause of death in the developing nations. In these countries, a child has a 50% chance of dying before the age of 7 years, primarily from a diarrheal disease. Even in the United States, diarrhea ranks among the principal causes of death in young children.

Acute diarrheal disease is caused by many different bacterial, fungal, parasitic, and viral pathogens. These organisms have distinct epidemiologic and clinical features that aid in diagnosis. Diarrhea exists in several epidemiologic forms. Epidemic diarrhea occurs during disasters, in association with contaminated food, and in outbreaks in hospital nurseries. Diarrhea often is a result of a breakdown in sanitation mechanisms which can be elucidated by careful study. Other diarrheal illness occurs without clear-cut evidence of breakdown of hygienic standards. Basically, all diarrheal disease is the result of oral contamination with material from other humans or from animals.

Table 30–1 lists the microorganisms implicated in diarrheal disease. All are seen in every society, but some are more common in developing nations because of poor sanitation.

EPIDEMIOLOGIC FACTORS

The transmission of diarrheal disease is primarily by the fecal-oral route. In most cases, this involves the ingestion of water or food contaminated with the feces of a carrier or of an active case. Occasionally, transmission of gastrointestinal infections may be via insect vectors such as flies or roaches that serve to transfer the infecting organism from feces to food. Major determinants in environmental exposure to enteric pathogens are personal hygiene, sanitary facilities, and the source of water. The type, severity, and frequency of diarrheal disease is determined by the geographical location of the person who is exposed to diarrheal pathogens and the season (Table 30–2).

PROTECTIVE ELEMENTS

Although general host factors such as age, nutritional status, and underlying diseases are important in protecting the host from gastrointestinal (GI) tract infectious disease, the GI tract itself has the most important role (Table 30–3). Organisms are ingested by way of con-

TABLE 30–1.

Etiologic Agents of Diarrheal Disease

Organism	Transmission/Vectors	Age Groups
Salmonella	Food, eggs, poultry, animals	All
Shigella	Family, custodial institutions, day care centers	Mainly children
Escherichia coli	Food, water	All
Vibrio cholerae	Water in tropics	All
Vibrio parahaemolyticus	Seafood, shellfish	All
Rotavirus	Family, institutions	Mainly children
Norwalk virus	Family, outings	All
Adenovirus	Family, institutions	All
Yersinia enterocolitica	Animal fecal material	All
Campylobacter	Food, animals, milk	All
Bacillus cereus	Food (rice, pasta)	All
Clostridium perfringens	Meats, poorly cooked	Adults
Giardia lamblia	Water/beavers	All
Entamoeba histolytica	Humans, institutions	All
Clostridium difficile	Nosocomial; follows antibiotic use	All
Cryptosporidium	Water/animals	All

TABLE 30–2.

Causative Agents of Diarrhea by Location

	United States (%)	Tropics (%)	Traveler's Diarrhea
Viruses			
Rotavirus	10–50	15–20	5–20
Norwalk	10–30	1–2	5
Bacteria			
Enterotoxigenic *Escherichia coli*	1–5	20–25	50
Campylobacter	1–20	5–15	1–5
Shigella spp.	1.0	8–10	1–20
Salmonella spp.	2–3	0–3	4–8
Aeromonas spp.	1–3	1–3	0–5
Clostridium difficile	1–5	1–3	0–1
Parasites			
Giardia	3–7	5–8	0.2
Cryptosporidium	0.5	1–5	0.5
Strongyloides	1.0	5	1.0
Entamoeba	1.0	5	1.0

TABLE 30–3.

Protective Factors in Gastrointestinal Infections

Factors That Protect	Factors That Predispose to Infection
Personal hygiene	Antacids
Gastric acidity	Large inoculum organisms
Indigenous intestinal	Decreased motility
flora	Immunoglobulin deficiency
Intestinal motility	
Local antibody	
Proteolytic enzymes	
Phagocytic cells	

taminated food or water, or, in the case of small children, by a direct fecal-oral route. Personal hygiene is the first and most important factor, as is the development of general sanitation in the community. The development of the flush toilet in England was probably the most significant reason cholera declined in that country in the 1800s.

The first body defense is the stomach. Enteric bacteria are destroyed at the **low pH** which develops in the stomach when food is ingested. Gastric surgery, which removes the potential acidification, as well as the use of antacids or H_2 histamine blockers such as cimetidine, ranitidine, or similar compounds, increases susceptibility to infection from enteric bacteria. pH alone is not critical since *Shigella* and *Salmonella* will survive in the stomach for several hours. The coating bacterial flora of the stomach, the lactobacilli and streptococcal species, play a role by competing with ingested organisms for attachment sites (Fig 30–1).

The **intestinal flora**, from the stomach to the termination of the colon, remains remarkably stable once established. Maintenance of the stability of the intestinal flora is related to the specific properties of the resident organisms which interfere with the establishment of invading microbial populations. Production of antibacterial

substances, bacteriocins, does not seem to be the mechanism by which this occurs. Rather there is competition for essential nutrients among closely related species. Toxic metabolites, such as short chain fatty acids, elaborated by the resident flora prevent establishment of new invading bacterial populations. For example, when concentrations of acetic, propionic, and butyric acids are low in the ileum, *Shigella* can attach to the mucosa and proliferate to high enough concentrations to invade. Bile acids deconjugated by anaerobes (cholic, chenodeoxycholic, and deoxycholic), are inhibitory to enteric bacteria, both aerobic and anaerobic, and probably play a role in maintenance of the normal bowel flora.

Bowel motility is an extremely important factor in protection since it moves bacteria along the intestine and prevents organisms from attaching to the epithelial barrier, proliferating, and penetrating cells or, when attached, from releasing toxin locally to alter the transport mechanism or to lyse intestinal cells.

There is an "unstirred water layer" over intestinal cells which retards the diffusion of solutes and the movement of infectious agents toward the mucosal epithelium. Intestinal mucus and the glycocalyx layer anchored to the plasmalemma of the epithelial cells interfere with attachment of pathogenic species.

Local immunity in the form of **secretory IgA** and other antibody is important in protection against viral, bacterial, and parasitic diseases. Attenuated viruses or bacteria can elicit a local antibody which prevents attachment of the organisms to the epithelial surface or aids in their destruction in the surface mucus. Furthermore, antibodies may protect against the absorption of intact organisms. Experimental studies with cholera have shown that intestinal antibody protects, whereas serum antibody is of little value. This is also true for *Shigella* and *Salmonella* organisms. How often antibody is formed to the toxins elaborated by organisms is not known.

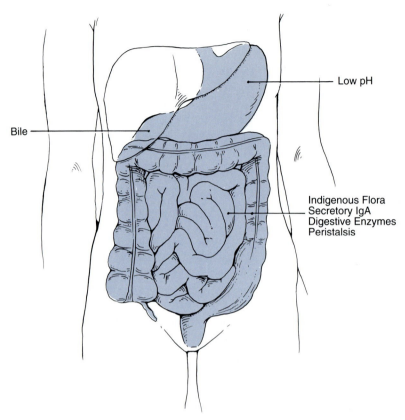

FIG 30–1.
Defenses of the gastrointestinal tract.

The digestive proteases in the intestinal lumen may also be protective. The enteritis necroticans (pig bel) of New Guinea occurs in natives who eat sweet potatoes with the result that they have a low level of intestinal proteases. If they ingest meat contaminated with *Clostridium perfringens* type C, they develop severe necrosis of the intestine, as this organism produces a toxin normally destroyed by intestinal proteases.

PATHOGENESIS OF BACTERIAL DIARRHEA

Enteric bacteria must attach to intestinal cells to cause diarrhea. There is active participa-

tion of both the bacterium and the epithelial cell. The bacterial factors involved in adherence are: intact and complete lipopolysaccharide, specific O-sugar repeat units, and a viable, metabolically active organism. The host cell factors involved in attachment of bacteria are: viable, metabolically active intestinal cells, intact glycolysis and microfilaments in the intestinal cell, and cyclic nucleotides in the intestinal cell.

Enterotoxicogenic *Escherichia coli* can be shown to adhere to intact intestinal microvilli. The organisms that cause diarrhea possess fimbrial adherence ligands. The fimbria (pili) are a filamentous surface protein. There are two major types of pili. The first is the common or type 1 pilus which is associated with mannose-sensitive nonspecific adherence to various body cells. The second group includes pili thought to mediate adherence to specific cells in specific species, the so-called colonization factor antigens.

Some *E. coli* adhere closely to epithelial cells lacking microvilli. These have been termed **enteroeffacing** or enteroeffacin. Human strains of enteropathogenic *E. coli* have been found to adhere to cells in culture with greater frequency than nonenteropathogenic *E. coli* strains.

BACTERIAL TOXINS THAT CAUSE DIARRHEA

Toxins have been shown to be involved in the capability of many organisms to produce diarrheal disease. The toxins can be classified as neurotoxins, enterotoxins, or cytotoxins (Table 30–4). Neurotoxins usually are ingested as preformed toxins and produce their GI effect via action on the central nervous system, not on the intestine directly. Enterotoxins affect the intestinal mucosa to cause loss of fluid. Cholera toxin is the classic example of an enterotoxin.

Some enteric pathogens produce cytotoxic products which cause local mucosal destruction that results in an inflammatory colitis. *Shigella dysenteriae*, *C. perfringens*, and *Vibrio parahaemolyticus* do this, but the best-studied example has been *Clostridium difficle*.

TYPES OF ENTERIC INFECTION

Basically, there are three ways that organisms can destroy the normal GI physiology. They can (1) cause a shift in the bidirectional flow of water and electrolytes in the small bowel as a result of enterotoxin action; (2) they can inflame the intestinal mucosa, ileal and colonic; and (3) they can penetrate through an intact mucosa to reach the reticuloendothelial system. Table 30–5 lists these types.

TABLE 30–4.
Bacterial Toxins Involved in Diarrheal Disease*

Neurotoxins
  Clostridium botulinum
  Bacillus cereus
  Staphylococcus aureus
Enterotoxins
  Vibrio cholerae (cAMP)
  Escherichia coli LT (heat-labile) (cAMP)
  E. coli ST (heat-stable) (cGMP)
  Salmonella enteritidis
  Citrobacter
  Aeromonas hydrophila
  Klebsiella
  Clostridium perfringens
  Shigella dysenteriae
  B. cereus
Cytotoxins
  Shigella spp.
  C. perfringens
  S. aureus
  Vibrio parahaemolyticus
  Clostridium difficile

*cAMP = cyclic adenosine monophosphate; cGMP = cyclic guanosine monophosphate.

SECRETORY DIARRHEA

Cholera is the prime example of a disease of the small intestine in which the enterotoxin elaborated by the organisms causes the small intestine to secrete salt and water via activation of the mucosal adenylate cyclase–cyclic adenosine monophosphate (AMP) system. Colonic water and electrolyte transport is unaffected, but diarrhea results since the volume of fluid elaborated by the small intestine overwhelms the absorptive capacity of the colon.

The mechanism of diarrhea due to enterotoxin-producing *E. coli* is similar although not exactly the same. In some cases *Salmonella* species, other than *S. typhi*, e.g., *S. typhimurium*, *S. enteritidis*, etc., also produce an enterotoxin which seems to inhibit Na^+ absorption and stimulate Cl^- secretion.

TABLE 30–5.

Three Types of Enteric Infection

	Mechanism	Site	Type
Luminal	Enterotoxin action; reduction of absorptive surface	Small bowel	Noninflammatory secretory diarrhea
Mucosal	Mucosal invasion	Colon	Inflammatory dysentery
Systemic	Intracellular survival	Illeum	Penetrating enteric fever

The properties of a virus that cause it to produce gastroenteritis are not known. Viral particles can be found in the absorptive epithelial cells of the upper small bowel during rotavirus and coronavirus infection. Morphologic studies in children infected with rotavirus have demonstrated mucosal changes with shortening and blunting of villi and increased infiltration of the lamina propria with mononuclear cells. Epithelial cells have altered shapes, and viral particles fill the endoplasmic reticulum of vacuolated cells. Studies of adult volunteers infected with the Norwalk agent also show damage of villous absorptive cells and polymorphonuclear and mononuclear leukocytes. Such changes have been associated with impaired absorptive function. Following infection with rotavirus, for example, there is a period of lactose intolerance due to alteration of mucosal surface lactase activity.

INVASIVE DIARRHEA (DYSENTERY)

Shigella and some *E. coli* organisms produce diarrhea only by local invasion after they have multiplied to a significant concentration within the colon. Diarrhea is the result of jejunal secretion superimposed on a defect in colonic absorption. The pathogenesis of the defect of jejunal transport is unknown, but it is possible that prostaglandins are released by the colonic lesions and that the prostaglandins affect the jejunum. The bacteria produce a cytotoxin, but it is the ability of the organism to invade as well as

produce toxin which is crucial. If mutants of *Shigella* are produced which produce toxin but cannot invade the mucosa, they will not cause diarrhea.

SYSTEMIC ILLNESS

The third type of enteric infection is best exemplified by *Salmonella typhi*. The organism penetrates intact intestinal mucosa in the distal small bowel and multiplies in the lymphatic and reticuloendothelial cells. Diarrhea may or may not be present, but when it is, there are usually fecal mononuclear cells. There is bacteremia during which bacteria lodge in other organs such as the gallbladder and lymph nodes and can persist for a long time. *Yersinia* and some *Campylobacter* organisms also produce this form of illness.

The number of organisms needed to produce infection varies, (Table 30–6). Thus only a few *Shigella* will infect, whereas it takes 100 million *Vibrio cholerae* organisms. This explains how easy it is for children to develop *Shigella* and why Western adults rarely develop cholera when visiting or working in countries in which cholera is endemic.

TRAVELER'S DIARRHEA

Diarrheal illness has plagued travelers for centuries. Various euphemisms such as GI trots, Casablanca crud, Aden gut, Turkey trot, Hong

TABLE 30-6.

Infective Doses of Enteric Pathogens

Organism	Infective Dose
Shigella	10^2
Campylobacter	10^5
Salmonella	10^5
Escherichia coli	10^8
Vibrio cholerae	10^8
Giardia	10-100 cysts
Entamoeba histolytica	10-100 cysts

TABLE 30-7.

Microorganisms Implicated in Traveler's Diarrhea

Microorganism	Incidence (%)
Escherichia coli, toxigenic	40-70
E. coli, invasive	0-4
Salmonella spp.	0-15
Shigella spp.	0-20
Vibrio parahaemolyticus	0-2
Giardia lamblia	0-2
Entamoeba histolytica	0-2
Rotavirus	0-4
Undiagnosed	10-35

Kong dog, Delhi belly, Aztec two-step, Montezuma's revenge, and turista are used to name the disease.

Typically, the traveler is well for the first 2 to 3 days, with the onset of illness beginning 4 to 6 days after arrival. The disease begins abruptly with abdominal cramps followed by watery diarrhea, numbering most often between three and eight stools per day, rarely more than 15 per day. By the second or third day, diarrhea usually has lessened and normal activity gradually resumes. The duration of illness is variable, but ranges between 2 and 5 days.

The leading pathogen in traveler's diarrhea has been enterotoxigenic *E. coli.* As noted in Table 30-7, many cases lack an etiologic diagnosis. In some cases, more than one potential pathogen is isolated from the diarrheal stool and it is difficult to assign a casual role to a specific organism. Special epidemiologic circumstances may produce a different range of pathogens. On cruise ships there have been outbreaks of *Shigella, Salmonella,* and *V. parahaemolyticus.* Travelers to the Soviet Union have experienced a high infection rate with *Giardia* and *Cryptosporidium.*

CHAPTER 31

Agents of Food-Borne Gastroenteritis

Fifteen student nurses living in a hospital residence hall experienced sudden onset of crampy abdominal pain and diarrhea between midnight and 8 A.M. Many of these students also complained of nausea and vomiting; most had headache, and all had low-grade fever. Stool samples or rectal swabs were obtained from each student for culture. All of the students reported eating scrambled eggs in the hospital cafeteria the previous morning, and all denied taking meals elsewhere. The symptoms continued for several days, but all recovered. *Salmonella derby*, a subspecies of *Salmonella enteritidis*, was recovered from 14 of the stool cultures. Samples of the scrambled eggs were not available for culture, but a rectal swab obtained from a food handler who served the eggs also grew out S. *derby*. One day after the initial attack six more student nurses became ill with the same symptoms. These students were unable to identify a shared food, but S. *derby* was recovered from their stools.

Food-borne gastroenteritis or bacterial food poisoning accounts for considerable morbidity throughout the world. In the United States in the 2-year period 1980–1981, more than 1,100 food poisoning outbreaks involving more than 28,000 people were reported to the Centers for Disease Control. The actual incidence was probably 10 to 100 times greater. The etiology was confirmed in about one third of the cases; of these 30% were caused by salmonella, 25% were due to *Staphylococcus aureus*, and about 15% were caused by *Clostridium perfringens*. *Clostridium botulinum* accounted for about 8% and less than 2% were caused by *Bacillus cereus*.

While many microbial agents can be acquired from food, this discussion is limited to those infections characterized by the acute onset of nausea, vomiting, cramps, and diarrhea occurring singly or severally within 72 hours of ingestion. Often the infection appears in two or more persons who have shared a meal.

SALMONELLA

The major clinical patterns of salmonella infection are acute gastroenteritis, bacteremia with or without localized infection, typhoid (enteric) fever, and the asymptomatic carrier state.

Gastroenteritis is characterized by the abrupt onset of nausea, vomiting, and diarrhea, occurring 8 to 48 hours after the ingestion of contaminated food. Low-grade fever for the first day or so is usual, accompanied by headache, and gripping abdominal pain. Bacteremia occurs in less than 4% of patients. The symptoms usually subside in 2 to 5 days. Salmonella bacteremia may occur in patients with hematologic diseases such as lymphoma, leukemia, sickle cell anemia, or AIDS. Localized abscesses can occur, such as pleural empyema, osteomyelitis, and infections of aortic aneurysms, vascular grafts, and prostheses. Typhoid fever is a multisystem disease and is discussed in Chapter 48.

The asymptomatic carrier state can occur following gastroenteritis and persist for several weeks. About 3% of typhoid patients become chronic carriers. Many of these patients have chronically infected gallbladders, complicated by cholelithiasis. Cure of the carrier state may require surgical removal of the gallbladder.

Salmonella are gram-negative, motile bacilli. They are classified in the large family of Enterobacteriaceae. Three groups are recognized: group I, *S. enteritidis*, containing more than 2,200 serotypes or subspecies that have a broad host range, and are involved in acute gastroenteritis; group II, *S. choleraesuis*, a single serotype adapted to swine, and causing abscesses in adults and gastroenteritis in children; and group III, *S. typhi*, a single serotype highly adapted to man, and the agent of typhoid fever. Serotyping is based upon the H (flagellar), and O (somatic) antigens. The O antigens consist of species-specific oligosaccharide chains attached to the cell wall lipopolysaccharide. Most strains of salmonella have multiple H and O antigens.

Group I serotypes are widely distributed in cattle, poultry, reptiles, and insects. Human infections are acquired by ingestion of contaminated poultry, eggs, meat, powdered food supplements, and shellfish or water contaminated by sewage. Infections have also occurred by direct contact with pet turtles and other reptiles. Hospital outbreaks have been traced to carmine red dye, derived from insects and used to color food, drugs, and cosmetics. Transmission may

also occur by food handlers who are asymptomatic carriers. *Salmonella choleraesuis* infections are acquired from pork products. The sources of *S. typhi* are limited to active cases or asymptomatic carriers; transmission occurs via the fecal-oral route. Flies with access to excreta containing salmonella may also serve as a vector of infection. Epidemics of typhoid fever may follow fecal contamination of the drinking water supply.

Ingestion of approximately 100,000 organisms are required to produce infection in healthy adults, but lower inocula may suffice in young children, the elderly, or debilitated persons. Salmonella are susceptible to a low pH and the presence of gastric acid is a major determinant in the development of disease. Factors reducing gastric acid secretion such as achlorhydria, antacid use, and the buffering action of some foods predispose to infection. Salmonella attached to epithelial cells by means of type I pili enter the cells by endocytosis and appear within membrane-bound vacuoles within the epithelial cell. Salmonella are invasive organisms which are able to penetrate the epithelial cells without destruction and reach the lamina propria, where an inflammatory response is elicited. The nature of this response appears to be important in determining the pathogenesis of disease and resultant symptomatology. Nontyphoid salmonella elicit a predominantly polymorphonuclear leukocytic reaction, leading to phagocytosis of the organism and containment of the infection in the lamina propria, resulting in gastroenteritis. The mechanisms of fluid secretion and diarrhea is not established but probably is related to prostaglandin stimulation. In contrast, *S. typhi* leads to a predominantly mononuclear response; the organisms enter the circulation and produce the bacteremia and systemic symptoms characteristic of typhoid fever.

Patients recovering from salmonella infection may develop humoral antibodies to the H and O antigens of the infecting strain but these antibodies are neither diagnostic nor protective.

The diagnosis of salmonella gastroenteritis depends upon the demonstration of the organism in the patient's stool by culture, antigen detection, or nucleic acid probe.

Antimicrobial therapy is not indicated in uncomplicated salmonella gastroenteritis. Most antibiotics prolong the carrier state and may predispose to bacteria, but fluoroquinolones can shorten the illness and often reduce fecal carriage.

STAPHYLOCOCCUS AUREUS

Staphylococcal food poisoning is actually an intoxication rather than an infection since it results from the ingestion of preformed toxin in food. Nevertheless, staphylococcal food poisoning is the second most commonly reported cause of gastroenteritis. The incubation period is very short: 1 to 6 hours. The onset is sudden with profuse vomiting, nausea, and abdominal cramps, often followed by diarrhea. Recovery is usually complete in 24 to 48 hours.

Most outbreaks occur in warm weather and are often associated with large social gatherings at which the offending food is served. Foods with a high starch, sugar, or salt content, such as cream or custard-filled pastries; ham; shrimp; and potato or macaroni salad, favor the growth of staphylococci. *Staphylococcus aureus* is described in Chapter 24.

The source of the organisms is invariably a food handler carrying an enterotoxin-producing strain of *S. aureus* in the nose or skin or with an insignificant infection, e.g., a paronychia (nail bed infection). The organisms are usually introduced directly into the food which typically does not undergo a terminal heat process, and is held for a number of hours at a warm temperature before it is served.

At least five immunologically distinct enterotoxins (a–e) have been identified. These are heat-stable proteins whose mechanism of action in humans has not been clearly defined. Animal studies suggest that the enterotoxin acts on the abdominal viscera which in turn stimulate the vomiting center in the brain via the vagus and sympathetic nerves.

The diagnosis is usually made on clinical grounds based upon the short incubation period and a history of ingesting a suspected food product. Specific identification can be made by demonstration of large numbers of *S. aureus* in the vomitus or suspected food.

CLOSTRIDIUM PERFRINGENS

In contrast to staphylococcal and salmonella gastroenteritis, *C. perfringens* food poisoning most frequently occurs in the fall and winter months. The incubation period is 8 to 24 hours and is followed by the onset of repeated bouts of abdominal cramps and watery diarrhea which persist for 24 hours. *Clostridium perfringens* is a gram-positive, spore-forming, anaerobic bacillus and is described in Chapter 29.

The foods involved are usually meat stews, poultry dishes, (most commonly turkey), or gravies that are precooked in large amounts, cooled, and subsequently reheated for serving. The food is contaminated with spores of *C. perfringens* from the animal's intestinal tract or from soil. Because of the bulk of the food, the internal temperature reached during cooking is inadequate to kill the spores, but serves to reduce the redox potential to a level that permits the surviving spores to germinate during the prolonged cooling stage, releasing the enterotoxin. The enterotoxin is a heat-stable protein component of the spore coat formed during sporulation. It exerts its maximal activity in the ileum where it inhibits glucose transport, damages the intestinal epithelium, and causes a loss of protein into the intestinal lumen.

The specific diagnosis is made by demonstrating large numbers of *C. perfringens* in the incriminated food.

BACILLUS CEREUS

Two types of illness, both mild and self-limited, are caused by this organism: an emetic form with a short incubation of 1 to 5 hours and characterized by vomiting and abdominal cramps and occasional diarrhea persisting for 8 to 10 hours; and a diarrheal form with an incubation period of 10 to 12 hours followed by watery diarrhea, abdominal cramps, and moderate nausea lasting about 12 hours. The two forms are explained by differences in the type of enterotoxin: the emetic form is caused by a heat-stable toxin, and the diarrheal type is caused by a heat-labile toxin.

Bacillus cereus is a large gram-positive, spore-forming aerobic bacillus. Relatively large numbers of organisms (more than 100,000/g) are needed to cause illness.

Foods are usually contaminated prior to cooking. The emetic form has been associated with fried rice prepared in Chinese restaurants from boiled rice inadequately cooled and rinsed, or from macaroni and cheese. Foods associated with the diarrheal form of illness include boiled beef, sausage, chicken soup, vanilla sauce, puddings, and mashed potatoes.

The heat-labile toxin associated with the diarrheal form stimulates cyclic adenosine monophosphate (AMP) in intestinal epithelial cells, resulting in increased secretion of water and electrolytes. The mode of action of the heat-stable emetic toxin has not yet been elucidated.

The diagnosis of *B. cereus* food poisoning is made by demonstrating large numbers of the organisms in the incriminated food.

Botulism caused by ingestion of *Clostridium botulinum* toxin is described in Chapter 22.

CHAPTER 32

Bacteria Causing Acute Secretory Diarrhea

A 42-year-old physician presented with profuse watery diarrhea, cramps, nausea, and malaise for the past 4 days. He had recently returned from a 2-week trip to Mexico. Symptoms developed 10 days after his arrival in Mexico. He stated that he did not drink tap water or iced beverages, but admitted to eating salads containing raw vegetables. Culture of his stool grew out *Escherichia coli*, which was later shown to be an enterotoxigenic strain.

Secretory diarrhea is the result of increased movement of water and electrolytes into the gut lumen as a result of biochemical alteration of small bowel mucosal cells. The increased secreted fluid of the small bowel exceeds the absorptive capacity of the colon. There are no inflammatory changes in the intestinal mucosa. In serious adult cases, intestinal fluid loss can exceed 1 L/hr, leading to marked dehydration. The majority of secretory diarrheas are caused by bacterial enterotoxins. Organisms producing enterotoxins include *Vibrio cholerae*, enterotoxigenic *E. coli* (ETEC), *Aeromonas hydrophila*, and certain noncholera vibrios.

VIBRIO CHOLERAE

Cholera is the prototype of noninvasive diarrheal disease. The etiologic agent is *V. cholerae*, a highly motile, slightly curved gram-negative rod that grows aerobically, preferably at an alkaline pH. The organism has flagellar H antigens and somatic O antigens. Three serotypes (Ogawa, Inaba, and Hikojima) based upon the O antigens, and a biotype *(El Tor)* are recognized.

The onset of cholera is abrupt, with nausea, vomiting, and profound diarrhea after an incubation period that averages 2 to 3 days. The stools are turbid and watery (rice-water), and can result in a fluid loss of 15 to 20 L/day with a concomitant escape of electrolytes (Na^+, K^+, HCO_3^-, and Cl^-). The diarrhea may cause a 10% loss of body weight within the first 12 hours of illness, and if untreated leads to dehydration, hemoconcentration, and hypovolemic shock. Electrolyte loss results in metabolic acidosis. The untreated case fatality rate can exceed 60% and is significantly higher in children. During epidemics, many *V. cholerae* infections are asymptomatic and are detected only by stool culture.

Cholera typically occurs in epidemics in Asia

and the Middle East; isolated cases occur in the United States. Cholera has recently caused a major outbreak in Peru and has spread up the west coast of South America. Water contaminated by sewage is the most frequent medium of transfer of the organism. The disease follows the ingestion of large numbers of *V. cholerae*. Even in epidemics, attack rates seldom exceed 15% because of the high numbers of organisms (1–10 million) required to initiate infection. Vibrios are extremely sensitive to acid, and the acid barrier of the normal stomach is an important defense mechanism. Persons with hypochlorhydria associated with antacid use or gastrectomy are especially susceptible to infection.

In the proximal small intestine, the organisms multiply and produce a potent enterotoxin. All pathogenic strains produce a single toxin, the production of which is chromosomally mediated. The factors permitting *V. cholerae* to penetrate the mucous layer, adhere to mucosal cells, and colonize the mucosal surface have not yet been identified, although certain enzymes produced by the organism have been implicated. These include mucinase, neuraminidase, and a hemagglutinin. It has been shown that the binding of *V. cholerae* to the intestine is calcium-dependent and inhibited by L-fucose. It is also possible that *V. cholerae* and other enterotoxigenic pathogens colonize the epithelial cell glycocalyx* rather than the plasma membrane itself.

The enterotoxin (choleragen) is a small protein composed of two major subunits, A and B. The A subunit containing the toxic activity is in turn composed of two fragments, A1 and A2, joined by a disulfide bond. The B subunit is responsible for the binding of the toxin to the cell membrane. The toxin is a globular molecule consisting of a ring of five B subunits surrounding an A subunit. The toxin is irreversibly bound via the B subunits to the GM_1 monosia-

---

*The glycocalyx is a filamentous carbohydrate-containing coat underlying the mucous layer and covering the epithelial surface.

loganglioside in the intestinal cell wall. After the toxin is bound, conformational changes occur in the toxin which, together with hydrophobic interactions within the cell membrane, permit the A subunit to penetrate the membrane. The disulfide bond linking the A1 and A2 fragments is reduced, releasing the A1 peptide. The A1 fragment activates the adenylate cyclase located on the inner surface of the cell membrane by an enzymatic reaction involving NAD, adenosine diphosphate (ADP)–ribose, adenosine triphosphate, (ATP), guanosine triphosphate (GTP), etc. This activation of adenylate cyclase blocks the influx of sodium and chloride across the brush border, while stimulating the outward secretion into the lumen of chloride and water.

The treatment of cholera is primarily replacement of water and electrolytes. Tetracycline diminishes the number of organisms in the gut reducing the fluid loss and eliminating the carrier state.

ENTEROTOXIGENIC *ESCHERICHIA COLI* (ETEC)

Diarrheal disease produced by enterotoxigenic *E. coli* (ETEC) causes considerably greater worldwide morbidity and mortality than cholera. The disease affects all age groups and is one of the major causes of diarrhea throughout the world. The incidence is greatest in the developing countries; 70% to 80% of cases of traveler's diarrhea in Americans traveling to South America, Africa, or the Middle East is due to ETEC. This organism is also responsible for many cases of "nonspecific" diarrhea in children.

Enterotoxigenic *E. coli* infection is more often associated with the consumption of raw vegetables in salads than with contaminated drinking water. The disease is a secretory diarrhea that is a milder version of cholera. The disease is less life-threatening in adults than cholera but it is life-threatening in young children because of fluid loss. In addition to the watery diarrhea, abdominal cramps are common, sometimes accompanied by nausea and anorexia. Symptoms last 5 to 10 days.

The ETEC strain is capable of producing two separate enterotoxins: a heat-labile toxin (LT) which is similar to cholera toxin, and a heat-stable toxin (ST). Both toxins are important in human disease, and strains of *E. coli* may produce one or the other or both. Strains that produce only the ST toxin are less common. The production of both toxins is under the control of transmissible plasmids.

The **LT toxin** has a molecular weight of 91,000 daltons and resembles cholera toxin immunologically and in its mode of action. Like cholera toxin, LT is inhibited by GM_1 gangliosides and has binding and activity subunits, the molecular structure of which remains to be determined. The intestinal receptor sites for LT toxin are the oligosaccharide side chain moieties of membrane glycoproteins and glycolipids. The specific activity of LT is 10 to 100 times less than cholera toxin in terms of adenylate cyclase activation and rate of fluid loss. This, together with the fact that *E. coli* strains produce much less enterotoxin in vitro than *V. cholerae* strains, may explain the milder nature of ETEC disease in humans. The LT toxin is antigenic and an LT serum antibody response is a regular feature of ETEC disease. LT is neutralized by cholera antitoxin, but LT antitoxin has only a weak effect against cholera toxin.

The **ST toxin** has a molecular weight of less than 6,000 daltons and is only weakly antigenic. The ST toxin does not cross-react with LT or cholera toxin, nor does it bind to ganglioside. The ST toxin has a rapid onset of action and probably produces hypersecretion by stimulating guanylate cyclase, leading to increased levels of cyclic guanosine monophosphate (cGMP). There are several *E. coli* ST toxins which differ in structure and in host specificity. Other enteric organisms (*Klebsiella, Enterobacter, Yersinia enterocolitica*) also elaborate ST toxins.

In order for enteric pathogens to produce disease, they must adhere to and colonize the intestinal mucosa. Thus, the ETEC strain must adhere to and colonize in the upper small intestine, as well as elaborate the enterotoxin if diarrhea is to be produced. For human strains, this adherence capacity is associated with a host species-specific **colonization factor antigen** (CFA) consisting of pili (threadlike proteins that serve to bind the organisms to the intestinal mucosa). These pili are distinctly different from the common pili present on non-ETEC species. The production of CFA is genetically encoded by the same plasmid that mediates LT or ST toxin production. At least three major CFAs have been identified in ETEC strains: CFA/I, CFA/II, and CFA/IV. CFA/I are complexes of fimbriae and *E. coli* surface-associated antigens. Volunteers challenged with ETEC strains lacking CFA did not develop diarrhea and shed the organism in 2 to 3 days. Other volunteers ingesting the ETEC strain with CFA developed diarrhea, carried the organism for 7 days, and produced antibody to LT toxin.

Protection against *E. coli* ETEC infection involves not only antitoxic immunity but immunity to colonization factor antigen as well.

AEROMONAS HYDROPHILA

Aeromonas hydrophila has been implicated as a cause of diarrheal disease, as well as of extraintestinal infections. Many extraintestinal infections involve wound, skin, bone, or muscle involvement, aspiration pneumonia, or septicemia following contact with a water source. About two thirds of the infections other than diarrhea occur in patients with malignancies, diabetes, or in persons with impaired hepatobiliary function. The role of *A. hydrophila* as a major cause of diarrheal disease is somewhat in question since the organism can be recovered from healthy persons as well as those with diarrhea.

Intestinal infections with *A. hydrophila* are

more prevalent in pediatric populations, and are characterized by watery diarrhea, mild fever, and occasional vomiting. About 20% of patients have stools containing blood and mucus. Diarrhea persists from a few days to 2 weeks.

Aeromonas are gram-negative, facultatively anaerobic bacilli, classified together with the vibrios in the *Vibrionaceae* family. The *A. hydrophila* complex contains three species, *A. hydrophila*, *A. caviae*, and *A. sobria* (the species most associated with diarrhea), but they are usually referred to collectively as *A. hydrophila*. *A. hydrophila* is widely distributed in the aquatic environment. Outbreaks of diarrheal disease occur most frequently during the warmer summer months.

Aeromonas hydrophila produces a variety of toxins and extracellular enzymes, some of which may act as virulence factors. Toxins include an extracellular heat-labile enterotoxin whose biologic activity resembles that of cholera toxin or *E. coli* heat-labile toxin (LT), but which is not neutralized by antibodies to those toxins. In contrast to cholera toxin, *A. hydrophilia* enterotoxin, is not decreased by prostaglandin inhibitors nor does it have the GM_1 tissue receptor. Other substances include a heat-labile cytotoxic beta hemolysin, an alpha hemolysin, proteases, elastase, peptidases, and a soluble hemagglutinin which may serve as the attachment mechanism to epithelial cells of the intestinal tract.

NONCHOLERA VIBRIOS

The noncholera vibrios include non-O1 *V. cholerae*, *V. mimicus*, *V. parahaemolyticus*, *V. hollisae*, *V. fluvialis*, and *V. furnissii*, which are involved in the production of diarrheal disease. Three additional species, *V. vulnificus*, *V. alginolyticus*, and *V. damsela*, are primarily agents of soft tissue infections and septicemia. With the exception of non-O1 *V. cholerae* and *V. mimicus*, all of the other species are halophilic, requiring sodium chloride and normally occurring in sea water and marine organisms. Non-O1 *V.*

cholerae are organisms that fail to agglutinate with cholera O1 antiserum. Some strains produce a cholera-like enterotoxin that can cause a mild to severe watery diarrhea. Nontoxigenic strains have been recovered from ear, wound, and respiratory and urinary tract infections and septicemia.

Vibrio mimicus has been associated with diarrheal disease in persons who have eaten raw shellfish, especially oysters. The diarrhea is watery and persists for about a week. Approximately 15% of this species produce an enterotoxin identical to cholera toxin. *Vibrio mimicus* has been recovered from ear infections in patients exposed to sea water. *Vibrio parahaemolyticus* produces a dysentery syndrome and is discussed in Chapter 33. *Vibrio hollisae* is strongly suspected of being an agent of diarrheal disease accompanied by fever and vomiting. The organism has also been isolated from the blood of a patient with serious liver disease. *Vibrio fluvialis* causes a cholera-like gastroenteritis characterized by watery diarrhea, vomiting, and abdominal pain and fever. Culture supernatants of this organism have enterotoxin activity. *Vibrio furnissii* can produce diarrhea, abdominal cramps, nausea, and vomiting. The disease has been associated with seafood. *Vibrio vulnificus* produces two clinical syndromes that differ from those caused by other *Vibrio* species. In persons with hepatic cirrhosis, the organism rapidly crosses the gut mucosa and invades the bloodstream, resulting in septicemia and the development of skin lesions that rapidly become hemorrhagic bullae and necrotic ulcers. The mortality is over 50%. In normal hosts, *V. vulnificus* can cause severe cellulitis, ulcers, and bacteremia following immersion of a superficial wound in warm sea water. *Vibrio alginolyticus* has been associated with cellulitis, otitis media, and otitis externa in fishermen and swimmers. *Vibrio damsela* has been recovered from leg or foot wounds.

The diagnosis of secretory diarrhea depends upon the recovery of the organism by cultures from the patient's stool.

CHAPTER 33

Bacteria Causing Acute Dysentery

A 4-year-old girl was brought to the clinic with fever, abdominal pain, and diarrhea. Two days previously, the child vomited, and then developed a fever of 40°C accompanied by a brief convulsion. Over the next 2 days, the child had frequent bowel movements, increasing to about 15 per day; the later stools contained mucus and were streaked with blood. On physical examination the child had a temperature of 38.8°C and showed evidence of abdominal tenderness and cramping. A smear of the stool stained with methylene blue revealed many polymorphonuclear leukocytes and a stool culture grew out *Shigella flexneri*.

The dysentery syndrome is characterized by the frequent passage of numerous small-volume bloody mucoid stools usually accompanied by fever, fecal urgency, and tenesmus (painful, long-continued and ineffectual straining at stool). Dysentery may be due to infection by some intestinal parasites such as *Entamoeba histolytica*, or more commonly by a group of bacteria that includes shigella, enteroinvasive *Escherichia coli* (EIEC), *Campylobacter jejuni*, *Vibrio parahaemolyticus*, *Plesiomonas shigelloides*, and verocytotoxin-producing *E. coli*.

SHIGELLA

Shigella are nonmotile gram-negative bacilli that primarily infect man. They are members of the family Enterobacteriaceae. There are four species or groups: *Shigella dysenteriae* (group A), *S. flexneri* (group B), *S. boydii* (group C), and *S. sonnei* (group D). There are more than 30 serotypes of groups A, B, and C; group D is a single serotype. *Shigella sonnei* infections are the most common in the United States and other industrialized countries, while *S. flexneri* is more frequent in developing nations. *Shigella boydii* is uncommon, and *S. dysenteriae* is rare in the United States.

Disease caused by *S. sonnei* tends to be milder than infections caused by *S. flexneri* serotypes. The most severe disease is produced by *S. dysenteriae* type 1. This species has been associated with several pandemics of dysentery in Asia and Central America that had a 10% to 20% mortality.

Shigella are worldwide in distribution and cause 10% to 20% of the cases of acute diarrhea, especially in children. There are 15,000 to 20,000 cases of shigellosis every year in the United States, almost 70% of which are in children under the age of 2 years. The highest incidence is between ages 1 and 4 years. In temperate climates, most cases occur during the summer months. The majority of cases are spread from person to person by the fecal-oral route. Transmission may also take place via contaminated food or water or by insect vectors such as flies. The opportunities for transmission are increased by crowding, poverty, and poor personal hygiene resulting from the nonavailability of water for washing. Shigellosis may become endemic in situations where people are crowded together, as in day care centers, nursery schools, kindergartens, institutions for retarded children, Indian reservations, and cruise ships. Shigellosis is an important cause of diarrhea in male homosexuals. The sole reservoir of shigella is man. The convalescent carrier state is short, seldom exceeding a month or so.

Shigella are the most virulent of the enteric pathogens; as few as 100 bacilli can cause disease. Three phenotypic properties of shigella are required for virulence: (1) the ability to survive gastric transit and proliferate in the intestinal lumen, (2) the capacity to invade intestinal epithelial cells, and (3) the ability to proliferate within epithelial cells after invasion. These determinants are present in both the chromosome and plasmids, and each appears to be necessary for full virulence.

Within 12 hours after ingestion, shigella multiply in the distal small intestine, reaching levels of 10^9/mL. By 24 to 96 hours, the large intestine is invaded. The organisms attach to the surface epithelial cell, enter the cells by endocytosis, and proliferate in the cytoplasm, causing cellular destruction. Multiplication continues in the lamina propria, but rarely progresses beyond the submucosa. Goblet cells disappear and epithelial cells are extruded at the luminal surface, leading to the formation of micro-ulcers. Inflammatory cells accumulate and crypt abscesses develop. The pathologic picture is one of acute inflammation and shallow ulcers on the mucosal surface.

Shigella produce a potent cytotoxin (Shiga toxin) that inactivates the 60S ribosomal subunit within the cell, inhibiting ribosomal protein synthesis, causing cell death, and presumably resulting in the dysentery syndrome. Shiga toxin also has enterotoxin activity affecting the proximal small bowel and causing watery diarrhea. Shiga toxin is also produced by other bacteria that cause diarrhea, including enteropathogenic *E. coli,* and some strains of *Vibrio cholerae.*

The incubation period for shigellosis is usually 1 to 3 days. Early in the infection there is a small-bowel phase, probably mediated by the toxin, which is characterized by voluminous watery stools, abdominal cramps, fever, and occasionally vomiting. In 25% to 50% of cases, the dysentery syndrome appears, with small liquid stools containing blood, mucus, or pus, accompanied by abdominal pain, tenesmus, and mucosal ulceration. Extraintestinal infections are rare. In most cases, the disease is self-limited and terminates in a few days. In young children, the elderly, and severely malnourished persons, severe infection may occur with dehydration, acid-base disturbances, and shock.

An uncommon but serious complication of bloody diarrhea is the **hemolytic uremic syndrome** (HUS). HUS is a triad of hemolytic anemia, acute renal failure, and thrombocytopenia. This syndrome occurs primarily in infants and young children, but cases of HUS have also been reported in the elderly. Many cases of HUS have been associated with *S. dysenteriae* serotype 1 infections, but the majority of cases are associated with gastrointestinal infections by verocytotoxin-producing *E. coli.* The pathogenesis of HUS remains to be elucidated, but damage to vascular epithelial cells by Shiga toxin appears to be the central event.

A rise in humoral and intestinal antibodies can often be demonstrated during shigellosis, and serotype-specific immunity follows the attack. Serum antibodies play little role in resistance, but the intestinal antibodies (coproantibodies) probably are more important in immunity. Intestinal antibodies develop earlier and disappear more quickly than serum antibodies.

An oral shigella vaccine has been developed that employs an attenuated streptomycin-dependent strain that is avirulent by virtue of its inability to proliferate or invade in the absence of streptomycin. This vaccine induces production of intestinal antibodies, probably IgA, that influence the ability of the shigellae to adhere to and penetrate epithelial cells.

The specific diagnosis of shigellosis depends upon the recovery of the organism from stool culture. A presumptive diagnosis can be made by microscopic examination of a drop of stool or mucus mixed with methylene blue on a slide and placed under a coverslip. Numerous polymorphonuclear leukocytes indicate inflammatory bowel disease.

Antibiotic treatment may shorten the duration of symptoms and the excretion of organisms in the stool. Drugs that reduce intestinal motility are contraindicated as they may prolong the duration of the diarrhea and the clinical illness, and the period of excretion of shigellae in the stool.

ENTEROINVASIVE *ESCHERICHIA COLI* (EIEC)

Certain strains of *E. coli* produce diarrheal disease indistinguishable from shigellosis. These strains do not produce an enterotoxin, and pili are not required to attach to and invade the mucosa. These strains resemble and share some somatic antigens with shigella. They are considerably less virulent than shigella, and the minimum infecting dose for humans is approximately 10^6 organisms. Genetic studies have shown that the EIEC strain may exchange plasmids and chromosomal regions associated with virulence with *S. sonnei* and *S. flexneri*.

CAMPYLOBACTER JEJUNI

The campylocbacters are a diverse group of small, gram-negative spiral organisms that grow best under microaerophilic conditions. They often occur in pairs, giving a sea gull–like appearance, and they possess polar flagella which impart a rapid linear or corkscrew motility. *Campylobacter jejuni* and related species (*C. doylei*, *C. coli*, and *C. laridis*) involved in human enteritis are thermophilic (capable of growth at 42°C).

Campylobacter jejuni is a major cause of acute diarrhea. In developing countries, the organism accounts for 30% of cases of diarrhea in children younger than 8 months, 6% of diarrhea in older children, and 2% of adult cases. In the United States, *C. jejuni* accounts for 5% to 10% of all cases of diarrhea—equal to the numbers produced by salmonella and shigella combined, with the highest incidence in young children.

Campylobacter jejuni is widely distributed in nature. Human infection has been traced to contact with poultry and dogs, but the mode of transmission is obscure. The organisms are commonly found in the gastrointestinal and genitourinary tracts of sheep, cattle, dogs, and chickens. Waterborne outbreaks have occurred and transmission among family members has been reported. The incubation period is 3 to 5 days. The most frequent pattern of disease is diarrhea accompanied by fever and abdominal pain. Stools typically contain blood and pus. It also can produce an ulcerative colitis type of illness. The disease is self-limiting and resolves after 3 to 5 days, but may persist for as long as 2 weeks. The numbers of organisms required to produce the disease is unknown; volunteers have become ill after ingesting only 500 organisms.

Flagella, lipopolysaccharide, and an outer membrane protein may play a role in the adherence of *C. jejuni* to intestinal epithelial cells. Strains of *C. jejuni* produce heat-labile enterotoxins that increase cyclic adenosine monophosphate (AMP) concentrations in cultured cells, and extracellular cytotoxins resembling Shiga toxin, but the pathogenic significance of these toxins remains to be established. *Campylobacter jejuni* penetrates the intestinal wall by an undefined mechanism. The site of infection appears to be the jejunum, ileum, and the colon. Histologic sections show an acute colitis with inflammatory infiltrates of the lamina propria and crypt abscesses.

In older children and adults, infection appears to impart immunity localized to the gut. Serum antibodies also develop during convalescence.

Campylobacter enteritis is specifically diagnosed by recovery of the organism from stool culture. It is effectively treated with erythromycin, or Fluoroquinolones. Untreated persons continue to excrete organisms for 2 to 7 weeks.

VIBRIO PARAHAEMOLYTICUS

This organism is a halophilic, curved, gram-negative rod found in sea water. The infection is associated with the consumption of raw, incompletely cooked, or contaminated seafood, especially in the summer. The incubation period is about 15 hours, but may be as short as 4 hours or as long as 3 days. The pathogenesis is not understood. The enteritis is characterized by explosive watery diarrhea, followed by severe abdominal cramping, nausea, and vomiting, sometimes accompanied by fever, chills, and headache. A dysenteric form occurs that resembles shigellosis, with fever, abdominal pain, and bloody mucoid stools.

PLESIOMONAS SHIGELLOIDES

Plesiomonas shigelloides is a gram-negative, rod-shaped bacterium, facultatively anaerobic, of the Vibrionaceae family. The infection is characterized by diarrhea, abdominal cramps, blood in the stool, vomiting, and fever. Most patients give a history of eating uncooked shellfish, usually raw oysters, in the 48 hours before the onset of symptoms. The average duration of symptoms in untreated patients is 11 days. Treatment with trimethoprim-sulfamethoxazole or tetracycline shorten the duration to 3 to 5 days.

CHAPTER 34

Other Bacterial Agents of Gastrointestinal Disease

A 75-year-old woman was admitted to the surgical unit for revision of a hip prosthesis. She was placed in a room with another patient who had diarrhea. The operation was without incident and cefazolin was administered prophylactically, and an indwelling catheter was placed postoperatively pending the return of bladder function. Three days later the patient showed evidence of a urinary tract infection and the antibiotic was continued beyond the perioperative period. Seven days after the surgical procedure the patient developed abdominal pain, fever to 38.8°C, and a leukocytosis. The following day she developed diarrhea. Microscopic examination of the stool revealed many polymorphonuclear leukocytes, and a test for *Clostridium difficile* toxin was positive. The catheter was removed, the cefazolin was discontinued, and the patient was treated with oral vancomycin. She became afebrile after several days and was subsequently discharged from the hospital.

CLOSTRIDIUM DIFFICILE

Diarrhea is a common and usually benign side effect of antibiotic therapy. Sometimes diarrhea is severe and the patient is found to have colitis. *Clostridium difficile* has been established as the most important cause of antibiotic-associated colitis. *Clostridium difficile* is a gram-positive, spore-forming anaerobic bacillus. The organism is widespread in the hospital environment, major sources being toilets, bedpans, floors, and the hands and stools of asymptomatic hospital personnel working in areas where there is a case of *C. difficile*. Approximately 3% of healthy adults have *C. difficile* in their stool; this increases to 15% to 20% of antibiotic recipients without diarrhea. Thirty percent to 70% of healthy children under 1 year of age are colonized with *C. difficile*. Unlike adults, this asymptomatic carriage in children is often associated with the presence of *C. difficile* toxin.

Clostridium difficile colitis occurs at all ages and it appears almost exclusively in association with antibiotic treatment. Alteration of the normal intestinal flora appears to be a critical factor for acquisition of *C. difficile* among those not colonized. The antibiotic inhibits those components of the colonic flora that would normally inhibit replication of *C. difficile* so that growth and toxin production of the pathogens are unchecked.

Symptoms of diarrhea and abdominal cramps may occur at any time during antibiotic therapy, but often appear several weeks after the drug has been discontinued. Large volumes of watery or mucoid stools, occasionally with evidence of blood, are characteristic. In severe disease, patients may have more than 20 episodes of diarrhea daily, continuing for several months. Additional findings include fever, leukocytosis, and abdominal tenderness. The characteristic lesion is a pseudomembrane composed of mucin, fibrin, acute inflammatory cells, and mucosal epithelial cells that have sloughed off. The pseudomembrane develops from a superficial ulceration.

It is believed that the pathogenesis of antibiotic-associated colitis is the result of toxin-mediated pathologic changes in the intestine, rather than the invasion of the intestinal mucosa by *C. difficile*. The organism produces two toxins: A and B. Toxin A causes hemorrhagic enteritis in the rabbit ileal loop assay, while the more potent toxin B is a cytopathic toxin. Most strains of *C. difficile* are toxigenic and produce both toxins.

Diagnosis of antibiotic-associated colitis can be made by assaying the stool for *C. difficile* toxin, and demonstrating pathologic changes in the colon by endoscopy.

Therapy of antibiotic-associated colitis is based upon eradication of *C. difficile* from the intestinal tract by the oral administration of vancomycin or metronidazole.

YERSINIA ENTEROCOLITICA

Yersinia enterocolitica and the closely related *Y. enterocolitica pseudotuberculosis* are gram-negative coccobacillary members of the *Enterobacteriaceae* family. These two species are closely related to *Y. pestis*, the etiologic agent of bubonic plague, but they seldom cause the rapidly fatal bacteremia associated with that organism. *Yersinia enterocolitica* comprises 57 serotypes and five biotypes; most human infections have been caused by serotypes O3, O8, and O9, and biotypes 2, 3, and 4. There are six serotypes of *Y. enterocolitica pseudotuberculosis* and four subtypes; the majority of human disease is caused by group O1 strains. The reservoir of *Yersinia* is primarily in wild and domestic animals and birds.

Infection in humans is associated with the ingestion of contaminated milk or milk products, water, or animal contact. *Yersinia* have been recovered from water, oysters, raw and pasteurized milk, and from wild and domestic animals. Two thirds of cases of *Y. enterocolitica* occur in infants and children; three fourths of *Y. enterocolitica pseudotuberculosis* infections involve 5- to 20-year-olds. Epidemics have been due to contaminated chocolate milk and other dairy products; person-to-person spread in institutions is also believed to occur.

The virulence of both organisms may be at least partially related to their peptide V antigen and lipoprotein W antigen, which enable the bacteria to resist phagocytosis. The ability of *Y. enterocolitica* to invade tissue is mediated by a plasmid. Most strains of *Y. enterocolitica* produce a heat-stable toxin that resembles the ST toxin of enterotoxigenic *E. coli* in stimulating guanylate cyclase resulting in enhanced cellular fluid secretion.

The organisms are ingested with food or milk. They penetrate the mucosa of the lower intestinal tract and enter the lamina propria where they multiply within mononuclear cells and lymphatic tissues producing foci of ulcerations, necrosis of mucosa at lymphoid follicles, and abscess formation. The terminal ileum is the site of maximal involvement. Hypertrophy of mesenteric lymph nodes and appendiceal lesions are common. The organisms spread from the gastrointestinal tract via the portal circulation to involve the liver and spleen with abscess formation, cholangitis, and peritonitis. The incubation period is 3 to 7 days.

The clinical manifestations of yersiniosis vary with age and the species. In children younger than 5 years of age, *Y. enterocolitica* usually causes either a self-limited gastroenteritis, characterized by an acute watery diarrhea, or colitis with fever, vomiting, abdominal pain, and stools containing blood and mucus. The disease lasts about 2 weeks. In older children, the organism causes acute mesenteric adenitis (pseudoappendicitis), a syndrome of fever, headache, joint pain, diarrhea, and diffuse abdominal pain. The localization of the abdominal pain to the right lower quadrant usually leads to laparotomy which reveals a normal appendix, but markedly enlarged and inflamed mesenteric lymph nodes. In adults, *Y. enterocolitica* infection is usually an acute self-limited dysentery. Extraintestinal yersiniosis includes septicemia, sometimes leading to metastatic abscesses. These complications seem to occur more frequently in infants and persons with hemoglobinopathies or cirrhosis. Postinfectious complications of *Yersinia* infection include reactive arthritis, inflammatory bowel disease, Reiter's syndrome,* and other autoimmune disorders. Patients who develop these complications are frequently HLA-B27-positive.

Diagnosis of yersiniosis is based upon the recovery of the organism from the stool. Many children and some adults with *Y. enterocolitica* enteritis also have pharyngitis. This may lead to confusion with streptococcal pharyngitis since children with streptococcal disease often have abdominal pain. Throat cultures should be taken if the patient has symptoms of pharyngitis. Blood cultures should also be obtained. Serologic tests are useful in diagnosing *Yersinia* infections. Agglutinating antibodies against the O antigen appear shortly after the onset of illness, but these antibodies cross-react with *Brucella*, *Vibrio*, *Salmonella*, and *Escherichia coli*, and therefore the patient's serum must be appropriately absorbed. Antibodies persist for 2 to 6 months.

There is no evidence that antimicrobial therapy is of any value in uncomplicated enterocolitis or mesenteric enteritis as these infections are generally self-limited. Patients with septicemia or other extraintestinal *Yersinia* infections need to be treated aggressively as the mortality is 50% with *Y. enterocolitica* and 75% with *Y. pseudotuberculosis*.

VEROCYTOTOXIN-PRODUCING *ESCHERICHIA COLI* (VTEC)

These organisms, also known as enterohemorrhagic *E. coli* (EHEC), are involved in hemorrhagic colitis, and the hemolytic uremic syndrome (HUS). These strains are distinguished by their failure to ferment sorbitol, their characteristic serotype (O157:H7 being the prototype and the most frequently isolated), and by their ability to produce cytotoxins resembling Shiga toxin. These Shiga-like toxins are termed verocytotoxins because of the vero (monkey kidney) cells used to assay their cytotoxicity. Two verocytotoxins, VT1 and VT2, are known to be associated with human disease. Enterohemorrhagic *E. coli* isolates from humans produce either VT1 or VT2, or both. Production of VTs is bacteriophage-mediated. The toxins interfere with protein synthesis causing cell death.

The reservoir of these organisms is believed to be cattle because of the high association of disease with ingestion of ground beef and raw milk or dairy products. The incubation period is 3 to 6 days (much longer than the 1 to 3 days associated with enterotoxigenic *E. coli* infections). All ages are affected, but increased risk has been associated with older age and previous gastrectomy.

---

*A disease of males in which initial diarrhea is followed by urethritis, conjunctivitis, and migratory arthritis.

Hemorrhagic colitis is a distinct clinical syndrome consisting of bloody diarrhea with little or no fever, and pus cells in the stool. The onset is sudden with severe abdominal cramps, followed by watery diarrhea. Within a short time, the diarrhea progresses to profuse bloody discharge resembling lower gastrointestinal hemorrhage. There is characteristically no fever. The lack of fever distinguishes hemorrhagic colitis from shigellosis, and dysentery due to *Campylobacter*, enteroinvasive *E. coli*, or amebas. The average duration of illness is 8 days. Milder cases occur but a high percentage of affected patients are hospitalized, indicating the severity of most cases. In one nursing home outbreak of hemorrhagic colitis, the mortality was over 30%.

Enterohemorrhagic *E. coli* are invasive but appear to produce disease by direct effect of the toxin on mucosal cells; the intense colitis may relate to the release of VT1 or VT2 during infection. As many as 20% of cases may develop HUS 1 week after onset of diarrhea. HUS was formerly believed to be primarily a disease of childhood, but cases also occur in the elderly. The syndrome is characterized by microangiopathic* hemolytic anemia, acute renal failure, and thrombocytopenia. Injury to vascular endothelial cells has been postulated to be the central event in the pathogenesis of HUS. Shiga toxin and the verocytotoxins have been demonstrated to damage vascular endothelial cells in vitro. It has been suggested that lipopolysaccharide may also play a role in the pathogenesis of HUS.

ENTEROPATHOGENIC *ESCHERICHIA COLI* (EPEC)

Enteropathogenic *E. coli* (EPEC) produce chronic diarrheal disease by destruction of microvilli and adherence to the damaged luminal surface of the intestine. These adherent strains

---

Microangiopathic refers to damage to small blood vessels.

do not produce enterotoxins, nor do they invade the intestinal mucosa. Typically the patients are infants and young children who develop protracted watery diarrhea that is sometimes accompanied by vomiting and fever. The pathogenesis appears to be penetration of the glycocalyx by the bacteria and close adherence to the mucosal cell surface causing disruption of the microvillous brush border. There is associated blunting of the villi, hypertrophy of crypts, histiocytic infiltrate in the lamina propria, and reduction in brush border enzymes.

HELICOBACTER PYLORI

Helicobacter pylori is a slow-growing, microaerophilic, curved or spiral gram-negative motile bacterium that was originally called *Campylobacter pyloris*. The organism produces large amounts of urease. The reservoir and transmission of *H. pylori* are unknown. The organism is present in the stomach of essentially 100% of type B (antral) gastritis in adults and children, and patients with duodenal ulcers, and in up to 70% of persons with gastric ulcers or nonulcer dyspepsia.

In the United States, *H. pylori* is uncommon in childhood and increases progressively during adulthood, reaching 50% to 60% by age 60 years. Infection is higher in black and Hispanic populations, and in developing countries *H. pylori* infection is even more common and is seen earlier in life. The organism is seldom present in the absence of gastritis or peptic ulcer. Persons infected with *H. pylori* develop serum antibodies to this organism; these antibodies are rarely seen in healthy persons less than 20 years old, but antibody prevalence progresses with age, reaching 50% in patients more than 60 years old.

Several mechanisms of pathogenesis have been proposed. The organism's potent urease output produces ammonia resulting in an alkaline microenvironment that protects the bacteria from gastric acid until it becomes established under the mucus layer. The bacteria attach to the surface of epithelial cells, the microvilli appear to become depleted and the organisms appear at and disrupt intercellular junctions, eliciting a leukocyte response and gastritis. Patients with high gastric acid output may develop gastric metaplasia in the duodenum, colonization by *H. pylori*, inflammation, and an ulcer. Alternatively, rapid urea hydrolysis at the intercellular junction could prevent the normal passage of hydrogen ions, causing backdiffusion, resulting in hypochlorhydria and tissue damage.

Helicobacter pylori infection may be diagnosed by examining biopsy specimens for urease activity, by culture, urea breath tests, or serologic techniques.

Treatment of *H. pylori* infection by antimicrobial agents or bismuth compounds results in clearance of the organism, clinical and histologic improvement, but there is a high relapse rate.

CHAPTER 35

Viral Agents of Gastroenteritis

A 4-month-old infant was brought to the emergency room because of profuse watery diarrhea. One week previously the infant had been admitted to the hospital for unexplained fever. The white blood cell count was found to be normal, blood and cerebrospinal fluid cultures were negative, and the child was sent home after 4 days. The mother reported that the baby, who was not breast-fed, was not taking its formula and cried constantly. Physical examination revealed a listless infant with sunken eyes, poor skin turgor, and a low-grade fever. Severe dehydration was confirmed by an elevated hematocrit, and an enzyme immunoassay (EIA) for rotavirus in the stool was positive. The infant was admitted, treated with oral glucose-electrolyte solution, and improved over the next few days.

It has been estimated that 40% of the 5 to 18 million deaths worldwide that occur annually due to diarrheal disease are caused by viruses. Most of the mortality (and morbidity) involves infants and children under 5 years of age. In the United States acute viral gastroenteritis is second only to the common cold in frequency. Viral gastroenteritis is usually a benign, self-limited disease, but deaths occur in infants, the elderly, and in debilitated persons. Death is related to dehydration and electrolyte imbalance, primarily hypernatremia and metabolic acidosis.

The major viruses that cause gastroenteritis are rotavirus, enteric adenoviruses, and the Norwalk viruses. Other viral agents involved in diarrheal disease are astroviruses, calciviruses, enteric coronaviruses, and other small round viruses.

The predominant site of viral infection is the proximal small intestine; the colon is not involved. The epithelial cells lining the small intestine are damaged and the absorptive villi are blunted, and consequently the diarrhea results from the loss of absorptive capacity and impaired sodium absorption. In addition, disaccharidases are depressed leading to increased carbohydrate in the intestine which pulls water and electrolytes into the lumen by osmosis.

Treatment of viral diarrhea is basically correction of dehydration and electrolyte imbalance. Oral glucose-electrolyte solution is commonly used, since glucose enhances sodium transport in the small intestine.

ROTAVIRUSES

Rotaviruses have a wheel-like appearance when viewed with the electron microscope. The double-stranded RNA genome is surrounded by two layers of polypeptides. The major outer capsid protein VP7 evokes neutralizing antibody. The group antigen is another glycoprotein, VP6. Group A rotavirus is the major etiologic agent in human disease, but occasionally other groups are involved.

In the temperate zone, community-acquired rotavirus infections occur in the colder months of the late fall, winter, and early spring. Rotavirus accounts for almost half of all diarrheal illness in children up to 2 years of age. Older adults are occasionally infected. Most transmission is person to person via the fecal-oral route, possibly by respiratory aerosols as well. Nosocomial outbreaks of rotavirus illness occur in pediatric units during the winter months. Rotavirus has been recovered from 36% of children with diarrhea; 25% to 35% of children without diarrhea have also been shown to excrete rotavirus in their stool.

The incubation period of rotavirus infection is 38 to 46 hours. The onset is sudden with fever and vomiting for 2 or 3 days followed by watery diarrhea and sometimes abdominal pain that persists for 3 to 8 days. Half of the patients show respiratory symptoms (rhinitis, pharyngitis, otitis media) at some time during the illness. Recovery is usually complete in 7 to 10 days. More severe and sometimes fatal infection is seen in the elderly.

Although rotavirus is sensitive to acid it can survive the pH of a stomach buffered by food. Replication takes place in the epithelial cells of the small intestine, selectively infecting the enterocytes of the mature villi. The infected villus tips are replaced by secretory crypt cells leading to impairment of glucose-coupled sodium transport. Abnormally low levels of lactase, maltase, and sucrase are common and most children develop lactose malabsorption intolerance that lasts several weeks.

Ninety percent of children acquire serum antibody against rotavirus by 3 years of age. Immunity is serotype-specific and related to neutralizing antibody levels. The protective effect is of short duration (less than 1 year) which explains recurrent attacks of gastroenteritis by the same serotype. Breast-fed infants are less likely to become infected with rotavirus, and they secrete rotavirus less frequently than infants fed by formula. Antirotavirus IgG and IgM are present in colostrum and milk; secretory IgA and trypsin inhibitor may also contribute to the protective effect of breast milk.

Several rotavirus vaccines are under development. These are administered orally to stimulate local intestinal IgA. The specific diagnosis of rotavirus infection can be made by visualizing the virus in the stool, or by detecting viral antigen in the stool by EIA or latex agglutination techniques. Treatment consists of fluid and electrolyte replacement.

ENTERIC ADENOVIRUSES

These agents are nonenveloped icosahedral viruses with a genome of linear, double-stranded DNA. The structure contains 252 capsomeres with hexons and pentons. The hexons contain antigens for group, subgroup, and type specificity. Serotypes 40 and 41 (previously called fastidious enteric adenoviruses) are the ones involved in gastroenteritis.

Enteric adenoviruses 40 and 41 are the second most important cause of infantile gastroenteritis after rotavirus and account for 5% to 20% of children hospitalized for diarrhea in the developed countries. The peak incidence is in children less than 2 years old. There are no seasonal peaks and cases tend to be endemic rather than epidemic. The mechanism of transmission is presumed to be person to person. The incubation period is 3 to 10 days. Diarrhea is the predominant symptom with or without vomiting. Respiratory symptoms are present in about 25% of the patients. The illness lasts about 8 days.

The pathogenesis is still not well understood. Immunity is related to antibodies directed against the common antigen and is believed to be acquired during childhood infection. Diagnosis is rarely possible since it requires viewing the virus in the stool by electron microscopy or detection of viral antigen in the stool by EIA.

NORWALK VIRUSES

Norwalk viruses are small round viruses that lack an envelope and cannot be cultivated in vitro. The nucleic acid is probably RNA. There are three or four strains or serotypes of Norwalk-like viruses. They are very resistant to acid. Unlike rotavirus, Norwalk agents affect older children and adults. Transmission may occur by water, food (especially shellfish and salads), fomites, aerosols, and person-to-person contact. Outbreaks have been associated with community water systems and have occurred in schools, nursing homes, recreational camps, and cruise ships.

The incubation period is 24 to 48 hours. There is sudden onset of nausea, sometimes with diarrhea and abdominal cramps. Vomiting is more prominent in children, diarrhea is more common in adults. Up to half of the patients experience headache, fever, chills, and myalgias. The illness lasts 12 to 60 hours. The virus replicates in the small intestine, causing blunting of the villi and moderate infiltration of the lamina propria by mononuclear cells. Susceptibility is poorly understood. Immunity is a paradox, since persons with the highest antibody levels are at greatest risk of infection.

Specific diagnosis can be made by visualizing the virus in feces by immunoelectron microscopy or by detection of viral antigen in the feces. These procedures are not generally available in clinical laboratories.

ASTROVIRUSES

Astroviruses are star-shaped agents whose nucleic acid type is unknown. There are at least five serotypes. Astroviruses are responsible for 3% to 5% of cases of infantile gastroenteritis. Children up to age 7 years are those most likely to develop symptomatic disease. Transmission is probably person to person. The incubation period is 24 to 36 hours. Vomiting is the most common symptom, often together with watery diarrhea, abdominal pain, and fever. Symptoms last 1 to 4 days. Little is known about immunity to astroviruses. Diagnosis may be made by direct visualization of the virus in feces. The virus can be isolated in cell culture and a rise in antibody titer between acute and convalescent sera can usually be demonstrated.

CALCIVIRUSES

Calciviruses are RNA viruses that have a Star of David configuration when viewed by electron microscopy. They have not been grown in cell cultures. Calciviruses primarily affect infants and young children. Nosocomial outbreaks have occurred. Transmission is person to person and by ingestion of contaminated shellfish, cold foods, and drinking water. Calciviruses have been recovered from the stools of healthy people. The incubation period is 1 to 3 days. Symptoms are primarily diarrhea and vomiting and last about 4 days. Immunity is probably acquired in childhood and is long-lasting. The virus may be detected in the feces by electron microscopy or by radioimmunoassay.

ENTERIC CORONAVIRUSES

Coronaviruses are round or pleomorphic, positive-stranded RNA viruses with club-shaped projections (peplomers) on their surface. Most cases of gastroenteritis or necrotizing enterocolitis occur in children less than 2 years old. In the United States outbreaks have occurred in the Southwest during the cooler, dryer months. The predominant features are diarrhea, vomiting, and fever lasting about 7 days. Patients often have at least one other enteric pathogen including *Salmonella*, *Shigella*, and *Campylobacter*. The diagnosis may be made by demonstrating the virus in the stool by electron microscopy or by a rise in the titer of specific antibody.

CHAPTER 36

Viral Hepatitis

A 20-year-old man with a history of intravenous drug abuse presented with weakness, malaise, nausea, anorexia, and right upper quadrant pain for the past 10 days. The previous day he awoke to find himself jaundiced, and passed some dark urine. Physical examination was remarkable only for a slightly enlarged and tender liver and multiple venipuncture marks on both forearms. Laboratory findings included a normal white blood cell count and markedly elevated bilirubin, alanine aminotransferase (ALT), and aspartate aminotranferase (AST) levels. Tests for hepatitis B surface antigens and antibody and hepatitis C antibody were all negative. He was sent home for rest and placed on a low-fat high-carbohydrate diet. He was seen again after several weeks and showed some improvement, and a repeated test for hepatitis C antibody was positive.

Hepatitis is an inflammation of the liver. Hepatitis may be caused by drugs, toxins, excess alcohol intake, bacteria, or viruses. Two herpesviruses, Epstein-Barr virus (EBV) and cytomegalovirus (CMV), may cause hepatitis as part of the infectious mononucleosis syndrome. The majority of hepatitis cases are caused by one of five hepatotropic viruses designated hepatitis A virus (HAV), hepatitis B virus (HBV), hepatitis C virus (HCV), hepatitis D virus, or delta agent (HDV), and hepatitis E virus (HEV). The reservoir of the human hepatotropic viruses is man. The hepatitides caused by the hepatotropic viruses are similar in many ways, but some differences in epidemiologic, immunologic, clinical, and pathologic characteristics exist among the five etiologic agents.

Many cases of hepatitis are asymptomatic. Overt infections are typically considered to have four stages: incubation period, preicteric phase, icteric phase, and convalescence. The incubation period varies from 2 weeks to 6 months. The onset may be sudden or insidious. Initial symptoms are nonspecific and may include malaise, weakness, anorexia, nausea, vomiting, and dull right upper quadrant pain. Some patients may complain of headaches, myalgias, chills and fever, and occasionally rash and arthritis. The liver may be enlarged and tender. These symptoms can persist for 3 to 10 days. The icteric phase begins with the appearance of jaundice and dark urine, and lasts for several weeks, after which time the patient begins to feel better.

Three biochemical tests are characteristically elevated in viral hepatitis: serum bilirubin, alanine aminotransferase (ALT; formerly called serum glutamic pyruvic transaminase, SGPT) and aspartate aminotransferase (AST; formerly serum glutamic oxaloacetic transaminase, SGOT). Other abnormal liver tests include elevation of alkaline phosphatase and gamma glutamyl transpeptidase. The diagnosis of viral hepatitis is made by serologic testing for specific viral antigens and antibodies.

HEPATITIS A VIRUS

Hepatitis A virus is the causative agent of **infectious hepatitis**. The agent is a small, nonenveloped virus with icosahedral symmetry and a single-stranded, linear RNA genome surrounded by a capsid composed of four polypeptides.

Transmission is primarily person to person by the fecal-oral route. Outbreaks have been traced to contaminated water and food (milk, sliced meat, shellfish, salads). Infection also occurs in persons exposed to children in day care centers, intravenous drug abusers, and male homosexuals.

The incubation period varies from 15 to 45 days and is dose-related; there is a shorter incubation with a larger infectious dose. The average incubation is 28 days. Two thirds of the cases remain asymptomatic. In symptomatic cases, the onset is abrupt with fever, malaise, nausea, and abdominal discomfort. Diarrhea is more common in children. These symptoms are followed in a few days by jaundice, which occurs in the majority of patients. The duration of symptoms is 1 to 3 weeks, but convalescence tends to be prolonged. Mortality is about 0.1%. Hepatitis A does not lead to a carrier state or to chronic hepatitis.

The pathogenesis of HAV infection is not completely understood. After a brief viremia, there is an initial phase of viral replication in the liver with the release of virus into the feces. HAV replication does not produce a cytopathic effect nor does it shut down macromolecular synthesis in host cells. The replicative phase is followed by a cytopathic phase with localized inflammatory cell infiltrates and developing immunity.

The initial humoral response involves IgM and probably IgG and IgA antibodies. The IgM response is short-lived (6–12 months) but the IgG persists for long periods, perhaps for life (Fig 36–1). These neutralizing antibodies have a primary role in preventing symptomatic reinfection, but other immune mechanisms such as interferon activation, natural killer cells, and T cell–mediated cytotoxicity may also be important in resistance.

HEPATITIS B VIRUS

Hepatitis B virus is the etiologic agent of **serum hepatitis**. HBV is a double-stranded, circular DNA virus composed of a nucleocapsid core antigen (HBcAg) surrounded by a lipoprotein coat containing a surface antigen (HBsAg). A soluble "e" antigen (HBeAg) is probably a constituent of the nucleocapsid. HBV infection is worldwide in distribution. In some areas of Asia, HBsAg carrier rates approach 15%; in the United States, the HBsAg carrier rate is 0.3%. HBsAg is found in almost all body fluids. The presence of HBcAg increases the infectivity of these fluids. Transmission is percutaneous or permucosal exposure to infective body fluids (blood, serum, saliva, semen, and vaginal fluids) by receiving unscreened blood or blood products, an accidental needle stick, or by sexual contact. Perinatal transmission is common in some parts of Asia.

The incubation period is 45 to 180 days; the average is 60 to 90 days. Approximately half of infected persons become symptomatic. The onset tends to be gradual with malaise, fatigue, and anorexia that lasts 1 to 4 weeks but which may persist for 6 months or longer. Approximately 20% of symptomatic patients develop jaundice. Recovery is slow. Five percent to 10% of patients fail to clear HBsAg and continue with chronic hepatitis that can progress to cirrhosis

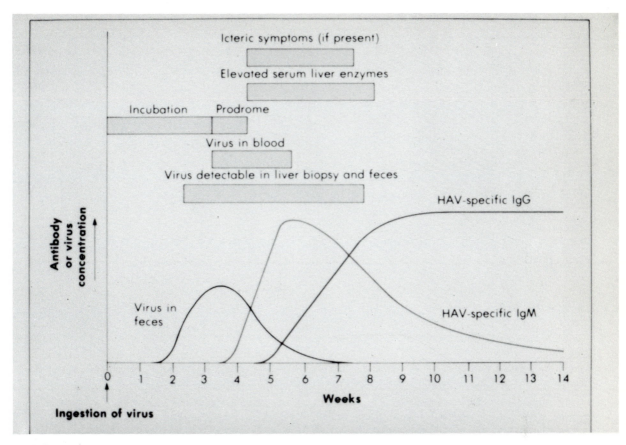

FIG 36–1.
Time course of HAV infection. (From Murray P, Kobayashi G, Thompson J, et al (eds): *Medical Microbiology.* St Louis, Mosby–Year Book, 1990. Used by permission.)

and hepatocellular carcinoma. An additional 0.5% to 2.0% develop fulminant hepatitis (complete destruction of liver cells) resulting in hepatic failure and death.

The immune response starts with the appearance of anti-HBc, followed by anti-HBe, and finally by anti-HBs. HBeAg is a marker of active viral replication and infectivity. The appearance of anti-HBe is a favorable prognostic sign indicating that viral replication has ceased and the patient is noninfectious (Figs 36–2 and 36–3).

Hepatitis immune globulin (HBIG) is available for temporary passive protection following exposure. Active immunity follows the adminis-

tration of hepatitis B vaccine. Two types of hepatitis vaccine are licensed in the United States: plasma-derived vaccine and recombinant vaccine. Recombinant vaccine is produced by a genetically altered *Saccharomyces cerevisiae* (brewer's or bakers' yeast) into which a plasmid containing a gene for HBsAg has been inserted.

HEPATITIS D VIRUS (HDV)

The hepatitis D virus, also known as the delta agent, is the cause of delta hepatitis. HDV is a viruslike particle consisting of a coat of HB-sAg surrounding an internal delta antigen, to-

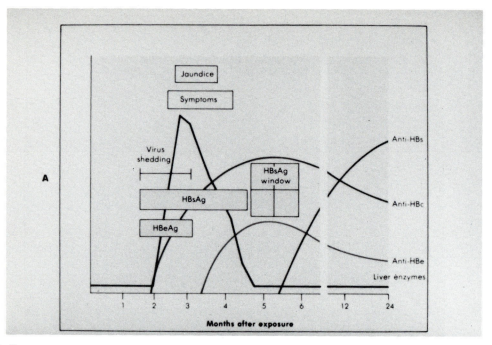

FIG 36–2.
The serologic events associated with the typical course of acute type B hepatitis. (From Murray P, Kobayashi G, Thompson J, et al (eds): *Medical Microbiology.* St Louis, Mosby–Year Book, 1990. Used by permission.)

gether with single-stranded linear RNA. The delta agent is a defective virus that requires coinfection with HBV for synthesis. The distribution of delta hepatitis is worldwide, with high prevalence in the Amazon basin of South America, Central Africa, southern Italy, and the Middle East.

Transmission is similar to HBV: percutaneous exposure to infected body fluids, and perinatal. The incubation period in man is not known; it is 2 to 10 weeks in experimentally infected chimpanzees.

Delta hepatitis can be a severe illness. Acute delta hepatitis has a mortality of 2% to 20%. There are two forms of acute delta hepatitis, depending on the stage of the underlying HBV disease: coinfection and superinfection. In coinfection the delta and HBV infections occur simultaneously. Most of these patients recover. Superinfection results when the delta infection occurs in patients with chronic HBV disease. More than 70% of cases of superinfection develop chronic hepatitis, and in most of these patients, cirrhosis and death follow.

The diagnosis of delta hepatitis is made by the presence of HBsAg and anti-hepatitis D in the patients' serum.

NON-A, NON-B HEPATITIS

It has been recognized for many years that the majority of cases of posttransfusion hepatitis were not caused by either HAV or HBV; these cases were designated as non-A, non-B (NANB) hepatitis. Recent studies have shown that NANB hepatitis actually includes at least two different agents and disease types. One of these agents, called hepatitis C virus (HCV), may account for more than 90% of all cases of posttransfusion

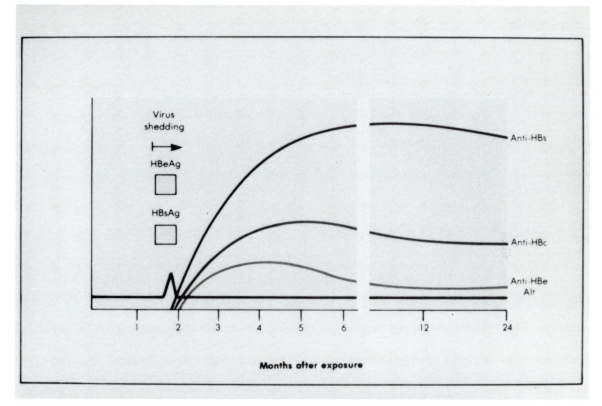

FIG 36–3.
Clinical, serologic, and biochemical course of a subclinical, asymptomatic hepatitis B virus infection. *HBsAG,* Hepatitis B surface antigen; *HBeAg,* hepatitis B e antigen; *Alt,* alanine aminotransferase; *anti-HBs,* antibody to *HBsAg; anti-HBc,* antibody to hepatitis B Core antigen; *anti-HBe,* antibody to HBeAg. (From Murray P, Kobayashi G, Thompson J, et al (eds): *Medical Microbiology.* St Louis, Mosby–Year Book, 1990. Redrawn from Hoofnagle JH: *Lab Med* 1983; 14:705. Used by permission.)

hepatitis (in countries where blood is screened for HBsAg). The other agent, called hepatitis E virus (HEV), is the cause of epidemic, enterically transmitted NANB hepatitis.

HEPATITIS C VIRUS

The hepatitis C virus is the major causative agent of all NANB hepatitis in the United States. The genome is single-stranded linear RNA. Transmission is percutaneous via contaminated blood or improperly sterilized syringes and needles. Originally associated with blood transfusion recipients, most cases now are seen with parenteral drug use and in dialysis patients. The incubation period varies from 2 to 26 weeks; the average is 8 weeks. The onset is insidious with nonspecific and gastrointestinal symptoms. About 25% of patients develop jaundice. The disease tends to be less severe than HBV hepatitis, but about half of the patients remain chronic carriers and there is a high incidence of severe complications, including cirrhosis and hepatocellular carcinoma. A few patients develop aplastic anemia. A unique characteristic of

TABLE 36–1.

Clinical Features of Acute Viral Hepatitis

Agent	Transmission	Incubation (days)	Onset	Jaundice	Carrier State	Chronic Hepatitis	Mortality
HAV	Fecal-oral	15–45	Acute	10%	No	No	0.1%–0.2%
HBV	Parenteral, sexual	30–120	Gradual	15%–20%	5%–10%	Yes	0.5%–2.0%
HCV	Parenteral, sexual	49–56	Gradual	25%	50%	Yes	1%–2%
HDV	Parenteral	21–90	Acute	Varies	Yes	Yes	Up to 30%
HEV	Fecal-oral	21–42	Acute	?	?	?	1%–2%

HCV infection is that ALT values rise and fall sporadically throughout the course of the disease. Diagnosis can be made by a serological test hepatitis C, but the antibody often does not develop for many weeks after acute infection. The antibody to hepatitis C, unlike the antibody to hepatitis A or B, is not protective.

HEPATITIS E VIRUS

Hepatitis E virus is a single-stranded linear RNA virus that is the major cause of epidemics of enterically transmitted NANB hepatitis. Epidemics have occurred in India, Burma, Nepal, the USSR, and North Africa. Transmission is by contaminated water and probably also person to person by the fecal-oral route. Most cases are in young adults. The onset is acute and the symptoms and severity are similar to HAV hepatitis. The mortality is 1% to 2% but may reach 10% in pregnant women in their third trimester. The clinical features of hepatitis caused by the hepatotropic viruses are summarized in Table 36–1.

PART VIII

Genital Infections

CHAPTER 37

Overview of Genital Infections

Genital infections are those that involve the penis, prostate, epididymis, testes, vulva, urethra, vagina, cervix, uterus, fallopian tubes, and ovaries. The causative agents include a number of bacteria, viruses, and fungi. These organisms are human pathogens and their reservoir is in infected persons. Transmission of genital infections is invariably by sexual intercourse with infected persons.

The manifestations of genital infection range from urethritis, characterized by burning on urination and the appearance of pus at the meatus, to the development of lesions on the external or internal genitalia. The various clinical presentations are listed in Table 37–1.

Several sexually transmitted diseases are not limited to the genitalia. In syphilis, only the primary stage is manifested by genital lesions, and there are no characteristic lesions in acquired immunodeficiency syndrome. Both of these infections involve multiple organ systems.

PRIMARY SYPHILIS

Syphilis is a multisystem disease caused by *Treponema pallidum,* a motile, spiral organism that is pathogenic only for humans. The organism enters the body during sexual contact via tiny breaks in squamous or mucous epithelium.

The incubation period is 14 to 21 days during which time the treponemes proliferate in the skin and enter the bloodstream and lymphatics.

Primary syphilis is characterized by the appearance of a single, indurated, nonpainful ulcer (chancre) on the genitalia. As the lesion evolves, the central area becomes necrotic, and healing takes place spontaneously in 3 to 6 weeks. There is painless enlargement of the inguinal lymph nodes. The coronal sulcus or the prepuce is the most common site in the male, and the labia in the female, but chancres of the cervix are also frequent. Primary syphilis may be atypical with skin lesions occurring on lips, breasts, mouth, and the anus in homosexuals.

Serologic testing may be negative in the first weeks of primary syphilis. The diagnosis depends upon the demonstration of the treponemes in the lesion by darkfield microscopy or direct fluorescent antibody staining. Treponemal and cardiolipin antibodies appear by the fourth week.

GRANULOMA INGUINALE

Granuloma inguinale, or donovanosis, is a chronic progressive disease of the external genitalia. The causative agent is *Calymmatobacterium granulomatis,* a gram-negative bacterium

TABLE 37–1.

Genital Infections: Clinical Presentations and Etiology

Clinical Presentation	Possible Etiology
Vaginal itching, burning, malodor	*Candida albicans*
	Trichomonas vaginalis
	Gardnerella vaginalis
	Mobiluncus spp.
Purulent or mucoid urethral or cervical discharge accompanied by burning on urination	*Neisseria gonorrhoeae*
	Chlamydia trachomatis
	Ureaplasma urealyticum
Painless chancre on penis, labia, vagina	*Treponema pallidum*
	C. trachomatis (lymphogranuloma venereum)
Painful papules, vesicles, ulcers on genitals	Herpes simplex virus
	Haemophilus ducreyi
Painless papules or warts on genitals	Papillomavirus
	Molluscum contagiosum virus
Inguinal lymphadenopathy	*H. ducreyi*
	C. trachomatis (lymphogranuloma venereum)
	Herpes simplex virus

that is not grown regularly on artificial media. The disease is rare in the United States, fewer than 100 cases per year, but it is fairly common in the Caribbean and other tropical areas. The reservoir is in infected persons and the disease is transmitted by sexual contact.

The incubation period ranges from 8 to 80 days. The initial lesion is a small subcutaneous nodule in the warm moist area of the genitalia, which breaks through to the surface to become a granulomatous ulcer that is frequently painless.

The diagnosis is made by visualizing Donovan bodies: intracellular clusters of "safety pin"–appearing organisms within the cytoplasm of large mononuclear cells in material from the lesion.

Herpesvirus and papillomavirus infections are discussed in Chapter 27.

CHAPTER 38

Neisseria gonorrhoeae

A 30-year-old woman complained of chills, fever, and a painful, swollen right knee for the previous 3 days. She also noticed that during the previous week blisters had appeared on both calves and on the left forearm, some of which had become hemorrhagic. On physical examination, she had a temperature of 38.8°C. The right knee joint was warm, swollen, and elicited pain on motion. Several hemorrhagic lesions, varying from 5 to 15 mm in diameter, were observed on both legs and on the left forearm. The remainder of the examination was within normal limits. Significant laboratory results included an elevated white blood cell count and erythrocyte sedimentation rate. The knee was aspirated and 5 mL of cloudy fluid were removed and cultured. Blood cultures and a cervical culture were also obtained, and she was admitted to the hospital. The joint fluid culture was negative, but one of the three blood cultures and the cervical culture were positive for *Neisseria gonorrhoeae*.

Neisseria gonorrhoeae is the cause of gonorrhea, a sexually transmitted disease. Gonorrhea is the most frequently reported infectious disease in the United States; in 1989, the number of reported cases was 297 per 100,000 population. It is estimated that less than 20% of the cases are reported. Factors predisposing to the high incidence of gonorrhea are the short incubation period, the high degree of transmissibility, little or no lasting immunity, and the large numbers of asymptomatic carriers. Man is the only natural reservoir of gonorrhea. The primary means of transmission is sexual intercourse with an infected partner. The risk of transmission from male to female is 50% per episode of vaginal intercourse; the female-to-male risk of infection is about 20% per episode. The highest attack rate is in young, sexually active adults in the 20- to 24-year-old age group.

The incubation period is 2 to 7 days. In males, the most common infection is acute urethritis, which occurs 2 to 5 days after exposure and is characterized by burning on urination and the presence of urethral exudate (Fig 38–1). Ten percent to 40% of males may remain asymptomatic urethral carriers for as long as 2 months after exposure.

Gonococcal infection in females may involve the cervix, urethra, or Bartholin's gland. The major symptoms are those of cervicitis or urethritis, vaginal discharge, intermenstrual bleed-

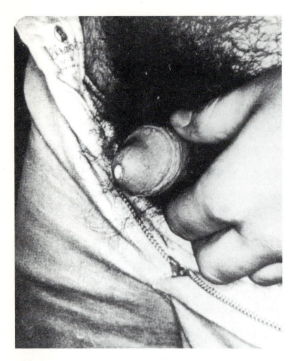

FIG 38–1.
Urethral exudate.

ing, or dysuria. Up to 80% of women may become asymptomatic carriers after being exposed to infection. The infection may extend to involve the fallopian tubes; gonococcal salpingitis can produce pelvic inflammatory disease resembling an acute surgical abdomen and result in tubal fibrosis, ectopic pregnancies, and infertility.

Gonococcal perihepatitis (Fitz-Hugh-Curtis syndrome) is the result of spread of infection from the fallopian tubes and peritoneum to the capsule of the liver. The major symptom is right upper quadrant pain.

Approximately 40% of women and homosexual men have gonococcal rectal infections but most of these are asymptomatic. A few patients have symptoms of acute proctitis with anal or rectal pruritis or bleeding. Pharyngeal infection is acquired by oral-genital contact. Most cases are asymptomatic, but occasionally infection is manifested as pharyngitis.

Conjunctivitis in adults is contracted from rubbing the eyes with fingers contaminated with genital secretions. In the newborn, conjunctivitis is acquired during the passage of the infant through an infected birth canal. Neonatal gonococcal conjunctivitis may lead to blindness unless promptly treated. Neonatal conjunctivitis in the developed countries has become uncommon as a result of prophylactic use of silver nitrate or erythromycin applied to the conjunctivae routinely after delivery, and the routine screening and treatment of pregnant women. In prepubertal girls, gonococcal vulvovaginitis is invariably the result of sexual molestation by infected adults.

Disseminated gonoccocal disease occurs in about 3% of untreated cases and is four times more common in females. Dissemination is more likely to occur during pregnancy or menstruation, possibly relating to changes in the pH and level of bactericidal enzymes in the cervical mucus. The most common form of disseminated disease is arthritis, often accompanied by hemorrhagic or bullous skin lesions. Gonococcal arthritis is the leading cause of infective arthritis in young adults. A rare but serious manifestation of disseminated gonoccocal disease is endocarditis, which occurs in about 1% of patients and usually involves the aortic valve.

Neisseria organisms are gram-negative, kidney-shaped cocci that characteristically occur in pairs with the flattened sides opposing. They are aerobic organisms that have a high level of cytochrome C oxidase (an enzyme that is useful for identification of this genus in the laboratory). Indigenous species (*N. sicca, N. flava, N. lactamica, Moraxella (Branhamella) catarrholis*, etc.) inhabit the mucous membranes of the upper respiratory and genitourinary tracts and seldom cause disease, except for respiratory disease due to *Moraxella*.

The two pathogenic species of this genus are *N. meningitidis*, the meningococcus; and *N. gonorrhoeae*, the gonococcus. Meningococci and gonococci have a number of characteristics that distinguish them from their nonpathogenic brethren besides their ability to produce disease. These two pathogens are more fastidious, i.e., they require enriched media such as heated blood (chocolate) agar supplemented with yeast extract; they grow only in the narrow temperature range of 35 to 37 °C and prefer a humid atmosphere enriched with 5% to 10% carbon dioxide. Most can grow on enriched agar containing colistin and vancomycin that inhibit the non-pathogenic *Neisseria* and many other members of the indigenous flora. They are very susceptible to drying. Both pathogenic species share a common outer membrane protein called H.8, and both species produce IgA protease.

Neisseria gonorrhoeae has a number of surface structural components that may play a role in the ability of the organism to produce disease. These include pili, outer membrane proteins, lipooligosaccharide (LOS), and peptidoglycan. Pili are hairlike filamentous appendages that can be seen by electron microscopy to extend from the bacterial surface. Pili are composed of repeating protein subunits (pilins) which are antigenic. A single gonococcal strain may produce pili of varying antigenic composition. Virulent fresh clinical isolates of *N. gonorrhoeae* have numerous pili and the colonies they form are small, opaque, and heaped up; these strains are designated Pil^+. Following about 24 hours of cultivation on laboratory media, chromosomal rearrangement causes phase variation to occur; nonpiliated organisms (Pil^-) predominate and the colonies become larger, flat, and translucent. Pil^- organisms are avirulent. Pili play a significant role in pathogenesis by participating in the attachment of the organism to nonciliated epithelial cells by overcoming the mutually repulsive negative electostatic forces between the surfaces of the gonococcus and the host cell. Pil^+ gonococci are more resistant to phagocytosis by neutrophils than Pil^- strains. Pil^+ strains are highly competent for the exchange of chromosomal DNA by transformation.

Several predominant proteins have been identified in the gonococcal outer membrane:

protein I (PI), which accounts for 60% of the protein in the outer membrane, and proteins II and III (PII, PIII). Protein I, present in all gonococci, functions as a porin by selectively permitting the passage of nutrient and waste molecules into and out of the cell. There is a possibility that protein I can move out of the membrane of the microorganism and into the membrane of the host cell, permitting a movement of molecules from the bacteria into the host tissues.

Production of the group of related proteins designated outer membrane protein II is genetically highly unstable. Strains with certain types of protein II produce opaque colonies; strains lacking this protein form transparent colonies. The presence of protein II enhances the attachment of the gonococci to certain mucosal cells and neutrophils, but strains with protein II have reduced adherence to fallopian tube cells. Most isolates from local mucosa contain protein II, but isolates from disseminated disease in normally sterile sites, e.g., blood, synovial fluid, and fallopian tubes, lack protein II. Protein II may be one of the binding sites for bactericidal antibody. Protein II is also involved in the stable adhesion of gonococci to host cell membranes, even in nonpiliated strains. Protein II–bearing strains have a tendency to clump in broth cultures; if these aggregates occur in vitro, they may act as "infectious units" by resisting phagocytosis.

Proteins I and II differ with respect to their resistance to cleavage by proteolytic enzymes, which may correlate with susceptibility to in vivo killing by serum enzymes. A third outer membrane protein (protein III, PIII) resembles protein I in that it is "surface-exposed," but its function in the pathogenesis is unknown. Protein III can stimulate blocking antibodies that reduce the bactericidal activity of serum against the gonococcus.

The LOS of *N. gonorrhoeae* differs from the lipopolysaccharide of other gram-negative bacteria in that it lacks the O antigen side chains. It has endotoxic activity, and mediates the loss of cilia and the death of uninfected cells adjacent to infected cells.

Peptidoglycan, which forms the rigid portion of the cell wall of the gonococcus, is formed rapidly, degraded into anhydrous peptidoglycan monomers, and released into the environment by gonococci. These monomers have ciliostatic activity and damage human fallopian tube mucosa with subsequent sloughing of ciliated cells, and may contribute to the inflammatory response in gonococcal infection.

The presence of IgA seems to be important in protecting mucosal surfaces from invasion by pathogenic bacteria. The ability of the gonococcus to produce an enzyme capable of hydrolyzing the immunoglobulin present on mucous membranes is thought to play a role in the pathogenesis of disease caused by these species, possibly by facilitating their adherence to epithelial cells and subsequent colonization.

There is evidence that iron has an important role in the virulence of *N. gonorrhoeae*, probably by influencing cellular functions. In order to obtain the iron required for growth, bacterial pathogens must compete with the host's iron-binding and storage proteins. These proteins occur in serum (transferrin), in mucosal secretions (lactoferrin), and in tissues (ferritin). Gonococci have mechanisms for utilizing the iron from the host's iron-binding proteins as well as from heme and hemoglobin.

PATHOGENESIS OF GONOCOCCAL INFECTION

Piliated gonococci have the ability to attach to sperm and this may represent the mechanism for transport throughout the female genital tract to establish infection in the fallopian tubes, or the epididymis in the male system. The contact of gonococci with human mucosal surfaces initiates a series of events leading to the attachment of the bacteria to the microvilli of nonciliated columnar epithelial cells.

Following attachment of the gonococci to the microvilli of columnar epithelial cells, the organisms enter these cells. (In the fallopian tubes, gonococci attach to the nonciliated cells while the ciliated cells slough off the mucosa.) The gonococci are transported in the phagocytic vacuoles to the base of the cell and the vacuoles are discharged from the cell, permitting the organisms to enter the subepithelial connective tissue. Here some gonococci are ingested by polymorphonuclear neutrophils and killed, but others survive and multiply, causing local disease. Tissue damage is primarily due to the lipid A of the LOS and the cell wall peptidoglycan. There is evidence that this damage potentiates the inflammatory response leading to the migration of leukocytes and the activation of complement.

Infection in prepubertal girls may result in vulvovaginitis, since the alkaline vaginal pH permits growth of the gonococci. In adult females the vaginal pH is acid owing to the fermentation of glycogen in epithelial cells by indigenous lactobacilli. The gonococcus is markedly inhibited by acid, and consequently, vaginal infection is uncommon.

Squamous epithelium as found in the vagina is less easily penetrated than the columnar epithelial layer of the urethra. Vaginal epithelial cells have been found to vary in their ability to bind bacteria during phases of the menstrual cycle.

HUMORAL IMMUNE RESPONSE TO GONOCOCCAL INFECTION

Patients with gonococcal infection have serum antibodies reactive with outer membrane proteins PI, PII, and PIII; with pili; and with LOS. Anti-PI antibodies may be bactericidal for the gonococcus. The role of anti-PII and anti-PIII antibodies is undefined. Antibodies to pili block pilus-mediated attachment to host cells. Men and women infected with the same strains of *N. gonorrhoeae* may have different immune responses.

In women, pili appear to be the predominant antigen in the immune response, while in men there are higher levels of other antibodies. Antibody against LOS can activate complement through the classic or alternative pathway; and can be chemotactic for polymorphonuclear leukocytes; anti-LOS IgM and IgG can be bactericidal, and IgA can block the IgG-mediated bactericidal activity. Specific IgA, IgG, and IgM have been found in cervical and vaginal secretions and urethral exudate in infected persons.

Gonococci, like other gram-negative bacteria, are susceptible to complement-mediated lysis. In the presence of specific antibody and complement, gonococci can be killed in the absence of phagocytic cells. The resistance of gonococci to complement-mediated killing appears to be important in the pathogenesis of infection because complement components from the blood can reach mucous membranes and underlying tissues during inflammation.

Virulent strains of gonococci resist killing by fresh immune serum more than avirulent strains. Outer membrane protein antigens with surface exposure may recognize naturally occurring antibodies that attach to gonococci and block complement-dependent lysis by serum bactericidal antibodies directed against the lipopolysaccharide. These blocking antibodies have been identified in the IgG fraction and may be important in the serum resistance of gonococci.

ANTIBIOTIC RESISTANCE

Prior to 1976 all gonococci were susceptible to penicillin. Since then penicillinase-producing strains of *N. gonorrhoeae* (PPNG) have been reported in the United States, England, and many other countries.

Two types of PPNG were originally described. The Far Eastern type, a proline-dependant auxotype, is also resistant to tetracycline. The plasmid for β-lactamase production in this type was 4.4 megadaltons. The West African

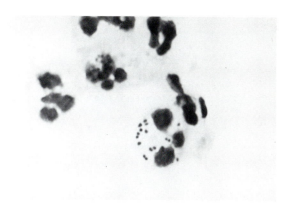

FIG 38–2.
Gonococci in exudate.

type, an arginine-dependent auxotype sensitive to tetracycline, carries a smaller 3.2-megadalton plasmid. By the mid-1980s both of these plasmid types were common throughout the world. The number of PPNG cases in the United States has increased steadily and has reached 10% to 40% in some metropolitan areas. Strains of chromosomally mediated penicillin and tetracycline resistance have also been rising in the United States.

DIAGNOSIS

A presumptive diagnosis may be made by visualizing gram-negative intracellular diplococci and leukocytes in a gram-stained smear of urethral or endocervical exudate (Fig 38–2). A definitive diagnosis depends upon the specific demonstration of *N. gonorrhoeae* in material from the patient by culture or by nucleic acid probe.

VACCINE

Attempts to produce a pili vaccine that would elicit antibodies inhibiting the attachment of organisms to urogenital cells have been frustrated by the strain variation in the antigenicity of the pili.

CHAPTER 39

Chlamydia

An 18-year-old male college student presented at the school infirmary complaining of mild but persistent urethral discomfort and a mucopurulent discharge. He had just returned from a 2-week holiday during which he had sexual intercourse with several girls. A Gram stain of the urethral exudate revealed many polymorphonuclear leukocytes, but no bacteria could be seen. Urethral scrapings were obtained for culture and he was started on tetracycline. The urethral culture was positive for *Chlamydia trachomatis.*

Chlamydia are coccoid bacteria about one-fourth the size of *Escherichia coli.* They resemble viruses in that they are strict intracellular parasites and cannot exist outside of avian or mammalian cells. They have a cell envelope similar to that of gram-negative bacteria and their cytoplasm contains both RNA and DNA. Chlamydia cannot generate their own energy but must use the adenosine triphosphate (ATP) of the host cell.

Chlamydia have a unique developmental cycle. There are two distinct forms of the organism: the **elementary body** and the **reticulate body.** The elementary body is spherical, about 200 to 300 nm in diameter, highly infectious, metabolically inactive, and seems to have surface ligands with a high affinity for normal configurations on the surface of host cells. The elementary body attaches to the host cell, possibly via sialic acid residues on the cell surface, enters the cell by endocytosis, and resides in the resulting phagosome separated from the host cytoplasm. Fusion of the phagosome with lysosomes is inhibited. After about 8 hours, the elementary body reorganizes into a larger reticulate body (800–1,000 nm in diameter) which is metabolically active but not infectious. The reticulate bodies replicate by binary fission and synthesize proteins and nucleic acids while inhibiting the macromolecular production of the host cell. As the reticulate bodies reproduce, the phagosome enlarges to form a microcolony (inclusion) within the host cytoplasm which can be visualized microscopically. The reticulate bodies eventually condense to form elementary bodies; the host cell lyses releasing the elementary bodies to infect other cells.

There are three species of chlamydia that infect humans: *C. trachomatis, C. psittaci,* and *C. pneumoniae.* All species share common antigens and the same reproductive cycle. *Chlamydia trachomatis* tends to produce localized infection in mucous membranes, while *C. psittaci* always produces a generalized infection.

Chlamydia come close to being the most successful parasite of all the microbial pathogens. Almost every species of bird and mammal is infected with chlamydia, in most cases an inapparent infection that does not severely damage the host. It is estimated that 10% to 20% of the world's human population is infected with chlamydia. The organism is highly infectious, easily transferred to new hosts, readily escapes immune responses, and rarely kills its host.

CHLAMYDIA TRACHOMATIS

Chlamydia trachomatis is the major cause of sexually transmitted disease in the United States today. It is estimated that every year approximately 3 million adults and adolescents in this country become infected with *C. trachomatis*. The organism is the cause of several different disease states: widespread **oculogenital infections** of adults; **lymphogranuloma venereum; neonatal conjunctivitis** and **pneumonia;** and **trachoma.** Chlamydial infections tend to become chronic and relapses are common.

Human strains of *C. trachomatis* can be divided into 15 different serotypes, which are associated with the above syndromes. Trachoma is caused by serotypes A, B, Ba, and C; lymphogranuloma venereum is caused by serotypes L-1, L-2, and L-3; and the oculogenital infections are caused by serotypes D–K. The group antigen shared with *C. psittaci* is located on the outer membrane of the organism and is a lipopolysaccharide. Species-specific antigens are proteins associated with the outer membrane.

OCULOGENITAL INFECTIONS

Nongonococcal urethritis (NGU) in males is estimated to be three times as common as gonococcal urethritis in the United States and Europe. About half of all cases of NGU are caused by *C. trachomatis*. The remaining cases are due to *Ureaplasma urealyticum*, herpesvirus, or are of unknown etiology.

The incubation period of chlamydial urethritis is 2 to 3 weeks and the symptoms are essentially the same as acute anterior gonococcal urethritis, namely, urethral discharge, dysuria, meatal itching, and occasionally fever. The urethral discharge tends to be scanty and mucoid, and the dysuria less severe and more chronic than in gonococcal urethritis. About 80% of patients with recurrent urethritis following penicillin treatment (postgonococcal urethritis) have chlamydia, since gonococcal and chlamydial urethritis may coexist. Epididymitis may occur, and proctitis is seen in homosexual males and heterosexual females.

Chlamydia trachomatis is a common cause of mucopurulent cervicitis. The infection is twice as frequent in women that use oral contraceptives, and may be asymptomatic or associated with cervical irritation. At least half of all females with gonorrhea also have cervical infection with *C. trachomatis*. Acute salpingitis occurs in 8% of women with chlamydial cervicitis, and carries a high risk of ectopic pregnancy and infertility.

Asymptomatic infection in pregnancy is associated with third-trimester spontaneous abortion, prematurity, low birth weight, and a tenfold increase in perinatal death. Four percent to 10% of pregnant women have cervical cultures positive for chlamydia, and there is a 50% probability that the infant will develop inclusion conjunctivitis, and a 10% chance of chlamydial pneumonitis. Pneumonitis or conjunctivitis occurs in 1 in 200 live births.

Chlamydia trachomatis is one of the causes of **acute urethral syndrome** in women. This infection, characterized by dysuria and frequency, may be confused with vaginitis or cystitis. Lymphogranuloma venereum (LGV) is an invasive genital tract infection caused by specific strains (serotypes) of *C. trachomatis*. LGV is endemic in tropical and developing countries, and is being seen with increasing frequency in the United States. This sexually transmitted disease is characterized by a 1 to 4-mm primary lesion on the external genitalia, which heals spontaneously in a few days, followed by inguinal lymphadenopathy. Over the next 1 to 4 weeks, the regional lymph nodes enlarge, become fluctuant, and eventually rupture. Headache, chills, fever, and myalgia are common. Proctitis may also develop.

Ocular infections due to *C. trachomatis* include two distinctly different syndromes: trachoma and inclusion conjunctivitis. Trachoma is a chronic disease, endemic in American Indians and developing countries. Trachoma is the major cause of preventable blindness in the world. Of the estimated 400 million people who have trachoma, 6 million are totally blind. The pathogenesis of trachoma appears to involve a massive B lymphocyte and plasma cell response in the conjunctiva and cornea. The role of chlamydial antigens and other immunologic responses is not known. The lymphoid follicles under the upper eyelid hypertrophy and the conjunctiva becomes inflamed and eventually scarred. This process causes the margin of the upper lid to turn in so that the lashes continually rub the cornea, producing scarring and blindness. Eye-to-eye transmission is the rule and infections are commonly acquired during infancy and early childhood.

In contrast to trachoma, inclusion conjunctivitis rarely leads to blindness. This is an acute follicular conjunctivitis that results from the introduction of infected genital discharges into the eye with the fingers during parturition. The conjunctivitis becomes more intense with ptosis and preauricular lymphadenopathy. Neonatal conjunctivitis develops between the 5th and 12th day of life and ranges from a mild infection to an acute purulent process. Chlamydial pneumonitis occurs during the first 3 months of life and is characterized by an afebrile course, tachypnea, and a staccato cough.

The pathogenicity of *C. trachomatis* is still not well understood. IgM, IgG, and IgA antibodies are detectable in infected persons. These antibodies can fix complement and neutralize the infectivity of chlamydia, but their role in immunity is obscure. Cell-mediated immunity also occurs. *Chlamydia trachomatis* can induce interferon production, but there is no evidence that interferon plays a role in resistance.

CHLAMYDIA PSITTACI

Psittacosis is primarily a disease of psittacine birds (i.e., parrots, parakeets, pigeons, and turkeys) that is transmissible to humans. The chlamydia are shed in the secretions from the eyes and nostrils and in the feces and remain viable in these dried materials. Man becomes infected by inhaling the organisms in these substances. The organism enters the bloodstream and spreads to the reticuloendothelial system. The incubation period is 7 to 14 days and the early symptoms are sore throat, chills, high fever, weakness, myalgia, and headache. The disease is a pneumonitis, and a nonproductive cough is common. Mild disease usually subsides in 2 to 3 weeks, but severe untreated pneumonia has a mortality of about 20%.

CHLAMYDIA PNEUMONIAE

In the mid-1980s a new chlamydial species was recovered from cases of acute respiratory disease. Initially thought to be a variant of *C. psittaci*, TWAR organisms (named for the laboratory designation of the first two isolates) are now considered to be a distinct species—*C. pneumoniae*. No bird or animal reservoir is known, and *C. pneumoniae* is believed to be a primary human pathogen. Transmission is person to person, probably via respiratory aerosols. The incubation period is unknown, but is probably long. Most cases occur outside the home. Epidemics take place in schools and closed population groups such as military units.

Chlamydia pneumoniae usually causes mild pneumonia or bronchitis in teenagers and young adults; many infections are asymptomatic. Severe pneumonia with death has been reported in older people, many of whom were hospitalized for a severe chronic illness such as a cardiopulmonary problem or kidney failure. *Chlamydia pneumoniae* probably accounts for 5% of all pneumonia, 5% of bronchitis, and 1% of pharyngitis. Pharyngitis, often accompanied by laryngitis, is a frequent early symptom. *Chlamydia pneumoniae* may be involved in 5% of sinusitis. Specific antibody to *C. pneumoniae* is very low in young children, increases in teenagers, and is present in about 50% of adults.

DIAGNOSIS OF CHLAMYDIAL INFECTIONS

Chlamydia trachomatis can be recovered from genital or ocular secretions by tissue cul-

ture. Direct antigen detection methods by fluorescent antibody or enzyme immunoassay are widely used. A nucleic acid probe is also available. Serology has little value in routine clinical practice. *Chlamydia psittaci* can also be cultured in a number of tissue cell lines, and the detection of a rise in titer of specific complement-fixing antibody is diagnostic. *Chlamydia pneumoniae* is difficult to grow in cell culture; the diagnosis is based upon specific antibody detected by microimmunofluorescence.

TREATMENT

Chlamydia are not susceptible to cell wall–active agents like penicillin or the cephalosporins. Tetracycline or erythromycin are the antimicrobials used in the treatment of chlamydial infections.

CHAPTER 40

Ureaplasma urealyticum

A marine recruit presented at sick call complaining of urinary urgency, burning on urination, and scrotal pain. On physical examination, there was marked tenderness of the right epididymis, and pus could be expressed from the meatus by urethral stripping. A Gram stain of the exudate revealed many polymorphonuclear leukocytes but no organism could be visualized. Culture of the exudate for *Neisseria gonorrheae* and *Chlamydia trachomatis* was negative, but *Ureaplasma urealyticum* was recovered.

Ureaplasma urealyticum is a member of the family Mycoplasmataceae which also contains the genus *Mycoplasma*. Mycoplasmas are the smallest free-living organisms. They are prokaryotes that differ from bacteria in lacking a cell wall, but like bacteria they can grow in artificial cell-free media. Mycoplasmas are pleomorphic, gram-negative, nonmotile, and facultatively anaerobic organisms that are widely distributed among plants and animals. In humans several species are indigenous to the oropharynx and the genital tract. The pathogenic species include *Mycoplasma pneumoniae, M. hominis,* and *Ureaplasma urealyticum*. Ureaplasmas were first re-

covered from men with nongonococcal urethritis as mycoplasmas that produced "tiny" colonies on the agar medium. They were initially called *T strains* (T for *tiny*) but subsequently were placed as a single species in the genus *Ureaplasma*.

Ureaplasma urealyticum prefers an acid environment, and produces a urease that breaks down urea to ammonia. Colonies appear in 24 to 48 hours on agar. At least 14 serotypes have been recognized in *U. urealyticum*.

The reservoir of *U. urealyticum* is the genital tract of sexually active men and women. The organisms are seldom present before puberty, except that up to one third of infant girls have their genitalia colonized by passage through the birth canal of an infected mother; this neonatal colonization rarely persists beyond 2 years of age. Transmission is via sexual contact, and results in colonization, which is frequently asymptomatic.

Because of the high colonization rate it has been difficult to associate *U. urealyticum* with specific syndromes. The organism is believed to be the etiologic agent of 10% to 40% of nongonococcal urethritis (NGU). (The majority of cases of NGU are due to *C. trachomatis*.) *Ureaplasma urealyticum* may cause epididymitis, prostatitis, and may be involved in male infertility. The organism has been shown to attach to the midpiece of sperm, markedly decreasing sperm motility.

In women, *U. urealyticum* has been associated with tubo-ovarian abscess and salpingitis, endometritis, and chorioamnionitis, and has been linked to perinatal problems such as spontaneous abortion, premature delivery, postpartum fever, and low-birth-weight infants. The neonate can develop pneumonia or meningitis.

Ureaplasmas have been implicated as one of the causes of urethral syndrome, characterized by dysuria, pyuria, and no demonstrable bacteria. Ureaplasmas have been isolated from normal ureters and kidneys; there is some evidence that some strains may be involved in the formation of urinary calculi.

Little is known of the pathogenetic mechanisms of ureaplasmas. The organism produces IgA protease which may facilitate colonization on mucous membranes. It is possible that cell damage could result from locally high concentrations of ammonia produced by the organism.

CHAPTER 41

Haemophilus ducreyi

A week after his arrival in the United States from Kenya, a college student presented with a painful ulcer on his penis and left inguinal lymphadenopathy. The swollen inguinal nodes were warm and tender. The student admitted to sexual intercourse with a prostitute shortly before departing Kenya. Direct Gram stain and darkfield examination of the ulcer were negative, but a culture of exudate from the base of the ulcer grew out *Haemophilus ducreyi*.

Haemophilus ducreyi, a gram-negative coccobacillus, is the etiologic agent of chancroid, a sexually transmitted disease characterized by single or multiple painful necrotizing ulcers on the genitals, often accompanied by swelling and suppuration of regional lymph nodes. *Haemophilus ducreyi* requires an enriched medium, a moist atmosphere supplemented with 5% to 10% carbon dioxide, and an incubation temperature of 33°C. Growth may take up to 9 days to appear. The organism has very limited biochemical activity. Virulence is lost on prolonged serial culture on laboratory media. The lipopolysaccharide of virulent strains differs from that of avirulent strains. The lipopolysaccharide seems to play a role in the susceptibility of *H. ducreyi* to the bactericidal activity of human serum; virulent strains are resistent to serum killing, while avirulent strains are susceptible to killing by serum.

The reservoir of *H. ducreyi* is in man. Transmission is by direct sexual contact with open lesions and pus from buboes. Chancroid is associated with low socioeconomic status and poor hygiene. Formerly considered to be common in developing countries, chancroid has become an important sexually transmitted disease in the United States. There have been nine large outbreaks in the United States since 1981. Chancroid is most often seen in non-white, uncircumcised men; only 10% of reported cases are in women, suggesting an asymptomatic carrier state. There is some evidence that chancroid is associated with an increased infection rate for acquired immunodeficiency syndrome (AIDS).

The incubation period is 3 to 7 days. The organism enters through a break in the integrity of the epithelium. The initial lesion is a small papule surrounded by a narrow erythematous zone. In 2 to 3 days a pustule forms and soon ruptures leaving an ulcer with ragged edges filled with yellow or gray purulent material. The ulcers are always painful and bleed easily when manipulated. About half of the patients develop painful, tender, inguinal lymph nodes (buboes), usually unilateral, which may become fluctuant and rupture leaving inguinal ulcers.

Men usually have single penile ulcers on the prepuce or coronal sulcus. Women often have multiple lesions at the entrance to the vagina on the labia, vestibule, and clitoris. Internal lesions, frequently painless, may occur on the vaginal walls or cervix.

The diagnosis of chancroid cannot be made clinically by the appearance of the ulcer, but requires culture of ulcer exudate. Chancroid lesions must be differentiated from ulcers caused by *Treponema pallidum* (syphilis), herpes simplex virus, or *Chlamydia trachomatis* (lymphogranuloma venereum).

The organisms produce β-lactamases and are often resistant to penicillins and to tetrocycline. Therapy is with ceftriaxone, trimethoprim/sufamethoxazole, or a fluoroquinolone.

CHAPTER 42

Agents of Vaginitis

Vaginitis is characterized by one or more of the following symptoms: increased volume of discharge; abnormal yellow or green color of discharge caused by increased concentration of polymorphonuclear leukocytes; vulvar itching or burning; introital dyspareunia; and malodor.

The major microbial causes of vaginitis are yeasts, *Trichomonas vaginalis*, and bacteria. The relative frequencies of these agents as causes of vulvovaginal symptoms varies markedly in different populations.

Yeasts are unicellular fungal organisms that reproduce by budding. Significant pathogenic genera include *Candida*, *Torulopsis*, and *Cryptococcus*. *Candida* are responsible for about one third of cases of vaginitis.

VAGINAL CANDIDIASIS

Candida are dimorphic fungi that normally grow as yeasts under most conditions, but have the ability to form pseudohyphae or true mycelia. *Candida albicans* is the most frequent agent of disease, but other species (*C. krusei, C. parapsilosis, C. tropicalis, C. guilliermondi, C. stellatoidea*) can also produce disease.

Candida albicans is a normal inhabitant of the alimentary tract and mucocutaneous sites such as the mouth and the vagina. The organism is present in the vagina of 5% to 10% of healthy, nonpregnant women; in 18% of nonpregnant women with a vaginal discharge; and in 30% of pregnant women.

The major cell wall constituent of *C. albicans* is mannan, a mannose glycoprotein. Other cell wall constituents include glucans and chitin. The cell wall composition of *C. albicans* varies in response to growth conditions in vitro and in vivo.

Candida albicans is responsible for about 80% of vulvovaginal yeast infections. Other species of *Candida* such as *C. tropicalis* are involved in about 15% of infection, and a related organism, *Torulopsis glabrata*, accounts for 3% to 16% of vaginal yeast infections.

Candidal vulvovaginitis is characterized by perivaginal pruritus and a thick, adherent discharge that contains curdlike matter. The vaginal walls are often erythematous. Recurrent infections are common, and are usually due to reinfection by new strains of *Candida*. The initiation of candidal disease is usually the result of overgrowth by the yeast which is apparently favored by high estrogen levels. The indigenous bacterial flora suppresses mucosal colonization by *C. albicans*, and suppression of the normal flora by antibiotics makes rats and mice more susceptible to gastrointestinal candidiasis. The attachment of *C. albicans* to mucosal epithelial cells is important in the pathogenesis of mucocutaneous candidiasis. The adherence rate of *C. albicans* and *C. tropicalis* exceeds that of less virulent *Candida* species; the germ tube phase (which initiates the conversion into pseudohyphae or mycelia) is 2 to 50 times more adherent than the yeast phase.

Mannans and mannoproteins are important constituents of the adhesin. Host cell ligands for the adhesin are probably membrane glycoproteins or glycolipids, but fibronectin and laminin may also play a role in attachment. Hyphal forms of *C. albicans* have less mannan and more chitin than the yeast phase.

Under certain conditions, the hyphae may invade the tissues, producing acute inflammation and tissue damage. Vulvovaginal candidiasis is more common in pregnancy, and with the use of oral contraceptives. Other predisposing factors are poorly controlled diabetes mellitus, treatment with broad-spectrum antibiotics, and acquired immunodeficiency syndrome (AIDS). The basis for the pathogenicity of *C. albicans* is not known, but the observation has been made that the hyphal form is usually seen in infection, whereas the yeast form is not generally associated with disease. In a number of *Candida* infections, it has been shown that the clinical onset of disease is preceded by transformation of the yeasts to the hyphal phase. Hyphal penetration of mucosal epithelial cells is believed to be the result of enzymatic lysis and mechanical force. Two hydrolytic enzymes of *C. albicans* that may act as virulence factors are phospholipase and an acidic carboxyl protease. It has also been demonstrated that receptors that can bind complement-derived opsonins are present on the surface of *C. albicans* yeast cells and pseudohyphae; these receptors may mask opsonic ligands and reduce uptake and killing of the pathogen by phagocytes.

The majority of people have antibodies to *C. albicans* in their serum and secretory globulins. However, those who have high levels of antibodies may have poor resistance to *Candida* infection. IgA antibodies found in oral and vaginal secretions could protect against infection by interfering with fungal colonization of mucosal surfaces. Cell-mediated immunity appears to be more important than humoral antibodies for defense against *C. albicans*. The importance of cell-mediated immunity is seen in the frequency of chronic mucocutaneous candidiasis in patients with genetic defects of T cell function.

C. albicans mannan can stimulate or suppress cell-mediated and humoral immune responses and may play a major role in immunosuppression leading to chronic mucocutaneous candidiasis.

TRICHOMONAS VAGINALIS

Trichomonas vaginalis is a highly motile protozoan that reproduces by binary fission. It is almost always acquired by sexual contact. The incubation period is 5 to 28 days. Males and approximately 25% of females are asymptomatic. Characteristic symptoms include vulvovaginal soreness, dysuria, and a discharge. *Trichomonas vaginalis* usually produces a profuse, yellow, purulent, homogeneous discharge which is often malodorous and may be frothy, presumably because of gas production by vaginal bacteria. The vaginal epithelium is inflamed, and petechial lesions may be present on the cervix.

BACTERIAL VAGINOSIS

Bacterial vaginosis is believed to be a noninflammatory synergistic, polymicrobial infection characterized by the massive overgrowth of certain bacterial species. These organisms include *Gardnerella vaginalis*, non-*fragilis Bacteroides* species, *Mobiluncus* species, and possibly *Mycoplasma hominis*. There is no evidence that the infection is sexually transmitted.

Gardnerella vaginalis is a nonmotile, pleomorphic, gram-negative coccobacillus that is

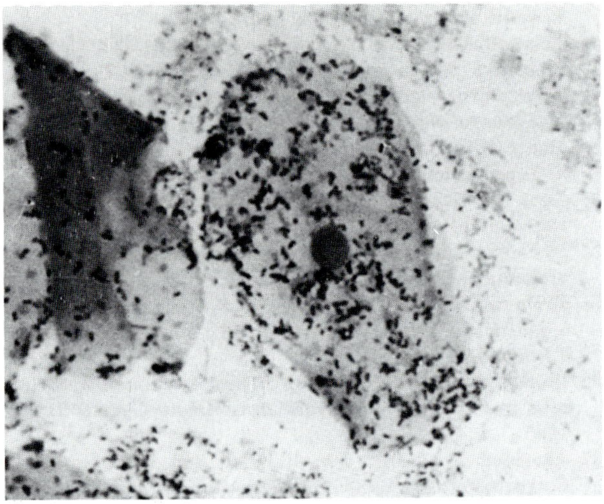

FIG 42–1.
Vaginal epithelial cells covered with *G. vaginalis* ("clue cells). Although *G. vaginalis* is gram-positive, the bacteria will typically appear as small gram-negative or gram-variable bacilli. *(From Holmes K, et al: Sexually Transmitted Diseases. New York, McGraw-Hill, 1984. Used by permission.)*

present in 40% to 70% of the vaginal flora of asymptomatic females of reproductive age. *Mobiluncus* are motile, curved, anaerobic gram-negative rods which have been recovered from the rectum and vagina of 80% of women with bacterial vaginosis. *Bacteroides bivius* and *B. capillosis*, anaerobic, gram-negative bacilli, are also frequently associated with bacterial vaginosis. The overgrowth of these bacteria is accompanied by a marked decrease in the numbers of *Lactobacillus* species, gram-positive bacilli that are the predominant vaginal flora of healthy women.

The infection is characterized by increased vaginal discharge that is typically grayish-white and homogeneous, a vaginal pH greater than 4.7, a "fishy" odor due to the presence of amines in the vaginal secretions, and the appearance of "clue cells," vaginal epithelial cells covered with

coccobacilli (Fig 42–1). At least 35% of women with bacterial vaginosis are users of intrauterine devices.

There is evidence that bacterial vaginosis can predispose to the development of acute salpingitis and other upper genital tract infections such as chorioamnionitis. In addition, there may be increased susceptibility to premature rupture of membranes, premature labor, and postpartum fever and endometritis.

The diagnosis of vaginitis cannot be made solely on clinical grounds. An accurate differential diagnosis requires determination of the vaginal pH, examination of a wet mount of vaginal secretions for yeasts, motile trichomonads, or clue cells, and testing of the secretions with 10% potassium hydroxide for generation of a fishy amine odor.

PART IX

Urinary Tract Infections

CHAPTER 43

Overview of Urinary Tract Infections

Urinary tract infections are among the most common infectious diseases of man, second only to respiratory infections in frequency. Nearly all urinary tract infections are bacterial, whereas most respiratory infections are viral. The largest single use of antibiotics is for the treatment of urinary tract infections. Many people have undiagnosed urinary tract infections; at autopsy 15% to 30% show some evidence of renal lesions, yet only 20% of this population are diagnosed during life as having urinary tract infections.

Bacteriuria, the presence of bacteria in the urine, is the hallmark of urinary tract infections. Bacteriuria may be asymptomatic, or associated with lower or upper urinary tract infection. Lower tract infection, also referred to as **cystitis,** is usually limited to the bladder. Upper tract infection involves the ureters and the kidneys (**pyelonephritis).** Urinary tract infection is designated as "complicated" when anatomic abnormalities, urinary calculi, or a foreign body is present, or in patients with pregnancy, diabetes, prostatitis, or other underlying diseases. Recurrent urinary tract infection may be due to reinfection, or relapse associated with persistence of the infecting organism.

EPIDEMIOLOGY

Approximately 1% of infants (mostly boys) have bacteriuria. In preschool children, the prevalence of bacteriuria is 0.5% in boys and 4.5% in girls. In children aged 5 to 15 years, the prevalence of asymptomatic bacteruria is less than 0.1% in boys and 1% increasing to 5% in girls. In adult men, the prevalence remains less than 0.1% until age 50 and then rapidly rises to 4% to 15%. In nonpregnant women, the prevalence increases about 1% per decade with age to 10% to 15%; 4% to 7% of pregnant women are bacteriuric. Among elderly institutionalized men, the prevalence of bacteriuria is 33%. The average urinary infection rate for women is 2.6 per patient-year with a range of 0.3 to 7.6 episodes per year, 73% of which are symptomatic. The ratio of cystitis to pyelonephritis episodes is 18:1.

PATHOGENESIS

The urinary tract is normally sterile, except for the first 2 to 3 cm of the anterior urethra and the vaginal introitus, which are colonized by a predominantly gram-positive flora that includes coagulase-negative staphylococci, diphtheroids, enterococci, viridans streptococci, lactobacilli, and anaerobes.

The first phase leading to infection is the "contamination" of the introitus and distal urethra with predominantly gram-negative fecal organisms. Factors that determine the outcome of the contamination episode are the numbers of organisms and their virulence, which has been associated with motility, the presence of pili, production of urease, and certain capsular antigens of *Escherichia coli*. These gram-negative species attach to the epithelial cells by various types of pili or other adhesins, colonize the periurethral region, and ascend into the bladder. This passage is expedited by the shorter female urethra. Entrance to the bladder may be precipitated by the mild urethral trauma of sexual intercourse or an improperly fitted or placed diaphragm. In males, entry of bacteria into the bladder is usually the result of instrumentation. Most gram-negative bacteria reach the bladder and kidneys by this **ascending route.** The exception to this are kidney infections, usually abscesses due to *Staphlycoccus aureus* or *Candida albicans*, which reach the kidney via the bloodstream from a distant focus. Bacteria multiply in bladder urine resulting in an inflammatory reaction.

Bacteria may ascend the ureters (especially if vesicoureteral reflux is present) to reach the renal pelvis and calyces and invade the renal parenchyma beginning with the medulla. The renal medulla is far more susceptible to infection than the renal cortex. It is postulated that the susceptibility of the medulla is due to its relatively low blood supply and hypertonicity, which depresses phagocytes, and ammonia, which inactivates complement. The normal kidney is resistant to infection, and bacteria reaching the kidney are cleared within about 7 days by phagocytes without inflammation or infection. Obstruction anywhere in the urinary tract mark-

edly interferes with renal clearance with resulting pyelonephritis. Other predisposing factors for pyelonephritis are preexisting renal disease, diabetes mellitus, hypertension, and pregnancy. Forty percent of pregnant women with bacteriuria develop pyelonephritis if untreated.

HOST DEFENSES OF THE URINARY TRACT

The most important defense mechanisms are the mechanical flushing action associated with micturition and the rapid turnover of mucosal epithelial cells. Urine is a relatively good culture medium, but the urea content, osmolality, and low pH are critical factors; the pH and osmolality of urine from pregnant women is more suitable for bacterial growth than urine from nonpregnant women, which in turn is a better growth medium than urine from men. Prostatic and periurethral secretions have an antibacterial effect, owing at least in part to IgA. Bacteria reaching the bladder are normally cleared within a few days by dilution and the flushing action of urine, as well as by the antibacterial action of the bladder mucosa. Additional host factors are those which interfere with bacterial adherence: the normal indigenous bacterial flora of the urethra, vaginal introitus, and periurethral region; urinary oligosaccharides; immunoglobulins and Tamm-Horsfall protein *; and mucopolysaccharides of the bladder mucosa (Fig 43–1).

PREDISPOSING FACTORS

The most important factors are those that interfere with complete emptying of the bladder,

*Tamm-Horsfall protein is a large glycoprotein produced by the cells in the ascending limb of the loop of Henle. It forms a slime in urine left standing overnight, and is the major constituent of the matrix of urinary casts. Its function is unknown. Antibodies to this protein are sometimes found in patients with obstructive kidney disease.

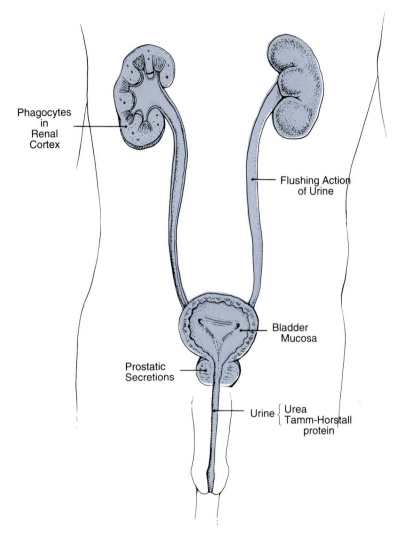

Phagocytes
in
Renal
Cortex

Flushing Action
of Urine

Bladder
Mucosa

Prostatic
Secretions

Urine $\left\{\begin{array}{l}\text{Urea}\\ \text{Tamm-Horstall}\\ \text{protein}\end{array}\right.$

FIG 43–1.
Defenses of the urinary system.

resulting in urinary stasis. This may be due to obstruction, secondary to congenital abnormalities, urinary calculi, prostatic hypertrophy, hydronephrosis, or neurogenic bladder. Urinary calculi also produce local irritation. Additional factors include sexual intercourse, which may lead to vaginal colonization; vesicoureteral reflux; and any type of instrumentation of the genitourinary tract. The risk of infection from catheterization of the bladder varies by type of patient. Only 1% to 2% of healthy young females who are catheterized develop infection, whereas 9% to 20% of hospitalized elderly men and women become infected.

The vaginal, periurethral, and uroepithelial cells of patients with recurrent urinary tract infections appear to have increased receptivity for bacterial attachment. There is some evidence that this increased receptivity may be due to a higher P fimbriae receptor density on the surface of the uroepithelial cells of these patients. It has been shown that women of blood groups B and AB who are nonsecretors of blood group substances have a significantly higher risk of developing urinary tract infections than do women of other blood groups or those who are secretors. Further studies have shown that 85% of high-risk women are of the P_2 phenotype (P_1). The possibility exists that histocompatibility antigens such as HLA-A3 may be a genetic determinant of increased susceptibility to urinary tract infections.

ETIOLOGIC AGENTS

More than 80% of urinary tract infections in women are caused by *E. coli*, and the remainder by other gram-negative bacilli and *Staphylococcus saprophyticus*. In men, about 80% of infections are caused by gram-negative bacilli, and the remainder by gram-positive organisms such as enterococci and coagulase-negative staphylococci other than *S. saprophyticus*.

CLINICAL MANIFESTATIONS

Cystitis is characterized by dysuria (painful urination), urinary frequency and urgency, and occasionally suprapubic tenderness. Cystitis is usually associated with significant bacteriuria (greater than 100,000/mL of urine) and pyuria (containing leukocytes). At least 20% to 30% of women with the symptoms of lower tract infec-

tion have urine that contains leukocytes but with low numbers of, or no bacteria. This presentation has been termed **urethral syndrome** or **dysuria-pyuria syndrome.**

Pyelonephritis is a syndrome of flank pain, fever, sometimes nausea and vomiting, costovertebral angle tenderness, and dysuria, urgency, and frequency.

Acute prostatitis is a febrile illness characterized by chills, low back and perineal pain, myalgia, arthralgia, dysuria, urinary urgency and frequency, and some degree of bladder outlet obstruction.

DIAGNOSIS

The hallmark of urinary tract infection is significant bacteriuria and pyuria. Microscopic examination of a drop of voided urine, preferably the first morning specimen, usually reveals leukocytes and bacteria. Various screening techniques for bacteriuria such as filtration, leukocyte esterase, nitrite determination, or bioluminescence detection of bacterial adenosine triphosphate, have sensitivities of about 90% for specimens containing bacterial counts greater than 100,000/mL, but quantitative urine culture is a relatively simple procedure. Women with urethral syndrome may have counts as low as 100 to 1,000/mL, or the urine may be sterile. In such cases, infection with gonococci, chlamydia, or herpes simplex virus should be considered.

In situations where contamination with fecal, urethral, or introital bacteria cannot be avoided, suprapubic bladder aspiration is a safe and simple alternative to catheterization.

CHAPTER 44

Uropathogenic Bacteria

A 23-year-old woman presented to her physician because of back pain, fever, and dysuria of 3 days' duration. One year previously, while on her honeymoon, she had an episode of cystitis for which she received a short course of sulfonamide and became asymptomatic within a few days. Six months later, she had a similar episode which again responded to antimicrobial treatment. The present episode began 3 days earlier when she noted dysuria, urgency, and blood-tinged urine. The next day, she had a fever and bilateral flank pain. On physical examination, she had a temperature of 38.8°C, and costovertebral angle and suprapubic tenderness. The urine contained many white blood cells, and a Gram stain of the urine revealed numerous gram-negative rods. Quantitative culture of the urine showed it to contain more than 100,000/mL of *Escherichia coli*.

Uropathogens are bacteria that are able to ascend the urinary tract, especially in the presence of challenging host defense mechanisms, and induce disease. *Escherichia coli* is the most common uropathogen, accounting for 85% of community-acquired urinary tract infections.

The remainder of community-acquired infections are caused by other Enterobactericeae such as *Proteus* and *Klebsiella* species, and by *Staphlyococcus saprophyticus*.

In hospitalized patients, *E. coli* still accounts for 50% of urinary tract infections, and other organisms such as *Enterobacter, Citrobacter, Serratia, Providencia, Pseudomonas, Enterococcus, Staphylococcus*, and *Candida* account for the remainder of cases.

ESCHERICHIA COLI

Escherichia coli are members of the *Enterobacteriaceae*, a large family of gram-negative, facultative bacilli that are widely distributed in soil, water, and the intestinal tracts of man and animals. A partial listing of the groups and numbers of species is given in Table 44–1. Many of these species contain multiple strains.

The major antigens of the Enterobacteriaceae family are the K antigens of encapsulated strains; the H (flagellar) antigens of motile strains; and the O antigens of the cell wall, a lipopolysaccharide-mucopeptide complex with side chains specific for each species. *Escherichia coli* is the organism most commonly recovered from clinical material. It is the etiologic agent of 90%

TABLE 44–1.

Partial Listing of Groups and Species of the Family Enterobacteriaceae

Group	No. of Species
Escherichia-Shigella	8
Klebsiella	7
Proteus	4
Enterobacter	13
Citrobacter	4
Serratia	10
Morganella	2
Providencia	5
Cedecea	5
Edwardsiella	4
Hafnia	2
Salmonella	12
Tatumella	1
Yersinia	11

of community-acquired urinary tract infections. Enterotoxigenic and enteroinvasive strains are responsible for a significant proportion of infectious diarrheal diseases. Extraintestinal infections caused by *E. coli* include neonatal meningitis, pneumonia, hepatobiliary infections, and abdominal and pelvic abscesses. *Escherichia coli* accounts for 40% of all nosocomial infections. Bacteremic *E. coli* infection has a fatality rate of 26%. *Escherichia coli* is antigenically complex. There are at least 155 somatic (O), 100 capsular (K), and 50 flagellar (H) antigens.

The invasive capability of *E. coli* has been correlated with its ability to resist killing by fresh normal human serum. Strains resistant to killing by neutrophils and by fresh human serum have a polysaccharide capsule designated as K1. The K1 capsule is unique among *E. coli* capsular polysaccharides in providing protection against serum killing. The K1 antigen is a polymer of *N*-acetylneuraminic acid, and has a negative charge, a neutral pH, and is immunologically identical to the capsular material of group B *Neisseria meningitidis*. The virulence of *E. coli* in extraintestinal invasive disease correlates very strongly with the presence of the K1 antigen. More than 70% of cases of *E. coli* neonatal meningitis are caused by strains with the K1 antigen.

Uropathogenic strains of *E. coli* usually originate in the colon. From the feces they colonize the uroepithelia of the vaginal introitus and the periurethral region. In some patients, this leads to bacteriuria, mucosal invasion, inflammation, and cell death, expressed clinically as cystitis or pyelonephritis. Strains causing urinary tract infections in patients without urologic abnormalities typically possess certain phenotypic virulence factors. In contrast, urinary tract infections in patients with predisposing medical or urologic conditions are often caused by fecal strains lacking these virulence factors. Virulence factors include serotypes associated with certain O and K antigens (O1, O2, O4, O6, O7, O8, O18, O25, O68, O75, K1, K5, K12, K13); resistance to the bactericidal action of normal human serum; production of hemolysin, aerobactin, and colicin V; and the capacity to adhere to and colonize the urogenital mucosa by means of protein adhesins that bind to receptors on the surface of epithelial cells.

Escherichia coli adhesin proteins are usually located on the distal tips of thin filaments termed *pili* or *fimbriae*, which are nonflagellar appendages, visible by electron microscopy and found on many strains. There are three classes of chromosomally encoded adhesins of uropathogenic *E. coli*: type 1 (common) pili, which can be produced by all *E. coli*; Gal-Gal pili; and X-binding adhesins.

Type 1 pili bind mannose-containing glycoproteins on uroepithelial surfaces, and play a role in establishing bladder infections. Type 1 pili also mediate bacterial hemagglutination; this reaction is inhibited by mannose and certain mannose-containing oligosaccharides. Tamm-Horsfall protein, a mannose-containing substance that occurs in urine, can entrap type 1 piliated *E. coli* and interfere with the ability of the organisms to colonize mucosa. When *E. coli* is grown in laboratory media, phase variation occurs with the loss of pili and the ability of the organism to adhere to uroepithelia. Phase variation can occur in vivo with the reappearance of type 1 pili.

Gal-Gal pili are associated with P fimbriae and bind α-galactosyl-1, 4-β-galactose, a saccharide component of some glycoproteins and glycosphingolipids that make up the antigens of the human P blood group system. Gal-Gal pili are present in 100% of *E. coli* isolates from the urine of patients with pyelonephritis and in 65% of patients with cystitis. These pili are probably essential for the production of pyelonephritis in most women with anatomically normal urinary tracts, whereas type 1 pili may be important in the production of cystitis. X-binding adhesins are heterogeneous among *E. coli* strains and can agglutinate erythrocytes in the presence of D-mannose and Gal-α-1, 4-Gal.

During both cystitis and pyelonephritis, it is probable that the lipopolysaccharide component of the O antigen plays an important role in inducing the local inflammatory response. Lipopolysaccharide also facilitates the ascent of *E. coli* to the kidneys by reducing ureteric peristalsis, resulting in relatively dilated, hypotonic ureters. Strains of *E. coli* with the complete O polysaccharide moiety are usually less susceptible to serum bactericidal activity (mediated through the classic and alternative pathways of complement) than rough strains. Serum resistance may also be associated with capsular K antigens.

Hemolysins are cytotoxic polypeptides that lyse erythrocytes. Hemolysins are believed to contribute to the spread of *E. coli* within the renal parenchyma by inducing membrane damage and acting as a pore-forming cytolysin. Hemolysin promotes microbial growth by releasing iron from lysed erythrocytes and other cells.

Aerobactin is a bacterial siderophore (an iron sequestration and transport system) which enables *E. coli* to grow in iron-poor environments such as dilute urine and complement-depleted serum. It is recognized as a virulence factor in strains causing pyelonephritis and

urosepsis (bacteremia) in noncompromised patients.

Colicin V is one of a group of plasmid-mediated proteins produced by strains of *E. coli* that inhibit other *E. coli* strains as well as other enterobacterial species. Colicins are used in typing *E. coli* strains.

In summary, the virulence of uropathogenic *E. coli* is the aggregate of these various factors.

KLEBSIELLA

Species of this nonmotile genus of gram-negative bacilli often possess a thick mucoid capsule, and are generally resistant to ampicillin and carbenicillin. They are frequently recovered from urinary tract infections, wound infections, bacteremia, and occasionally from meningitis. *Klebsiella* is a common cause of nosocomial infections. *Klebsiella pneumoniae* can cause a primary pneumonia (Friedländer's pneumonia) which was most frequently seen in older men, especially men suffering from alcoholism, diabetes, or chronic obstructive pulmonary disease. Within the past decade, *Klebsiella* has accounted for less than 1% of cases of community-acquired pneumonia, but is a common cause of nosocomial pneumonia. It also causes bacteremia, wound, and nosocomial urinary infection.

ENTEROBACTER

Most commonly, *E. aerogenes* and *E. hafnia* are recovered from urinary tract infections. *Enterobacter gergoviae* has been isolated from wound and urinary tract infections, and *E. sakazakii* has been the agent in some cases of neonatal meningitis. *E. cloacae* causes many types of nosocomial infection and outbreaks of nosocomial bacteremia have resulted from the administration of intravenous fluids contaminated with *E. cloacae* or *E. agglomerans*.

PROTEUS, MORGANELLA, AND PROVIDENCIA

These highly motile gram-negative bacilli are often recognized in the laboratory by their characteristic swarming on moist agar plates (rather than forming discrete colonies). All *Proteus* and the closely related *Morganella* species are potent producers of urease, and can grow at an alkaline pH.

Proteus mirabilis is a common agent of community-acquired urinary tract infections. The organism can split urea to ammonia, resulting in a highly alkaline urine. The high urinary pH predisposes the patient to the formation of urinary calculi by inducing the precipitation of salts normally present in the urine. The alkaline urine also diminishes the efficacy of many antimicrobial agents used in treating urinary tract infections. *Proteus mirabilis* can infect wounds, often in combination with other bacterial species. Indole-positive species (*P. vulgaris*, *M. morganii*) are more often seen in hospitalized patients.

Providencia species can cause nosocomial wound and burn infections. The organisms may become endemic in burn or intensive care units, and are often multiply resistant to antibiotics. All species of *Proteus*, *Morganella*, and *Providencia* can cause urinary infections and septicemia.

SERRATIA

Many strains of *Serratia* produce a pink or red pigment. Before the pathogenic potential of these organisms was recognized, they were widely used as tracer or indicator organisms in studies of aerosol dissemination or water supplies. *Serratia marcescens* are important causes of nosocomial infections and are of serious concern because they are often resistant to antimicrobial agents. They have caused pneumonia in association with contaminated respiratory equipment, and they also cause wound and urinary tract infections, and septicemia. They are resistant to many antimicrobial agents.

NONFERMENTERS

Approximately 15% of the aerobic gram-negative bacilli recovered from clinical specimens are nonfermenters. These gram-negative organisms are widely distributed in water and soil, and many species are commonly present in the hospital environment. Some genera are part of the indigenous flora of man and animals and include *Pseudomonas*, *Acinetobacter*, *Flavobacterium*, *Alcaligenes*, and *Kingella*. Only two species are primary pathogens: *Pseudomonas mallei* and *P. pseudomallei*, the etiologic agents of glanders and melioidosis, respectively. The remainder of the nonfermenters are opportunistic pathogens. *Pseudomonas aeruginosa* is the species most frequently encountered in clinical material. Urinary tract infections caused by this organism are common in hospitalized patients following instrumentation or catheterization with indwelling catheters.

STAPHYLOCOCCUS SAPROPHYTICUS

Staphylococcus saprophyticus is, after *E. coli*, the second most frequent causative agent of acute primary, nonobstructive urinary tract infections in young persons, both female and male. The organism is a gram-positive coccus, one of several species of coagulase-negative staphylococci. The main reservoir of *S. saprophyticus* is not known, but the organism is found in the normal urethral flora of some persons. There is a seasonal variation in *S. saprophyticus* urinary tract infection with peaks during late summer and early autumn. The mechanism of spread is not known, and the pathogenesis is poorly defined. The adhesin for *S. saprohyticus* is a lactosamine structure that binds to an oligosaccharide receptor on the surface of uroepithelial cells.

Patients with urinary tract infections caused by *S. saprophyticus* usually present with symptomatic cystitis. There is evidence that spread to the kidneys occurs in approximately one-half of all cases. The organism is a urease producer. The urine sediment of patients infected with this organism has a typical microscopic appearance, with leukocytes, erythrocytes, and numerous cocci occurring both in clumps and adhering to cellular elements and casts.

PART X

Oral Infections

CHAPTER 45

Overview of Oral Infections

The microbial flora of the mouth is complex. The oral cavity is not a uniform environment but rather consists of several sites, such as the tongue, tooth surfaces, gingival crevices (sulci), and saliva. These sites and saliva have their own characteristic microflora.

The infant's mouth is sterile in utero and at birth and a consistent oral flora is not established until after the third month of life. By 1 year the flora is essentially the same as an adult's.

Adult saliva contains 5 to 6 billion microorganisms per milliliter, divided among approximately 30 species, mostly derived from the dorsal surface of the tongue. Viridans streptococci, *Peptostreptococcus*, *Veillonella*, *Lactobacillus*, *Corynebacterium*, and *Actinomyces* account for more than 80% of the total bacterial flora. The predominant bacterial species from various sites of the oral cavity are given in Table 45–1.

Multiple factors regulate the microbial flora of the mouth. The selective adherence characteristics of each bacterial species, and local environmental conditions such as pH, oxidation-reduction potential, and the presence or absence of teeth determine the composition of the bacterial flora at each site. Additional factors that modulate the oral flora are diet and nutrition, oral hygiene, smoking habits, antimicrobial therapy, hospitalization, pregnancy, the presence of dental caries or periodontal disease, and genetic

or racial factors. Phagocytosis and the composition of saliva (ionic strength; mineral, protein, and carbohydrate content) are additional determinants of the qualitative and quantitative composition of the oral flora. Saliva contains both inhibitory substances (lysozyme and specific immunoglobulins) and stimulatory factors for microorganisms.

The complex host-parasite relationship that exists within the oral cavity involving regulatory factors and a concentrated and varied microbial population often becomes unbalanced with the resulting development of oral infection. These infections may involve the soft tissues of the mouth; the teeth; or the salivary glands, especially the parotid glands. Additionally, the mouth may be involved in a wide variety of systemic viral, bacterial, and mycotic infections.

APHTHOUS STOMATITIS

Stomatitis is a general term for inflammation of the oral mucosa. The buccal or labial mucosa, palate, tongue, floor of the mouth, and gingivae may be involved.

Aphthous stomatitis is the most common cause of recurrent oral ulcers. Characteristically, small ulcers appear in the anterior portion of the oral cavity on the buccal and labial mucosa, the

TABLE 45–1.

Predominant Cultivable Bacteria From Various Sites of the Oral Cavity*

Type	Predominant Genus or Family	Total Viable Count (Mean %)			
		Gingival Crevice	Dental Plaque	Tongue	Saliva
Facultative					
Gram positive cocci	Streptococcus	28.8	28.2	44.8	46.2
	S. mutans	(0–30)	(0–50)	(0–1)	(0–1)
	S. sanguis	(10–20)	(40–60)	(10–20)	(10–30)
	S. mitior	(10–30)	(20–40)	(10–30)	(30–50)
	S. salivarius	(0–1)	(0–1)	(40–60)	(40–60)
Gram positive rods	Lactobacillus	15.3	23.8	13.0	11.8
	Corynebacterium				
Gram negative cocci	Branhamella	0.4	0.4	3.4	1.2
Gram negative rods	Enterobacteriaeae	1.2	ND	3.2	2.3
Anaerobic	Peptostreptococcus	7.4	12.6	4.2	13.0
Gram positive cocci					
Gram positive rods	Actinomyces				
	Eubacterium	20.2	18.4	8.2	4.8
	Lactobacillus				
	Leptotrichia				
Gram negative cocci	Veillonella	10.7	6.4	16.0	15.9
Gram negative rods	Fusobacterium	1.9	4.1	0.7	0.3
	Bacteroides, pigmented	4.7	ND	0.2	ND
	Bacteroides, nonpigmented	5.6	4.8	5.1	2.4
	Campylobacter	3.8	1.3	2.2	2.1
Spirochetes	Treponema	1.0	ND	ND	ND

ND = not detected.
*From Mandell GL, Douglas Jr RG, Bennett JE (eds): *Principles and Practice of Infectious Disease*, ed 3. New York, Churchill Livingstone, 1990, p 517.

floor of the mouth, or the tongue. The ulcers are grayish-yellow with a raised erythematous margin, and are very painful. Ulcers persist for several days to 2 weeks and heal spontaneously. The cause of aphthous stomatitis is not known; there is some evidence that it is an autoimmune phenomenon.

ACUTE HERPETIC GINGIVOSTOMATITIS

Herpes stomatitis is an acute inflammatory infection of the oral mucosa caused by herpes simplex virus type 1 (HSV-1). (Herpes simplex viruses are described in Chapter 27.) Herpes stomatitis is the result of primary HSV-1 infection and occurs mainly in children between 6 months and 5 years of age. In neonates or immunosuppressed patients, infection may disseminate to the lungs, liver, and other viscera. Transmission of the infection is by contact with HSV-1 in the saliva of carriers.

The incubation period is 2 to 12 days. Primary infection with HSV-1 may be mild and inapparent, but in 10% of persons it may be of moderate severity with the abrupt onset of fever, anorexia, irritability, and gingivostomatitis. The gums become hyperemic, swollen, and bleed easily. Vesicular lesions commonly appear on the tongue, the inner surface of the lips, and the buccal and sublingual mucosa. The vesicles quickly rupture leaving tender, shallow, yellowish-gray indurated ulcers. The anterior cervical and submandibular lymph nodes are enlarged and tender. The ulcers heal in 4 to 7 days. The cause of primary infection in adults is essentially the same but less severe.

Regardless of severity, primary HSV-1 infection is followed by lifelong persistent infection. The virus remains latent in the trigeminal ganglion until reactivation, resulting in recurrent infection. Reactivation may be precipitated by trauma, exposure to sunlight, fever, menstruation, or emotional stress.

Recurrent infection commonly results in **herpes labialis** (fever blisters or cold sores) and occurs in up to 50% of adults. The brief prodrome of pain, burning, tingling, or itching is followed by raised papules, usually on the vermilion border of the lip. Within hours the papules become vesicles which become pustular and burst within 2 days, leaving a scar. Healing is complete within 6 to 10 days.

ACUTE NECROTIZING ULCERATIVE GINGIVITIS

Acute necrotizing ulcerative gingivitis (ANUG, Vincent's infection, fusospirochetosis) is an ulcerative necrosis of the gums, particularly of the marginal gingivae and interdental papillae. It is characterized by the sudden onset of gingival bleeding, severe pain, and halitosis. Culture and microscopic examination of lesions invariably demonstrate a mixture of anaerobic bacteria that usually includes *Bacteroides intermedius, Fusobacterium nucleatum,* and spirochetes such as *Treponema denticola, Borrelia vincentii,* and *Selenomonas*. All of these organisms are normal indigenous flora of the gingival sulcus.

Predisposing factors to ANUG are erupting molars and dental trauma, resulting in devitalized tissue susceptible to invasion by the mixture of anaerobes. Other factors are excessive smoking, malnutrition, metabolic disturbances, and physical or emotional stress.

GANGRENOUS STOMATITIS

Gangrenous stomatitis (noma, cancrum oris) is an acute, rapidly progressive, gangrenous infection involving the tissues of the mouth and face. Children are most often affected, and malnutrition and severe debilitation are predisposing factors. The initial lesion is a small, painful vesicle on the mandibular gingiva in the molar or premolar region. A necrotic ulcer develops and involves deeper tissues, progressing into a painful cellulitis of the lips and cheeks. Excessive sloughing of necrotic tissues exposes underlying teeth and bone. Gangrenous stomatitis resembles ANUG in that fusospirochetal bacteria such as *Borrelia vincentii, F. nucleatum,* and *Bacteroides melaninogenicus* are recovered from the lesions, but the noma lesions are much more focal and destructive, and involve deeper tissue.

ACTINOMYCOSIS

Actinomycosis is a chronic infection characterized by inflammatory induration and sinus formation. The infection is due to *Actinomyces israelii*. A similar organism, *Arachnia propionica,* causes a similar infection. Actinomycosis is characterized by chronic suppuration, necrosis, and fibrosis. *Actinomyces* and *Arachnia* are gram-positive, filamentous, branching bacteria that are normally present in the mouth, vagina, and intestinal tract.

Cervicofacial actinomycosis is invariably the result of trauma such as the extraction of a tooth or an open mandibular fracture. After 1 or 2 weeks, painful indurated swelling appears over the jaw. As the swelling increases, fistulas appear on the surface and drain pus. The pus usually contains small yellow particles (sulfur granules). When crushed between a slide and a coverslip and examined microscopically, sulfur granules are seen to consist of a tangled mass of gram-positive branching filaments.

Pulmonary actinomycosis involves the lungs, pleura, and the chest wall. Abdominal actinomycosis can be mistaken for appendicitis or carcinoma of the cecum. Tubo-ovarian actinomycosis is associated with the use of intrauterine devices.

ORAL CANDIDIASIS

Oral candidiasis (thrush) is an inflammatory infection of the oral mucosa by yeasts of the genus *Candida*. The most frequently recovered species and the most pathogenic is *C. albicans*, but other species (*C. guilliermondi, C. krusei, C. parapsilosis, C. stellatoidea, C. tropicalis* and *C. pseudotropicalis*) may be involved. These organisms are all constituents of the normal flora of the mouth, vagina, and lower intestinal tract. They are organisms of relatively low pathogenicity and are present in low numbers.

Candidiasis is distinguished by creamy white, adherent, curdlike patches on the oral mucosa. They are nonpainful, but firmly adherent; when removed, the underlying mucosa is painfully raw and bleeds easily. Predisposing factors may be local and associated with poorly fitting dentures causing mucosal damage; topical antibiotics or steroids; heavy smoking; or radiation therapy to the head and neck. Systemic predisposing factors include systemic antibiotics, various intravascular catheters, prosthetic cardiac valve surgery, and immunosuppression. In the newborn, elderly, and in immunocompro-

mised patients, pain during eating may interfere with nutrition. Neonatal thrush has been related to maternal vaginal candidiasis at the time of delivery.

Continued mucosal invasion by *Candida* may extend to involve the esophagus. Oral and esophageal candidiasis are often seen in patients with acquired immunodeficiency syndrome. The common symptoms of esophageal candidiasis are painful and difficult swallowing, substernal chest pain, nausea, and vomiting.

HAND-FOOT-AND-MOUTH DISEASE

Hand-foot-and-mouth disease is a mild exanthematous infection of children caused by group A coxsackieviruses, especially A16. The disease is most common in children from birth to age 4 years. The reservoir of the virus is man and domestic animals, including dogs. Transmission is by direct contact with respiratory discharges and feces of infected persons and asymptomatic carriers. The incubation period is 3 to 5 days and the initial symptoms are low-grade fever, sore mouth, and refusal to eat.

Oral lesions start as small red macules in the pharynx, on the soft palate, buccal mucosa, gingivae, and tongue. Vesicles form and may coalesce to form bullae. Some vesicles are absorbed; others form painful, shallow ulcers. The rash is maculopapular becoming vesicular. Vesicles appear on the back of the hands and lateral margins of the feet. They are not painful or pruritic and usually disappear in 3 to 4 days. The acute phase of the infection may be accompanied by abdominal pain, diarrhea, cough, headache, and chest pain. Outbreaks occur predominantly in the summer and early autumn. There is a high attack rate; almost half of contacts develop clinical illness.

CHAPTER 46

Agents of Dental Caries and Periodontal Disease

Dental caries (decay) is a disease characterized by the progressive demineralization of the teeth caused by acids produced by certain of the resident oral bacteria. Caries is the greatest cause of tooth loss in children and young adults. Carious lesions can develop almost as soon as the teeth erupt. The initial lesions are usually in fissures or pits of the deciduous molars. With increasing age, the mineral content of the tooth surface becomes somewhat less susceptible to decay. There is a distinct relationship between the consumption of sucrose in the diet and the prevalence of dental caries.

AGENTS CAUSING DENTAL CARIES

Streptococcus mutans is the major etiologic agent in human dental caries. *Streptococcus mutans* is one of the viridans group of streptococci, a gram-positive coccus that occurs in chains, and a member of the indigenous oral flora. Other bacteria implicated in dental caries are other species of viridans streptococci *(S. salivarius, S. mitis, S. sanguis), Lactobacillus,* and *Actinomyces (A. viscosus, A. naeslundii).*

Streptococcus mutans possesses several characteristics, including sucrose metabolism, that contribute to its cariogenicity. One of these virulence-associated traits is the presence of a surface enzyme, glucosyltransferase, which splits sucrose into fructose and dextrose and provides energy for the synthesis of extracellular insoluble polyglycans such as dextrans and levans.

A cleaned tooth surface rapidly becomes coated with a pellicle, a thin organic film of salivary proteins and glycoproteins. This pellicle mediates the attachment and colonization of the tooth surface by oral bacteria. Initially, streptococci and lactobacilli adhere, followed by various anaerobes, to form a soft, insoluble, and extremely adherent deposit termed **plaque.** Plaque consists almost entirely of bacterial cells together with their extracellular polyglycans. Plaque eventually becomes calcified to form **calculus.** The adsorption of *S. mutans* to the pellicle-coated hydroxyapatite component of enamel is reversible in the absence of sucrose metabolism by the bacterium. In the presence of sucrose there is an irreversible binding of *S. mutans* to the tooth surface via the glucan. Sucrose is also eventually metabolized via the glycolytic pathway to copious amounts of lactic acid, resulting in the dissolution of enamel and dentine with caries formation. Demineralization of the enamel is followed by proteolysis of its organic matrix. When the carious process reaches the dentine of the root surface, the tooth becomes sensitive to touch, temperature, or osmotic changes engendered by foods. The infection may extend into the pulp chambers of the tooth and via the root canals involve the periapical region, with abscess formation.

Saliva provides some protection against caries, primarily through its buffering action and also by its content of lysozyme and secretory IgA. Plaque is not flushed away by the saliva. Additional protection against caries is provided by the ingestion of fluoride (1 mg/day) while the teeth are forming until the permanent dentition is completely erupted. The fluoride combines with hydroxyapatite to form fluorapatite, a less soluble compound.

PERIODONTAL DISEASE

Gingivitis is an inflammation of the gums characterized by redness surrounding the teeth, swelling of the interdental papillae, and bleeding on minimal trauma. Gingivitis usually begins at puberty and during pregnancy, suggesting endocrine factors. The main cause of gingivitis is poor oral hygiene, leading to the accumulation of subgingival plaque. The swelling deepens the crevices between the gums and the teeth, forming gingival pockets where more plaque accumulates. The connective tissue underlying the gingival pockets loses collagen. Tissue destruction is probably mediated by various enzymes such as protease, collagenase, hyaluronidase, chondroitin sulfatase, and also lipopolysaccharide (endotoxin) produced by the plaque bacteria. As gingivitis progresses there is resorption of the alveolar bone around the neck of the teeth, leading to a loss of the periodontal ligament and fur-

ther deepening of the gingival sulci to form periodontal pockets. The teeth become loosened and may fall out. This condition is termed **periodontitis.**

The organisms involved are the anaerobic gram-negative bacilli that include *Bacteroides forsythus, Porphyromonas (Bacteroides) gingivalis, Fusobacterium nucleatum,* and *Eikenella corrodens,* together with spirochetes such as *Treponema denticola. Treponema denticola* produces tissue-damaging enzymes, immunosuppressive substances, metabolic products, endotoxins, and antigens, all of which are potentially harmful.

A somewhat different form of the disease, termed **juvenile periodontitis,** is seen in adolescents, and is characterized by rapid bone loss affecting the incisors and the first molars. Plaque and calculus are minimal. The bacteria involved in juvenile periodontitis are somewhat different from those involved in the adult disease, and include species of *Capnocytophaga* and *Actinobacillus actinomycetemcomitans. Capnocytophaga* are slow-growing gram-negative capnophilic, filamentous rods. Under appropriate conditions, the organisms glide across the surface of agar media forming pink or yellow colonies with fingerlike projections. *Capnocytophaga ochraceus, C. sputigena,* and rarely *C. gingivalis* are inhabitants of normal gingival sulci, but they have been found in large numbers in patients with juvenile periodontitis. These organisms, as well as other species of *Capnocytophaga,* can cause sepsis in patients with granulocytopenia. *Actinobacillus actinmycetemcomitans* is a small, anaerobic, gram-negative rod that can cause endocarditis. Many patients with juvenile periodontosis have antibodies to *A. actinmycetemcomitans* and defects in neutrophil function.

CHAPTER 47

Mumps and Bacterial Parotitis

MUMPS

Mumps (infectious parotitis) is an acute viral disease characterized by swelling and tenderness of the salivary glands, most commonly the parotid, and low-grade fever. Mumps virus is one of the paramyxoviruses and resembles the parainfluenza viruses. Paramyxoviruses are spherical particles and have an outer envelope with spikes enclosing a nucleocapsid of protein and negative, single-stranded RNA. The surface of mumps virus contains the hemagglutinin-neuraminidase (V) and the cell fusion–hemolysis (F) glycoprotein antigens. The RNA-protein-soluble (S) antigen is associated with the nucleocapsid. There is only one serotype of mumps virus. Other viruses that can cause parotitis include parainfluenza, influenza, lymphocytic choriomeningitis viruses, coxsackie virus groups A and B, echovirus, and Epstein-Barr virus. Man is the sole reservoir of mumps virus. The infection is transmitted by respiratory aerosols and saliva of infected persons.

Mumps is uncommon in infants less than 1 year of age on the basis of passively transferred maternal antibodies. Most cases of mumps occur in children less than 14 years old, but all ages are affected. Epidemics have occurred in military camps and other closed populations, and

prior to the availability of mumps vaccine, occurred every 2 to 5 years.

The incubation period is 2 to 3 weeks, usually 18 days. Approximately one third of susceptible persons have an inapparent infection. In persons developing clinical disease, there may be a brief prodrome of low-grade fever, anorexia, malaise, and headache, lasting a day, followed by swelling of the parotids and earache. Typically, one gland swells during the first 2 days and then both swell. The swelling is maximal over a 2- to 3-day period and disappears by 7 to 10 days. The orifice of Stensen's duct is frequently red and edematous. Citrus fruits or other foods stimulating salivation cause pain on ingestion.

The most common extrasalivary gland manifestation of mumps is aseptic meningitis, a relatively benign infection that may occur at any stage of, or in the absence of, parotitis. Symptoms of fever, headache, vomiting, and nuchal rigidity usually resolve in 3 to 10 days with complete recovery. Mumps infection of the central nervous system is present in about half of all cases, but only 1% to 10% show clinical symptoms. Mumps encephalitis is a rare complication and is considerably more serious (see Chapter 20).

Twenty percent to 30% of postpubertal men

with mumps develop orchitis, usually during the first week of parotitis. There is abrupt onset of testicular pain and tenderness, fever, chills, headache, and vomiting. Epididymitis commonly accompanies the orchitis. Symptoms resolve in 7 to 14 days, and sterility is rare. The pain of orchitis is largely due to the swelling of the affected testicle within the inelastic tunica albuginea. Oophoritis occurs in 5% to 7% of postpubertal women with mumps and is manifested by fever, nausea, vomiting, and back or lower quadrant pain.

Pancreatitis with vomiting and severe epigastric pain occurs in less than 10% of patients with mumps. The abdominal muscular spasm and the clinical syndrome may be confused with appendicitis. Other rare extrasalivary gland complications include thyroiditis, prostatitis, hepatitis, nephritis, myocarditis, and thrombocytopenia.

Following contact of a susceptible person with the saliva of an infected person, the mumps virus attaches to and invades the epithelial cells of the respiratory tract. Viral multiplication continues in the upper respiratory tract, the cervical lymph nodes, and occasionally the conjunctivae, causing edema, increased vascular permeability, lymphocytic infiltration, and eliciting IgA secretion. The virus eventually enters the bloodstream and infects the salivary glands and other organs. The parotid swelling is caused by interstitial edema. Virus is present in the saliva and in the urine 6 days before swelling occurs. Viremia and virus in the saliva continue for 3 to 10 days after the onset of infection. Virus is present in the cerebrospinal fluid of about half of the cases.

The earliest antibodies to appear are those directed against the S antigen. These are present at the onset of clinical symptoms and then decline rapidly. Anti-V titers appear later and continue to rise to a peak several weeks after the beginning of clinical disease. Neutralizing antibodies appear during convalescence and persist for many years. Lifelong immunity follows mumps, even after inapparent infection. Delayed-type hypersensitivity to mumps antigen develops 3 to 12 weeks after mumps infection and can be elicited by a skin test. The mumps skin test is often used as a measure of general delayed hypersensitivity. The diagnosis of mumps is largely clinical. Virus is readily recovered from saliva and urine, but this is seldom necessary. A definitive diagnosis may be made by demonstrating at least a fourfold rise in titer between acute and convalescent sera as measured by complement fixation, hemagglutination inhibition, enzyme-linked immunosorbent assay (ELISA), or neutralization tests.

A live attenuated mumps virus vaccine for active immunization has been widely used in the United States since 1968. A single injection elicits neutralizing antibody and immunity to infection. Hyperimmune mumps globulin has been used to provide passive protection to exposed susceptible persons with varying success.

BACTERIAL PAROTITIS

Bacterial parotitis, also known as suppurative, pyogenic, or surgical parotitis, is an acute inflammation of the parotid glands caused by one or several species of bacteria. The infection is seen in debilitated, often elderly patients, commonly as a postoperative complication. The most important predisposing factor is dehydration, which may be the result of diarrhea or vomiting, severe sweating, or inadequate fluid replacement. Dehydration results in a reduction of salivary flow, permitting bacteria from the oral cavity to ascend Stensen's duct and infect the gland. Salivary stasis may also be the result of treatment with anticholinergics, antihistamines, diuretics, or other drugs.

The onset is sudden, with swelling of the parotid, usually unilaterally, and purulent drainage from the duct. The commonest cause is *Staphylococcus aureus*, but various streptococci, *Haemophilus influenzae*, *Pseudomonas aeruginosa*, or *Escherichia coli* may be involved. Occasionally the infection is polymicrobial. The infection generally subsides in 5 to 7 days with antimicrobial therapy and rehydration.

Bacterial parotitis can be a serious threat in patients with underlying diseases such as poorly controlled diabetes mellitus, neoplastic diseases, renal failure, or a recent cerebrovascular accident. The organisms may cause a septicemia leading to fatal septic shock.

PART XI

Multisystem Infections

CHAPTER 48

Overview of Multisystem Infections

The microorganisms discussed in this section are all primary pathogens. They all have sufficient virulence to produce disease in otherwise healthy immunocompetent persons. These organisms are not normally present in the indigenous flora and consequently all of them are acquired exogenously. The reservoir of these organisms varies. In some cases, such as typhoid fever and the agents of viral exanthems, the source of the organism is persons with clinical or inapparent infections, or carriers. Other organisms, such as the agents of anthrax, plague, tularemia, and brucellosis, are primarily animal pathogens. Man becomes infected by direct contact with infected animals, or indirectly via an insect vector.

Bacterial Infections
Typhoid fever
Brucellosis
Plague
Tularemia
Anthrax
Melioidosis
Rat-bite fever
Cat-scratch disease

Rickettsial Infections
Epidemic typhus fever
Murine typhus
Scrub typhus
Rocky Mountain spotted
 fever
Rickettsialpox
Ehrlichiosis

Spirochetal Infections
Syphilis
Yaws
Pinta
Relapsing fever
Lyme disease
Leptospirosis

Viral Infections
Varicella
Measles
Rubella
Erythema infectiosum
Arthropod-borne viral
 fevers
Ebola-Marburg disease

CHAPTER 49

Bacterial Agents of Multisystem Infections

A 26-year-old previously healthy woman returned to her native village in Mexico for a brief visit. Two weeks after her return to the United States she experienced the gradual onset of fever, malaise, and anorexia. Her physician prescribed a 5-day course of an antibiotic, believed to be a cephalosporin. She took the medication for about 3 days and felt better. Two weeks later, the fever recurred, accompanied by chills, a continuous dull frontal headache, and constipation. Physical examination showed her to be an acutely ill young woman with a temperature of 40°C, dry skin, a pulse rate of 80 beats per minute, and a blood pressure of 120/70 mm Hg. Moist rales were heard in both lungs. Her abdomen was distended and tender in both lower quadrants. The edge of the liver and the spleen could be palpated. Her white blood cell count was 4,000/mm^3 with 30% neutrophils, 66% lymphocytes, and 4% monocytes. Erythrocytes were 3.5 million/mm^3; hemoglobin, 10 g/dL; platelets, 150,000/mm^3.* Three blood cultures were obtained from which *Salmonella typhi* was subsequently recovered.

TYPHOID FEVER

Typhoid fever is an acute systemic bacterial infection with a prolonged course and frequent complications. Typhoid fever is caused by infection with *Salmonella typhi*. Clinically similar syndromes (paratyphoid fever) are caused by *S. paratyphi A, S. schottmuelleri (paratyphi B)*, and *S. hirschfeldii (paratyphi C)*. Typhoid and paratyphoid fevers are collectively called enteric fevers because they all involve Peyer's patches in the intestines.

*Normal values: white blood cell count: 5,000–10,000/mm^3, with 40%–60% neutrophils, 20%–40% lymphocytes, 4%–8% monocytes; erythrocytes: 4.3–5.5– million/mm^3; hemoglobin: 12–16 g/dL; platelets: 200,000–500,000/mm^3.

The incubation period of typhoid fever is 1 to 3 weeks, but it is influenced by the size of the infective dose: the larger the dose, the shorter the time of incubation. The onset is insidious with sustained fever, headache, anorexia, relative bradycardia,* nonproductive cough and bronchitis, constipation more often than diarrhea, and involvement of lymphoid tissues. There is diffuse lower quadrant abdominal discomfort with tenderness and distention. The liver and spleen can often be palpated. Crops of periumbilical erythematous maculopapular lesions, 2 to 4 mm in diameter, that blanch on pressure (**rose spots**) may be seen in less than 10% of the patients. Rose spots are transient and disappear within a day or so. Laboratory findings include anemia and transient leukocytosis followed by leukopenia, relative neutropenia, and thrombocytopenia. If untreated, the fever lasts 2 to 3 weeks after the onset of symptoms; other symptoms resolve in an additional week, but weakness persists for several weeks. The untreated patient usually sustains significant weight loss over the course of the disease. Relapse occurs in up to 10% of untreated cases and 20% of treated cases. The case fatality rate in untreated cases is 10% but can be reduced to less than 1% with appropriate antibiotic therapy. Intestinal hemorrhage or perforation occur in about 3% of patients, usually in the third week of the disease. These complications are the result of necrosis and ulceration of the lymphoid tissue of the ileocecal region.

Salmonella are motile, facultative, gram-negative bacilli that are members of the *Enterobacteriaceae* family. Salmonella can be separated into three groups, based upon their host range: group I, *S. enteritidis*, containing more than 2,200 serotypes or subspecies that affect a broad range of animals as well as man; group II, *S. choleraesuis*, primarily affecting swine but occasionally causing disease in man; and group III, *S. typhi*, a single serotype highly adapted to

man. Salmonella are also divided into groups based upon their somatic O antigens. Further classification utilizes their flagellar H and envelope K antigens. *Salmonella paratyphi A* is in group A; *S. schottmuelleri* is in group B; *S. hirschfeldii* is in group C; and *S. typhi* is in group D. The latter two organisms have a unique K antigen, a highly polymerized polysaccharide designated Vi because of its role in the *virulence* of the organism. *Salmonella typhi* and the paratyphoid salmonella only affect man.

The reservoir of *S. typhi* is man: patients, and especially carriers. The carrier state can follow clinical or inapparent infection and may persist for long periods of time, especially in middle-aged women with chronic cholecystitis. In areas of the world where *Schistosoma haematobium* infection is endemic, patients convalescing from typhoid fever may shed the bacteria in their urine.

Transmission of typhoid fever is primarily by food or water contaminated with the feces or urine of infected persons. Shellfish taken from waters contaminated with sewage, and foods contaminated by the hands of food handlers who are carriers are additional mechanisms for transmission. Flies with access to unscreened privies can contaminate food with fecal material containing typhoid bacilli.

Following ingestion of *S. typhi* the organisms pass through the stomach to reach the proximal small intestine. Survival through the low pH of the stomach is facilitated by the buffering action of foods. During the long incubation period the organisms penetrate the mucosal epithelium and are ingested by mononuclear cells of intestinal lymph follicles. The salmonella are able to survive and multiply within the mononuclear cells, and are carried by the cells from the mesenteric lymph nodes to the thoracic duct and eventually to the bloodstream. This transient primary bacteremia serves to seed the liver, spleen, and bone marrow, where the bacteria continue to multiply within macrophages. This ability for intracellular survival and multiplication is characteristic of some salmonella and cer-

*Relative bradycardia refers to a slow pulse despite an elevated body temperature.

tain other organisms such as *Mycobacterium tuberculosis, Yersinia pestis, Brucella, Francisella tularensis,* and *Histoplasma capsulatum.* When the macrophages of the reticuloendothelial tissues are no longer able to contain the multiplying salmonella, the organisms again enter the bloodstream with the onset of fever and other symptoms. This sustained bacteremia persists for about 3 weeks, with seeding of the kidneys, gallbladder, and intestine. Fever increases during this time with patients becoming acutely ill. During the second week, salmonella appear in the urine. In the gallbladder the organisms multiply in the bile, reinfecting the intestine. In the intestine, the Peyer's patches become inflamed and ulcerated, and salmonella appear in the feces by the second or third week of disease.

Antibody titers to the H and O antigens increase during the third and fourth weeks. The organism disappears from the bloodstream and the patient begins to feel better. Two complications—intestinal hemorrhage and perforation of the bowel near the ileocecal valve—account for most of the 10% mortality in untreated disease. Relapse is common. The definitive diagnosis of typhoid fever is based upon the recovery of *S. typhi* from the blood. During the first week of disease blood cultures are positive in more than 80% of patients, unless they have received antimicrobial therapy. The single most effective specimen is bone marrow, and should be obtained if blood cultures are negative. Urine cultures are often positive during the second week of disease and stool cultures become positive during the second and third weeks.

Serologic diagnosis is based upon rises of antibody titers to O and H antigens. A greater than fourfold rise in group D O antibody between serum obtained in the first and in the third to fourth week of disease is suggestive of acute infection but is not completely reliable since the antibody response may have been due to infection with group D salmonella other than *S. typhi.*

Various typhoid vaccines have been used for many years, but the immunity engendered by them can easily be overwhelmed by a large inoculum of the organism. At the present time, a live, attenuated oral vaccine appears to be the most effective.

BRUCELLOSIS

Brucellosis (undulant fever) is an acute, prolonged, febrile, systemic disease caused by infection by one of several species of *Brucella. Brucella* are small, gram-negative, aerobic coccobacilli. They are nonmotile and require an atmosphere supplemented with carbon dioxide and an enriched medium for growth. Growth is slow; blood cultures may require prolonged incubation (up to 30 days) to become positive, and colonies take up to 5 days to appear on solid media. Humans can be infected by any of four species: *B. melitensis* (the most virulent), *B. abortus, B. suis,* or *B. canis.*

Brucellosis is primarily a disease of domestic animals, including cattle, swine, and goats, which constitute the reservoir for human infection. In these animals the disease is primarily genitourinary, with a high incidence of abortion, and the organisms are frequently shed in the milk. Humans become infected by contact with infected animal tissues or ingestion of milk from infected animals. In the United States more than half of the cases result from occupational exposure to infected animals—abattoir workers, meat inspectors, veterinarians; most of the remainder of cases are due to consumption of unpasteurized dairy products.

The incubation period is usually 1 to 3 weeks, but may be as long as several months. The onset is insidious with continuous or intermittent fever; chills; headache; profuse sweating, especially in the evening; weakness; and generalized aching. Symptoms may continue for weeks or months if untreated, with significant weight loss.

Complications occur in up to 30% of cases, the most common being osteomyelitis. Other complications include gastrointestinal (nausea, vomiting, diarrhea, abnormal liver function tests); epididymo-orchitis; and neurologic (depression, meningioencephalitis). Endocarditis, the most common cause of death, is uncommon, occurring in less than 2% of cases.

After entering the body by abraded skin, ingestion, or inhalation (laboratory infections), the brucellae are ingested by phagocytic polymorphonuclear neutrophils. Many organisms are able to survive within the neutrophils with the production of adenine and 5'-guanosine monophosphate which inhibits the antibacterial myeloperoxidase-peroxide-halide system by interfering with the degranulation of the peroxide-positive granules of the neutrophil. Surviving organisms are carried to the regional lymph nodes, and eventually, via the lymph and the thoracic duct, enter the bloodstream. The organisms reach the reticuloendothelial components of the liver, bone marrow, and especially the spleen, where they multiply within the macrophages. When macrophages become activated, the intracellular organisms are killed, releasing endotoxin from the bacterial cell walls. Eventually, small granulomas develop at these reticulendothelial sites with episodic release of bacteria into the bloodstream. These releases of bacteria and endotoxin may be responsible for the recurrent chills and fever associated with brucellosis.

Brucella infection results in the development of both humoral and cell-mediated immune responses. Immunoglobulins appear during the first weeks of disease, followed by delayed-type hypersensitivity. IgM antibodies appear initially and decline after about 3 months; IgG antibodies begin to rise during the second week of disease and remain elevated for 1 year or more.

The diagnosis of brucellosis often depends upon the demonstration of IgM and IgG antibodies by the agglutination method. False-negative tests may be due to the prozone phenomenon (masked by the zone of antibody excess); such false-negative reactions can be avoided by

routinely diluting the serum to greater than 1:320. Blocking substance in serum can also mask the agglutination reaction. These incomplete or blocking antibodies have been associated with chronic brucellosis. Such antibodies can be detected by the indirect Coombs' test, which detects antibody on the patient's erythrocytes. Blood cultures should be taken and incubated with carbon dioxide for up to 4 weeks. Biopsy specimens of bone marrow, liver, or lymph nodes may also yield the organism. Treatment of brucellosis is with trimethoprim/sulfamethoxazole. Other agents are tetracycline plus streptomycin and the new fluoroquinolones. There is a 10% to 20% relapse rate irrespective of the drug used as therapy.

PLAGUE

Plague is an acute systemic disease caused by infection with *Yersinia pestis* and characterized by the sudden onset of fever and local lymphadenitis. Plague is primarily a disease of rodents and small mammals; human disease results from the bite of an infected flea. *Yersinia pestis* is an ovoid, gram-negative, nonmotile bacillus, classified with the *Enterobactericeae*. The organism grows readily on laboratory media and often exhibits a bipolar, "safety pin" appearance when viewed microscopically, especially if stained with Giemsa or Wayson stain.

The virulence factors and mechanisms of *Y. pestis* are multiple and complex. Most are plasmid-mediated and several are temperature-dependent. V and W antigens are proteins that are involved in the spread of the organisms through the tissues as well as their resistance to phagocytosis. The V and W antigens are not synthesized at 20 to 25°C (the temperature of the flea), but are produced within macrophages at 37°C. Similarly, a chromosomally mediated capsular antigen, fraction 1, that confers antiphagocytic protection to the organism, is only synthesized at 37°C. Other temperature-dependent factors are coagulase and fibrinolysin enzymes which may be involved in the dissemination of the bacteria within the body. The cell wall contains a lipopolysaccharide with the properties of endotoxin, and a protein murine toxin, lethal for mice, is located in the cell envelope.

Epidemics of plague have been the most devastating outbreaks in human history. In the 6th century of the present era, a plague epidemic that lasted 50 years killed more than 100 million people, and the "black death" in the 14th century devastated Europe, killing 25% of the population.

Most human cases occur in the developing countries of Asia, Africa, and South America. In the United States most cases are in the southwestern states of New Mexico, Arizona, Colorado, Utah, and California, usually during the summer and fall months when people are outdoors and come into contact with rodents and their fleas.

Plague is epizootic in wild rodents (ground squirrels, prairie dogs, mice, wood rats) and is spread by the bite of their fleas. This is known as wild or **sylvatic plague.** Humans, usually children, may occasionally contract the disease by being bitten by fleas while handling dead rodents, or when pet dogs or cats carry rodent fleas into the household. Small mammals such as bobcats may become infected by ingesting infected rodents.

The reservoir of urban plague involving humans is in urban and domestic rats, and is transmitted by the tropical rat flea, *Xenopsylla cheopis.* The infection is transmitted to man when a flea, deserting a dying rat, bites a human. The bubonic and septicemic forms of plague are not usually transmitted person to person. Man-to-man transmission by human fleas, *Pulex irritans,* is important in the Andean regions of South America. Persons who develop secondary plague pneumonia (about 5% of cases) shed *Y. pestis* in their respiratory secretions and can transmit the disease by the airborne aerosol route.

The incubation period of **bubonic plague** is 2 to 10 days. There is sudden onset of fever, chills, tachycardia, headache, and prostration, followed within a few hours by the appearance of the bubo. Buboes are grossly swollen and intensely painful lymph nodes, usually in the groin, axilla, or neck. In untreated cases, buboes may become fluctuant and suppurate. Patients may become agitated or delirious, and seizures are common in children. Some persons develop purpuric skin lesions containing blood vessels occluded by fibrin thrombi, resulting in hemorrhage and necrosis and gangrene of distal extremities. Death may occur in 2 to 4 days. About 25% of cases develop **septicemic plague** in which there is a massive bacteremia, sometimes in the absence of the lymphadenitis. In approximately 5% of patients, the organisms reach the lungs hematogenously with the development of plague pneumonia. **Pneumonic plague** is highly fatal: exposed persons have become ill and died on the same day.

After the flea feeds on an animal infected with *Y. pestis,* the blood clots in the foregut of the insect owing to the production of coagulase by the bacteria. This clotted blood blocks the flea's ability to swallow and the bacteria continue to multiply in the clotted blood. A blocked flea may regurgitate thousands of plague bacilli onto the skin of its next host while attempting to ingest another blood meal. Organisms growing at the flea's temperature do not produce fraction 1 or V and W antigens. When a person is bitten, the injected bacteria are engulfed by polymorphonuclear leukocytes and macrophages; they are destroyed by the neutrophils, but survive the intracellular environment of the mononuclear cells where they replicate at the body temperature of the host and produce V and W antigens and fraction 1. Organisms released when the mononuclear cells lyse are fully virulent and resistant to further phagocytosis. The organisms enter the bloodstream and seed distant lymph nodes, skin, lungs, spleen, liver, and the central nervous system. The case fatality rate for bubonic plague is more than 50%. Untreated septicemic or pneumoinc plague is nearly always fatal. Death may be due to disseminated intravascular coagulation and shock associated with endotoxemia.

The definitive diagnosis of plague is based upon the demonstration of *Y. pestis* in the blood, sputum, or other body fluids by culture. Buboes should be aspirated by injecting and recovering 1 mL of sterile saline into the bubo. The aspirate should be stained and cultured. A provisional diagnosis may be made by demonstrating the ovoid bipolar staining bacilli in the aspirate. A formalin-killed plague vaccine is available for persons who live or work in close proximity to rodents, or who travel to hyperendemic or epidemic regions.

Treatment is with streptomycin, gentamicin, or tetracycline. Close contacts of pneumonic plague should receive chemoprophylaxis with tetracycline.

TULAREMIA

Tularemia (rabbit fever, deer fly fever) is a zoonotic bacterial disease caused by *Francisella tularensis*. In humans the disease is characterized by high fever and severe systemic symptoms which may persist for weeks or months. *Francisella tularensis* is a small, gram-negative, nonmotile pleomorphic coccobacillis. It is aerobic and nutritionally fastidious, requiring glucose and cysteine or sulfhydryl compounds for growth. The organism will usually not grow on the media routinely employed in the clinical laboratory; growth may take place on chocolate agar (used for gonococci) or on charcoal-yeast extract agar (used for *Legionella*). Small colonies appear in 24 to 48 hours at 37°C. *Francisella tularensis* is surrounded by a capsulelike substance containing carbohydrate, protein, and a large amount of lipid, composed of a unique fatty acid. The antigenic components include a polysaccharide antigen, a protein antigen that cross-reacts

with *Brucella*, and an endotoxin-like substance. Two epidemiologic variants that differ slightly biochemically are *F. tularensis* biovar *tularensis* (Jellison type A, Nearctica), which is highly virulent and found predominantly in North America in ticks and rabbits; and *F. tularensis* biovar *palaearctica* (Jellison type B), less virulent and occurring in rodents and insects in Europe and Asia.

The reservoir of *F. tularensis* is in lagomorphs (rabbits, hares), muskrats, beavers, and many other species of mammals, birds, fish, and invertebrates (ticks, deer flies, mosquitoes). Transmission to man is the result of direct contact with the blood or tissues of an infected animal, the bite of an arthropod (ticks, deer fly), ingestion of inadequately cooked meat from an infected animal or contaminated water, or inhalation of dust from contaminated soil. Laboratory infections may result from the inhalation of aerosols. As few as 10 to 50 organisms are sufficient to produce tularemia in humans if injected or inhaled. At least half of all cases occur in Texas, Oklahoma, Arkansas, Missouri, and Tennessee.

The incubation period is 2 to 10 days, usually 3 days. The onset is abrupt with high fever, chills, fatigue, and additional symptoms that relate to the portal of entry of the organism. The most common form (80% of cases) is the **ulceroglandular,** characterized by an indolent ulcer on the hand or finger and painful adenopathy of the regional lymph nodes. The enlarged nodes may suppurate. This syndrome may be confused with plague or sporotrichosis. The **typhoidal syndrome** (10%–30% of cases) is characterized by fever, weight loss, diarrhea, vomiting, dehydration, mental confusion, and meningismus. Pneumonia may occur in 40% of these patients. This is the most serious form of the disease. The **oculoglandular** type of tularemia follows contamination of the eye and accounts for 1% to 5% of patients. Usually only one eye is involved, with photophobia, lacrimation, decreased visual acuity, conjunctival erythema and ulceration, and enlargement of the cervical and periauricular lymph nodes. Pneumonia is a common complication in all forms of tularemia.

Francisella tularensis is said to be able to penetrate the unbroken skin. The organism probably enters through microabrasions, mucous membranes, or by the bite of an arthropod. There is a bacteremia that seeds the organs of the reticuloendothelial system. The organisms are able to survive intracellularly for long periods of time in mononuclear cells. Focal areas of necrosis develop in these organs. These lesions often evolve into granulomas.

The case fatality of tularemia caused by the type A organism is 5% to 15% in the untreated patient, and up to 30% in the untreated typhoidal type. Appropriate antimicrobial treatment reduces the mortality to 1% to 3%. The case fatality due to the type B organism is negligible. There is a live attenuated vaccine that provides good protection against respiratory tularemia and which modifies the signs and symptoms of the ulceroglandular type. Natural infection and vaccination result in the production of specific and long-lasting humoral and cell-mediated immunity. The serum antibodies recognize the antigens of the carbohydrate capsule, while the T lymphocytes recognize the membrane polypeptide antigens. The crucial protective mechanism is cell-mediated immunity.

The diagnosis of tularemia is usually made serologically. *Francisella tularensis* is not usually visualized in Gram stains of ulcers, sputum, or lymph nodes, and cultures of clinical specimens are generally negative, since the organism fails to grow on ordinary laboratory media. Agglutinin titers usually become positive by the second week of illness and reach a maximum by 4 to 8 weeks. Sera from these patients usually cross-reacts with *Brucella abortus* antigens, but the nonspecific cross reaction disappears with high dilution of the serum.

Treatment with antibiotics such as streptomycin or tetracycline is highly effective.

ANTHRAX

Anthrax is an acute bacterial disease of animals caused by infection with *Bacillus anthracis*, and is occasionally transmitted to man. *Bacillus anthracis* is a large, gram-positive, spore-forming rod. It is nonmotile, encapsulated, and characteristically occurs in chains resembling bamboo. The organism is aerobic and grows readily in ordinary laboratory media.

The virulence of *B. anthracis* is associated with two factors: a polypeptide capsule and an exotoxin. The capsule is composed of D-glutamic acid, and interferes with phagocytosis. There is also evidence that the capsular material neutralizes the activity of an anthracidal factor normally present in tissues. Anthrax toxin is composed of three proteins: edema factor, lethal factor, and protective antigen. The binding of protective antigen to cell surface receptors produces a new type of receptor that is recognized by the edema and lethal factors. When the bound edema factor enters the cytoplasm it interacts with a heat-stable substance, probably calmodulin, to form adenolate cyclase. The resulting increases in cyclic adenosine monophosphate (cAMP) cause the edematous response in skin and presumably other effects in the tissues.

The primary reservoir of anthrax is in ruminants, especially goats, sheep, and cattle, but horses, pigs, and other animals may be affected. Man becomes infected by cutaneous contact with infected animal material, by inhalation of dust containing spores of *B. anthracis*, or rarely, by ingestion of contaminated tissues. In the United States, anthrax is an occupational disease. Eighty percent of the cases are considered industrial and are due to contact with imported goat hair, hides, or wool. The remaining cases are agricultural and occur in farmers, ranchers, and veterinarians who have contact with animals sick or dead of anthrax.

There are three clinical forms of anthrax in man: **cutaneous** (malignant pustule), accounting for 95% of cases (see Fig 25–1), **pulmonary** (woolsorter's disease), representing 5% of cases, and gastrointestinal, which is very rare. In the cutaneous form of anthrax, a painless pruritic lesion resembling a pimple appears after an incubation period of 2 to 7 days. The pustule develops a surrounding area of erythema which becomes vesicular. After a few days, the vesicles coalesce and break down, leaving the small doughnutlike lesion 1 to 2 cm in diameter, containing fluid that is initially straw-colored, then turning dark, and teeming with anthrax bacilli. The lesion soon resembles an ulcer crater with a black eschar at the base, surrounded by an area of edema. Most of the lesions occur on exposed parts of the body: hands, arms, neck, or head. Untreated infections may spread to the regional lymph nodes, eventually entering the bloodstream. The bacillemia is followed by toxemia which occurs late in the disease and is responsible for most of the pathologic changes. Untreated cutaneous anthrax has a case fatality rate of 5% to 20%, but death is rare with effective antimicrobial treatment.

Pulmonary anthrax begins as a mild and nonspecific upper respiratory infection. Within 3 to 5 days there is rapid progression of a fulminating pneumonia, fever, and shock, septicemia, and meningitis are frequent complications. Untreated pulmonary anthrax is uniformly fatal; if treated promptly the mortality can be reduced to 20%. A cell-free vaccine is available for high-risk persons. The diagnosis of anthrax is based upon a history of occupational exposure and the demonstration of *B. anthracis* in edema fluid or sputum by microscopic examination and culture. *B. anthracis* has become resistant to many of the older antibiotics due to the presence of plasmids mediating β-lactamases and other enzymes that inactivate antibodies.

MELIOIDOSIS

Melioidosis is an uncommon disease caused by infection with *Pseudomonas pseudomallei.*

Clinical manifestations range from a rapidly fatal septicemia to inapparent infection. *Pseudomonas pseudomallei* is a small, gram-negative, aerobic, motile bacillus. When stained with Wright's, Giemsa, or Wayson stain, the bacteria show a bipolar safety pin appearance. The organisms grow on ordinary laboratory media; after prolonged incubation (14 days) colonies are cream to orange in color, wrinkled, and have a pungent, earthy odor. The organism is a saprophyte that has been found in certain soils and waters of South-East Asia and northern Australia. The disease is rare in the Western Hemisphere.

Transmission to man may occur through skin wounds or abrasions contaminated with soil or water, by the ingestion or aspiration of contaminated water, or by inhalation of dust from soil. The incubation period varies widely from 2 days to several months or years.

The clinical forms of melioidosis are extremely variable and include an acute septicemic form, a subacute pulmonary form, chronic forms, and a mild, self-limited febrile illness. The acute septicemic form is characterized by the sudden onset of high fever, chills, and a cough with hemoptysis. Physical examination may show pneumonia, lung abscess, and enlargement of the liver and spleen. There may also be profuse watery diarrhea and a rash. The patient becomes comatose and dies in septicemic shock. The subacute form is predominantly a pneumonitis, lung abscess, or empyema, and may simulate pulmonary tuberculosis. Chronic forms include abscesses of the lungs, liver, spleen, or subcutaneous tissues. Abscesses may form fistulas. The organism can reactivate in the lung years after the initial diseases.

The diagnosis of melioidosis should be considered in all febrile patients who have been in an endemic region. Because of the protean nature of the symptoms, definitive diagnosis depends upon the demonstration of *P. pseudomallei* from clinical material. Exudates and all body fluids (except stool) should be cultured and examined microscopically. Blood cultures may become positive in 24 hours.

Treatment is with trimethoprim/sulfamethoxazole.

RAT-BITE FEVER

Rat-bite fever is an uncommon febrile disease transmitted by the bite of a rat or other small rodent. The syndrome may be due to either of two different bacteria: *Streptobacillus moniliformis* or *Spirillum minus*. In the United States, rat bite fever is caused by *S. moniliformis;* most of the *S. minus* infections occur in Asia.

Streptobacillus moniliformis is a highly pleomorphic, facultatively anaerobic, nonmotile gram-negative rod. It frequently appears microscopically as long filaments with bulbous swellings resembling a string of beads. The organism is best visualized by staining with Giemsa or Wayson stain. *Streptobacillus moniliformis* requires a medium enriched with blood or serum, and a humid atmosphere enriched with carbon dioxide at a temperature of 35°C. In broth, "puffball" colonies appear in 2 to 6 days, and cottonlike colonies can be seen in 3 to 4 days on agar plates. *Spirillum minus* is a gram-negative, spiral organism that stains poorly, and is best demonstrated in blood, exudate, or body fluids by darkfield microscopy. Blood specimens may be stained with Wright's or Giemsa stain. The organism cannot be cultivated on artificial laboratory media.

Both *S. moniliformis* and *S. minus* are commonly present in the oropharyngeal flora of rodents, including both wild and laboratory rats, squirrels, and gerbils. Infection by both organisms is transmitted to man by the bite of a rodent. In the case of *S. moniliformis* the vehicle of infection has also been milk or water contaminated by rodents.

The incubation period of *S. moniliformis* infection is 2 to 10 days. There is abrupt onset of fever, chills, headache, vomiting, and severe migratory arthralgias and myalgias. Within 2 to 4 days, a morbilliform or petechial rash appears on the palms, soles, and extremities, and half of the patients develop arthritis, commonly involving the knees. The fever generally subsides spontaneously and the remaining symptoms resolve within 2 weeks. When the infection has been due to ingestion of the pathogen (Haverhill fever), vomiting and pharyngitis are prominent symptoms. Complications of *S. moniliformis* infection include abscesses of any organ. The mortality of untreated disease is 7% to 10%.

Diagnosis of *S. moniliformis* infection is made by demonstration of the organism in blood, joint fluid, or exudate, by staining, and by culture. Specific agglutinins appear within 2 weeks after the onset of symptoms and reach a maximum titer within 1 to 3 months.

The incubation period of *S. minus* infections (spirillum fever, sodoku) is 1 to 3 weeks. The clinical appearance is similar to *S. moniliformis* infections, except that a macular red-brown rash spreads from the initial bite lesion. Complications and arthritis are rare.

CAT-SCRATCH DISEASE

Cat-scratch disease is usually a benign, self-limited illness characterized by regional granulomatous lymphadenitis and fever. There is evidence that the disease is caused by a previously unknown bacterial agent. The organism is a small, pleomorphic, gram-negative bacillus that is seen in biopsied affected lymph nodes by staining with an impregnation silver stain (Warthin-Starry) and by culture in biphasic medium. This medium consists of slants of brain-heart infusion agar overlaid with broth and incubated in air at 30 to 32°C. When inoculated with a ground-up suspension of the lymph node, growth appears in the broth in 1 to 6 days, and colonies on the agar in 2 to 9 days.

The reservoir of the organism is unknown.

More than 90% of all cases have been transmitted by scratches, bites, or licks of cats, usually newly acquired kittens or strays, rather than long-term household pets. Family outbreaks have occurred in households with cats. Cases have also followed bites or scratches by dogs or monkeys. Eighty percent of cases occur in children.

The incubation period is 3 to 14 days. The primary lesion is an erythematous, crusted papule that is most often found on the fingers, hand, or wrist. Two to 3 weeks after the primary lesion, regional lymphadenopathy appears, typically draining the site of inoculation. Splenomegaly is present in 12% of patients, and 1% to 2% have severe symptoms of encephalopathy, pneumonitis, osteomyelitis, and hepatic or splenic necrotizing granulomas. The lymphadenopathy usually resolves spontaneously in 1 to 4 months. Rarely, children with cat-scratch disease experience the sudden onset of fever and encephalitis. If the inoculum involves the eye, there may be conjunctivitis or ocular granulomas with periauricular lymphadenopathy (Parinaud's syndrome).

The diagnosis of cat-scratch disease is based on a history of animal contact; a positive skin test, utilizing an antigen prepared from the pus of patients with cat-scratch disease (Hanger-Rose antigen); characteristic histopathologic findings in biopsied lymph nodes; and the presence of silver-staining pleomorphic bacteria in lymph node suspensions.

An opportunistic infection with the bacterial agent causing cat-scratch disease may be responsible for bacillary **epithelioid angiomatosis,** an unusual vascular proliferative lesion seen in patients with acquired immunodeficiency syndrome or in transplant patients. The focal diffuse cutaneous involvement in some of these patients suggests bacteremia with dissemination to multiple skin sites or internal organs.

Treatment has been successful with tetracycline and recently with ciprofloxacin.

CHAPTER 50

Spirochetes

A 27-year-old sailor presented at sick call with a rash over his entire body, including the palms and soles. It did not itch. He also had a painless, indurated, ulcerlike lesion on his penis. He complained of headache, muscle aches, and malaise. On physical examination he was found to have a temperature of 38.8° C and generalized lymphadenopathy. Darkfield examination of material from the penile lesion showed spiral organisms resembling *Treponema pallidum*, and a serologic test for syphilis was positive.

Spirochetes are slender, coiled organisms that differ from other bacteria in having a flexible cell wall. One or more fibrils (axial filaments), which originate from subterminal attachment disks, are intertwined around the spirochete. An envelope enclosing the organism and the axial filaments is a triple-layered membrane similar to that of gram-negative bacteria. Spirochetes are motile by flexion of the cells (coiling and uncoiling of a spring), movement along a helical pathway (corkscrew), end-over-end tumbling, or a combination of these. Although spirochetes are gram-negative, many are so thin and stain so poorly that a special technique—darkfield microscopy—is necessary to visualize them. With the darkfield microscope, a special condenser is used that prevents light from directly entering the objective. Instead, light is shown obliquely through the drop of fluid specimen on the slide. Any particles, e.g., spirochetes, suspended in the fluid are illuminated by reflected light so that the observer sees brightly lighted spirochetes in a darkfield.

Some spirochetes are free-living in nature, others are members of the indigenous flora of the mouth, intestine, and vagina, and a few are agents of human disease. These pathogens are included in three genera: *Treponema*, *Leptospira*, and *Borrelia*. Each of these genera contains pathogenic and nonpathogenic species and has its own distinctive features, its specific antigenic characteristics, and causes one or more characteristic diseases (Table 50-1).

Treponemes are small gram-negative spiral organisms, 10 to 13 μm long with tight regular spirals. They are difficult to visualize with the light microscope because of their extreme narrowness. Treponemes have an outer membrane consisting of a lipid bilayer; the actual composition of the membrane is unknown. Treponemes have three to eight piroplasmic flagella that orig-

TABLE 50–1.

Pathogenic Spirochetes

Genus	Species	Disease
Treponema	*T. pallidum*	Syphilis
	T. pertenue	Yaws
	T. carateum	Pinta
Leptospira	*L. interrogans* (many serotypes)	Leptospirosis
Borrelia	*B. recurrentis*	Relapsing fever
	B. burgdorferi	Lyme disease
	B. vincenti (together with *Fusobacterium* and other organisms)	Acute necrotizing ulcerative gingivitis (Vincent's angina)

inate from each end of the cell. When viewed with the darkfield microscope, they exhibit a characteristic motility with bending, flexing, and rotation around their longitudinal axis. The pathogenic treponemes include *T. pallidum*, the cause of syphilis; *T. pertenue*, the agent of yaws; and *T. carateum*, the etiologic agent of pinta.

Treponemal diseases share similar characteristics: they tend to run a subacute to chronic course with intervals of remission and relapse; they occur predominantly among people living under poor hygienic conditions; lesions often involve the skin and bones; the same type of antibodies are present; and they respond promptly to penicillin therapy.

SYPHILIS

Syphilis is a chronic infection caused by *T. pallidum* that involves multiple organ systems. Humans are the sole host of *T. pallidum* and sexual contact is the usual means of transmission. Syphilis is the third most commonly reported infectious disease in the United States; there are about 200,000 new cases each year. It is most prevalent in young adults in large urban centers; 60% of the cases occur in persons between 15 and 25 years of age. Congenital syphilis results from the transplacental passage of the organism from a maternal infection.

Treponema pallidum is a thin, delicate organism about 7.5 μm long. It does not survive for long outside the human host and is very susceptible to drying, heat, air (oxygen), and other physical and chemical agents. The organism has an outer protective layer or capsule, composed of acidic mucopolysaccharide that appears to be vital to treponemal survival. This capsule may be antiphagocytic, may limit antibody access, and may explain the oxygen sensitivity of *T. pallidum*, since acidic mucopolysaccharides irreversibly depolymerize in the presence of oxygen. The organism penetrates the intact skin or mucous membrane during sexual contact, multiplies, and rapidly spreads to the regional lymph nodes. The spirochetes enter the bloodstream within hours to be transported to other tissues. Within infected tissue, *T. pallidum* localizes perivascularly.

Attachment to host tissues is an important initial step in the pathogenesis of syphilis. Two receptors are involved: the surface receptor within tissues and the specific site on the organism. It is believed that the cell receptor that mediates treponemal attachment is the outer surface layer of acidic mucopolysaccharide (hyaluronic acid and chondroitin sulfate), distributed uniformly as an intact layer over the cell surface. In tissue cultures as many as 200 attached treponemes have been observed per individual cell. It has been postulated that *T. pallidum* attaches to host tissue by elaborating a mucopolysaccharidase that reacts with the tissue cell mucopolysaccharide, possibly attaching at the inner surface of capillaries. Capillary endothelial cells would be split apart, permitting the treponemes access to the perivascular area, eventually leading to obliterative endarteritis with a cutoff of the blood supply, necrosis, and ulceration.

Acquired syphilis has three symptomatic stages: primary, secondary, and tertiary. Primary syphilis is characterized by the appearance of a lesion—the chancre—that appears at the site of inoculation usually on the genitalia 3 to 4 weeks after infection, (Figs 50–1 and 50–2). Genital lesions are typically indurated and painless, but extragenital lesions (lips, breast, etc.) are often quite painful. Regional lymphadenopathy is usually present. The chancre persists for 1 to 5 weeks and heals spontaneously. *Treponema pallidum* is mostly extracellular within lesions. Unattached organisms are engulfed by polymorphonuclear leukocytes, macrophages, and activated T lymphocytes, and removed,

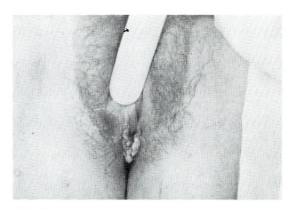

FIG 50–2.
Syphilitic chancre.

which may explain the healing of the chancre. A small number of treponemes are intracellular within a wide variety of cell types and remain virulent. These intracellular organisms may explain the chronic and relapsing nature of syphilis.

Secondary syphilis occurs about 6 to 8 weeks later, and is characterized by headache, generalized arthralgias, malaise, and lymphadenopathy, followed by a generalized rash (Fig 50–3). The rash is dry, does not itch, and often involves the palms and soles. Localized patches of baldness may appear giving a moth-eaten appearance. In moist areas like the axillae or the anogenital region, flat, papular lesions—condylomata lata—may appear. Mucous patches often occur in the mouth, the throat, or the cervix, and about 5% of patients complain of some eye symptoms that are due to iritis or retinitis. The rash persists for 2 to 6 weeks and then heals spontaneously. About one fourth of the patients have at least one cutaneous relapse. Secondary syphilis is the most contagious stage of the disease. The dry skin lesions, the condylomata, and mucous patches are all heavily infected with *T. pallidum*.

It has been suggested that secondary syphilis might be the result of immunosuppression of the host defenses that were involved in the healing of primary syphilis. The treponemal mucopolysaccharide capsular material could interfere

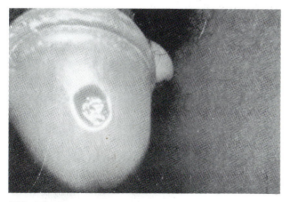

FIG 50–1.
Syphilitic chancre.

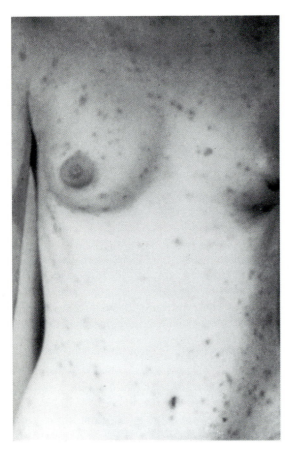

FIG 50–3.
Secondary syphilis—rash.

with the production of antibodies to treponemal mucopolysaccharidase by plasma cells and B lymphocytes, and inactivate helper and killer T lymphocytes and macrophages. Intracellular organisms could then emerge and begin to multiply extracellularly.

The lesions of secondary syphilis heal within 4 to 12 weeks and the disease enters the latent stage. The latent stage may last a few years or the entire lifetime of the patient. There are no clinical signs or symptoms, and about two thirds of the patients go through life with little or no physical inconvenience. Latent syphilis of greater than 4 years' duration is considered to be noninfectious except in pregnant women who may transmit the disease to their fetus.

The remaining one third of untreated cases go on to develop tertiary (late) syphilis with destructive lesions, and about one fourth of these will die as a result of the disease. Tertiary syphilis may take the form of gumma formation (late benign), aortitis, or involve the central nervous system. Gummas are granulomatous lesions that may occur in skin, bones, joints, or any other tissues. These highly destructive lesions contain few treponemes and it is generally believed that gumma formation is a hypersensitivity phenomenon, possibly a response to mucopolysaccharide material within host tissues. Circulating immune complexes may represent an additional factor in the pathogenesis of lesions.

Aortitis results from continued multiplication of the treponemes in the media of the aorta, causing necrosis and eventual production of an aneurysm. Eighty percent of the mortality in tertiary syphilis is due to cardiovascular complications such as aortic insufficiency or rupture of an aneurysm. Neurosyphilis is the result of continual multiplication of treponemes in the central nervous system and accounts for 20% of the deaths associated with tertiary syphilis. Neurosyphilis may be asymptomatic, meningovascular, or involve the parenchyma of the brain manifested by paresthesias, ataxia, autonomic system dysfunction, optic nerve atrophy, pupillary abnormalities (Argyll Robertson pupil), personality changes, and psychosis.

Congenital syphilis involves multiple organ systems and must be differentiated from other neonatal diseases. The stage of syphilis in the mother often determines the effect on the fetus. If the mother has primary or secondary syphilis, the infant is frequently dead at birth. If she has latent or tertiary disease, the baby may develop congenital syphilis, or may escape infection. It is believed that the fetus is safe from infection until about the 18th week of gestation, at which time cellular changes (atrophy of the Langhans' layer) permit treponemes to cross the placenta. Early congenital syphilis occurs from birth to 2 years old and is characterized by mucocutaneous lesions, rhinitis, and other symptoms. The mucous discharges are highly infectious. The earlier the onset of disease, the poorer the prognosis. Late congenital syphilis is characterized by bone and joint involvement, cranial neuropathies, and interstitial keratitis, which can lead to blindness if untreated.

Immunity develops following syphilitic infection. Protective, neutralizing antibodies can be demonstrated, but there is evidence that untreated cases harbor infectious treponemes for a number of years after the primary infection. A number of antibodies develop during the course of syphilis that have diagnostic usefulness. About 2 to 3 weeks following infection, a specific antibody appears, directed against the surface of the treponeme. This treponemal antibody persists for many years (regardless of therapy). It is found in IgG, IgM, and IgA, and, in the presence of complement, immobilizes and kills the spirochete. Approximately 4 to 6 weeks after infection (1–3 weeks after the appearance of the primary chancre), a nonspecific antibody develops that reacts with cardiolipin, a phospholipid component associated with mitochondrial membranes of human and animal tissues. This cardiolipin antibody may be the result of tissue damage and is also found in other diseases (viral infections, malaria, leprosy, collagen-vascular diseases, etc.) Cardiolipin antibodies usually disappear with antisyphilitic treatment.

The diagnosis of syphilis is based upon the clinical presentation, microscopic detection of the spirochetes, and serologic testing. The reliability of diagnosis based solely on the examination of primary genital lesions ranges from 42% to 78%. Examination of material obtained from a chancre by darkfield microscopy requires expertise in distinguishing *T. pallidum* from the numerous commensal spirochetes of the oral, genital, and rectal mucosa. The sensitivity of this procedure is about 75%. A much more sensitive (73%–100%) and specific (100%) procedure is direct immunofluorescence, utilizing monoclonal antibody against *T. pallidum*.

Serologic testing utilizes treponemal and nontreponemal tests. Nontreponemal tests (VDRL, rapid plasma reagin) utilize a cardiolipin antigen and are rapid, inexpensive, rather insensitive in primary, latent, and late syphilis, but useful in screening and to monitor the effectiveness of therapy. Biologic false-positives occur in less than 1% of the general population but are more common in the elderly, drug addicts, and patients with chronic infections or autoimmune diseases. Positive results obtained with a nontreponemal test must be confirmed with a specific test. Specific treponemal tests (the fluoresent treponemal antibody absorption test and microhemagglutination assay—*T. pallidum*) are more sensitive in primary, latent, and late syphilis, but are more expensive and laborious.

Therapy with penicillin G is still effective, but treatment of nervous system syphillis has been shown to require high doses of penicillin intravenously for at least 10 days.

NONVENEREAL TREPONEMATOSIS

The nonvenereal or endemic treponematoses occur exclusively in underdeveloped populations of tropical and arid regions, and include yaws, pinta, and bejel. All three are nonfatal but potentially debilitating diseases that are transmitted person to person by direct skin or mucous membrane contact. They are characterized by a primary superficial lesion at the site of inoculation and secondary, hematogenous satellite lesions of the skin. Destructive granulomas of skin, subcutaneous tissues, bones, and joints are tertiary manifestations of yaws and bejel, and pigmented skin changes are the tertiary lesions of pinta. The endemic treponematoses were once widespread throughout the rural tropics and subtropics, but they have been greatly reduced or eradicated locally by mass treatment campaigns with penicillin. The diagnosis of these infections is based upon their clinical appearance, the demonstration of the treponemes in lesions by darkfield microscopy or direct immunofluorescent staining, and by serologic tests for syphilis.

YAWS

Yaws is a communicable disease of the humid tropics caused by *T. pertenue* and characterized by chronic relapsing benign lesions separated by periods of latency, and late destructive lesions of skin and bone. Yaws occurs in rural Africa, Southeast Asia, Australia, the Caribbean, and the Atlantic coast of South America.

The incubation period of yaws is 3 to 5 weeks. The primary papilloma usually occurs on the lower leg, face, or arm in children, becoming up to 8 cm in diameter. After the treponemes disseminate to the skin (weeks or months), secondary lesions occur. These are multiple, circular, raised, red-yellow, granular lesions that produce a yellow discharge and form black scabs, eventually healing and leaving scars (Fig 50–4). Bone pain may be severe, reflecting osteitis. This stage of disease is followed by a 3-year latent period. Tertiary lesions commonly occur after puberty and include destructive, bony lesions of the hands, feet, and cranium.

PINTA

Pinta is a chronic contagious disease caused by *T. carateum* and characterized by pigmented skin lesions. Pinta occurs primarily among the primitive Indians of tropical Central and South America. About half of all cases are in children. After an incubation period of 3 days to 2 months a pruritic red papule appears, usually on the hand or foot. This primary lesion slowly spreads, becoming raised and scaly, and persists for years. Six to 12 months after the appearance of the primary lesion, widespread pruritic macules erupt, appearing in crops and coalescing, eventually becoming pigmented (Fig 50–5).

BEJEL

Bejel (endemic syphilis) is a nonvenereally transmitted disease caused by *T. pallidum* subsp. *endemicum.* Bejel occurs in the cooler, drier climates of the Middle East, Botswana,

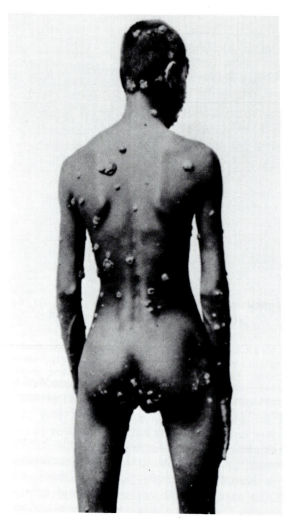

FIG 50–4.
Yaws. The elevated papillomatous nodules characteristic of early yaws are widely distributed and painless. They contain numerous spirochetes easily demonstrable by darkfield examination. (From Binsford CH, Connor DH (eds): *Pathology of Tropical and Extraordinary Diseases: An Atlas,* vol 1. Washington, DC, Armed Forces Institute of Pathology, 1976. Used by permission.)

Rhodesia, Central Australia, and Bosnia. Most cases are seen in young children. Transmission is by direct contact of mucous membranes or by fomites. The incubation period is 2 weeks to 3 months. The initial lesions are usually mucous patches in the mouth, followed by moist papules

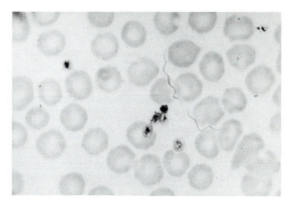

FIG 50−6.
Borrelia in blood.

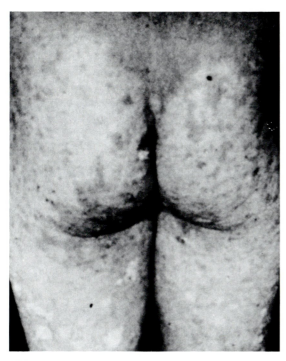

FIG 50−5.
Pinta. Note the marked variation in pigmentation with the presence of several achromic areas which cannot be distinguished from vitiligo. Depigmentation is commonly seen as a late sequela of any of the treponemal diseases. (From Binford CH, Connor DH (eds): *Pathology of Tropical and Extraordinary Diseases: An Atlas,* vol 1. Washington DC, Armed Forces Institute of Pathology; 1976. Used by permission.)

in skin folds and drier lesions on the trunk and extremities. Late manifestations after a latent period are inflammatory or destructive lesions of the skin, long bones, and nasopharynx.

BORRELIA

Borrelia are relatively large spirochetes with irregular coils. They are gram-negative and stain well with Wright's or Giemsa stain (Fig 50−6). They can be cultured in special media that supply the long chain fatty acids they require for growth. A characteristic of *Borrelia* is the frequency with which mutations occur that deter-mine the surface antigens. Seven antigens have been identified that are outer envelope proteins. Species pathogenic for man include *B. burgdorferi*, the agent of Lyme disease, and several other species that cause relapsing fever.

RELAPSING FEVER

Relapsing fever is an acute disease caused by one of several species of *Borrelia* transmitted by the bite of an arthropod and characterized by an initial febrile episode, an apyrexial interval, and relapses of fever and other symptoms. There are two forms of relapsing fever: epidemic (louse-borne) caused by *B. recurrentis* and its variants, and endemic (tick-borne) caused by one of about 15 species of *Borrelia*.

Epidemics of louse-borne disease occur in Asia, Africa, and South America. The infection is transmitted by the bite of the human body louse, *Pediculus humanus*. Man is the reservoir of this form of relapsing fever. Epidemics are associated with overcrowding, poor personal hygiene, and malnutrition, conditions that often follow large-scale disasters. *Borrelia* are ingested by the louse when it takes a blood meal from an infected person. The spirochetes multiply within the louse, and are transmitted when the louse is crushed when biting an uninfected person. Lice remain infected for life. The incubation period is approximately 8 days. There is an abrupt onset of high fever (often to 40.5° C); shaking chills; severe headache; lethargy or delirium; severe muscle, bone, and joint pain; and weakness, nausea, and vomiting. Eye pain and cough are common symptoms. The initial febrile episode lasts for about 5 days during which time there is spirochetemia. The fever resolves by crisis (suddenly) and is followed by an afebrile period of approximately 9 days, during which time 8% of the patients develop a petechial or macular rash. The fever returns for about 2 days with milder symptoms. The case fatality is up to 40% in untreated persons; 3% to 4% in treated patients. Death is often due to myocarditis.

Endemic tick-borne relapsing fever is widespread in Africa, Asia, the Middle East, and in North and South America. In the United States, relapsing fever is endemic throughout much of the Western States and is caused by *B. hermsii* or *B. turicatae*, transmitted by ticks of the genus *Ornithodoros*. These ticks inhabit rodent burrows and are reclusive, usually feeding at night for short periods. They can survive for up to 20 years without feeding, and *Borrelia* may remain viable and infective within them for months to years. The reservoir of the spirochete is in various species of wild rodents. Ticks infect by irrigating the feeding puncture with contaminated saliva.

The clinical manifestations of endemic relapsing fever are similar to the epidemic form of the disease with the following differences: the initial febrile attack is shorter (3 days); the afebrile interval is shorter (7 days); there may be up to three relapses; rash is more common (25%); and the case fatality rate is much lower (2%–5%). The fever and other manifestations are believed to be due to an endotoxin associated with the organism. The relapses characteristic of this disease are due to the repetitive mutations of the organism during the course of the infection, presenting a variety of antigens to the host. Antibody formed to the predominating spirochetal population applies selective pressure that permits variants with a different antigenic composition to emerge. The antibody produces a crisis phenomenon when large numbers of *Borrelia* lyse and release endotoxin.

The diagnosis of relapsing fever is based on the demonstration of *Borrelia* in the blood. During febrile episodes, spirochetes can be found in the blood of 70% of the patients. Repeated examination of the blood by thick and thin smears stained with Wright's or Giemsa stain can increase the yield. It is rare to see organisms in blood smears taken during afebrile intervals. Therapy of *Borrelia* is with tetracycline or one of the newer cephalosporins.

LYME DISEASE

Lyme disease is a multisystem disorder caused by a spirochete, *B. burgdorferi*, and transmitted by the bite of a tick. Lyme disease was first recognized in 1975 as an outbreak of arthritis in Old Lyme, Connecticut. Some of the manifestations of Lyme disease were observed in Europe for many years. The disease occurs primarily in three regions of the United States: the East Coast (Massachusetts to Maryland); the Midwest (Wisconsin and Minnesota); and the Far West (northern California, southern Oregon, western Nevada). Lyme disease has also been reported from 27 other states, including Texas, Arkansas, and North Carolina. In Europe, cases have been reported in France, Austria, Germany, southern Scandinavia, and Russia. In the eastern and midwestern United States, the disease is transmitted by the deer tick, *Ixodes dammini*. Other ticks (including dog ticks) are involved in Southern and Western States, and in Europe. Approximately 14,000 tick bites are reported each year in the Eastern States. It is estimated that 30% of these ticks are infected with *Borrelia*.

The life cycle of the tick starts when adults feed and mate, usually on deer. The adults leave the host, the female lays eggs and dies. The eggs hatch in the fall and the larvae infect small mammals, such as field mice. The following spring, usually during May, the larvae mature to the nymph stage. The nymphs feed on deer, other animals, and humans, eventually maturing to adults. Infection occurs when the spirochetes are injected as the tick feeds. The incubation period ranges from 3 to 32 days. Less than 50% of patients recall the tick bite. The spirochetes migrate to the skin, producing a lesion, erythema chronica migrans (ECM) (Fig 50–7), that is pathognomonic for Lyme disease, but is absent in 15% to 30% of the patients. The spirochetes enter the bloodstream and disseminate to the lungs, spleen, liver, joints, and the central nervous system. The organisms are predominantly extracellular.

Lyme disease is a three-stage disease, resembling syphilis in many respects. In stage 1, the ECM lesion starts as a small papule at the site of the tick bite. The papule expands over several days to form a large annular lesion with partial central clearing. Multiple secondary erythematous lesions develop over the next few days. In addition to the ECM, patients may develop hepatitis, orchitis, interstitial pneumonia, or conjunctivitis. Prominent symptoms are intermittent headache, neck pain and stiffness, migratory muscle and joint pain, and nausea and anorexia. Stage 1 lasts approximately 4 weeks.

Stage 2 is characterized by central nervous

system and cardiac involvement. Approximately 15% of untreated patients develop neurologic disease about 1 month after the onset of ECM. Cranial palsies that usually affect the facial nerve (Bell's palsy) may persist for weeks or months, and peripheral radiculoneuritis affecting the upper extremities or the thorax is common. These manifestations may be accompanied by aseptic meningitis. Eight percent of patients develop endomyocarditis about 3 weeks after the onset of ECM, with variable heart block and congestive heart failure. Stage 2 can last from days to months.

Stage 3 is characterized by synovitis and arthritis. Fifty percent to 60% of untreated patients develop arthritis within a few weeks to 2 years after the appearance of ECM. Large joints are affected with effusions leading to swelling, and 10% of these patients develop chronic, destructive disease with erosion of cartilage and bone. Other late manifestations are chronic atrophic acrodermatitis (rare in the United States), and severe, chronic, central nervous system disease with encephalitis, demyelinating syndromes, and psychiatric disorders. Stage 3 may last for months or years, and resembles tertiary syphilis in the long latency period and few spirochetes in the tissues. Circulating immune complexes are present in most patients with Lyme disease and it is thought that they play some role in the pathogenesis of this disorder.

The cultivation of *B. burgdorferi* requires a complex medium that is not generally available in clinical laboratories, and although the organism has been recovered from ECM lesions, blood, and cerebrospinal and synovial fluid, isolation is not the diagnostic method of choice. The laboratory diagnosis of Lyme is based primarily upon serologic tests and a specific immune response is usually detectable within a few weeks of the onset of disease, by enzyme-linked immunosorbent assay (ELISA), or indirect immunofluorescence. Caution must be used in the interpretation of serologic tests that have not yet been standardized. False-positive results are as-

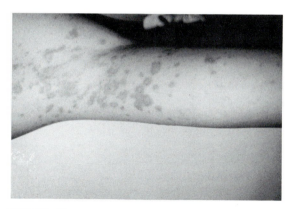

FIG 50–7.
Lyme disease. Erythema chronicum migrans.

sociated with syphilis or other spirochetal infections such as periodontal disease, infectious mononucleosis, rheumatoid arthritis, or systemic lupus erythematosus. True-positive results may be due to previous asymptomatic Lyme disease and may not relate to the present clinical problem. Most patients with the complications of stage 2 or 3 have positive test results.

The early administration of antibiotics may abolish the antibody response. Therapy with amoxicillin, doxycycline, or ceftriaxone has been effective particularly in central nervous system illness. There is presently a tendency to over-diagnose Lyme disease in patients who have other diseases or vague, unexplained symptoms.

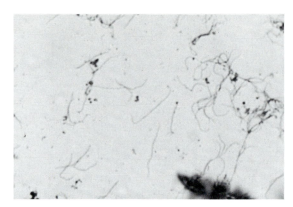

FIG 50–8.
Leptospira.

LEPTOSPIROSIS

Leptospira are aerobic spirochetes with closely wound spirals and hooked ends (Fig 50–8). They are not readily stainable. The pathogenic species is *L. interrogans*, which contains 18 serogroups (formerly designated as species, e.g., *L. icterohaemorrhagiae*, *L. canicola*, *L. autumnalis*, etc.) and 150 serotypes. The organism is a pathogen of wild or domestic animals (dogs, cats, cattle, swine, horses, rodents) and is excreted in the urine of infected animals. The organism can survive in neutral or alkaline water for several weeks.

Humans become infected by coming into contact with water that has been contaminated with animal urine. The organism enters the body through abraded skin, the conjunctiva, or the upper respiratory tract. In the United States, leptospirosis was an occupational disease of sewer and abattoir workers who had contact with rat urine, but in recent years the disease has occurred primarily in young adults in the warm weather months who swim or are otherwise exposed to contaminated water. The incubation period is about 10 to 14 days. The onset is abrupt with fever, chills, severe muscle aches, and often, a nonproductive cough which may be accompanied by nausea, vomiting and diarrhea. The most common sign is conjunctival suffusion.

Leptospirosis is typically a biphasic illness. The individual febrile period lasts 3 to 10 days and is followed by an afebrile interval of several days that coincides with the appearance of IgM antibodies. The second febrile period may be accompanied by aseptic meningitis and iridocyclitis. A more severe form of leptospirosis (Weil's syndrome) is manifested by jaundice, hemorrhages, and disturbances in consciousness, and is associated with liver or kidney dysfunction. The mortality rate is 2% to 10%, but rises sharply to 33% in men over 60 years of age. Death is usually due to liver or kidney failure or myocarditis.

Therapy with penicillin or cephalosporins such as cefotaxine or ceftriaxone has been shown to decrease morbidity and mortality.

CHAPTER 51

Rickettsia and Rickettsia-Like Organisms

A 49-year-old man presented with fever, rash, and intense headache. He was born in Poland but had resided in the United States for the past 10 years. Five days earlier, there was an abrupt onset of chills, and fever to 39.4° C, accompanied by intense headache that persisted day and night and was unrelieved by aspirin. His temperature fluctuated between normal and 39.4° C. A Weil-Felix test was negative, but a complement fixation test for *Rickettsia prowazekii* was positive and he was started on tetracycline. His symptoms disappeared within 4 days.

The family Rickettsiaceae contains four genera pathogenic for man: *Rickettsia*, *Coxiella*, *Rochalimaea*, and *Ehrlichia*. All are small, nonmotile, gram-negative coccobacilli, barely visible with the light microscope. They stain poorly with the Gram stain, but they can be visualized with special stains (Gimenez or acridine orange). The cytoplasm contains both RNA and DNA. With the exception of *Rochalimaea*, they are obligate intracellular organisms that infect arthropods. Vertebrate hosts are infected by the bite of the parasitized arthropod. The various pathogenic species are listed in Table 51–1.

RICKETTSIA

Four groups of rickettsia are pathogenic for man: the spotted fever group, including *R. rickettsii* and *R. akari*; the typhus group, including *R. prowazekii* and *R. typhi*; *R. tsutsugamushi*; and *Coxiella burnetii*. These groups differ in size, extracellular behavior, intracellular location, and antigenic composition.

Rickettsia have the enzymes for electron transport, the tricarboxylic acid cycle, and other metabolic capabilities, but the increased permeability of their cytoplasmic membrane to nucleotides requires them to utilize certain host metabolites for survival. In the absence of vertebrate hosts, rickettsia are maintained in arthropods from generation to generation by transovarial passage. With the exception of the louse, the arthropods are not harmed by the rickettsia. Human infection is an accidental interruption in the transmission cycle.

Rickettsia enter the cell by attaching end on

TABLE 51–1.

Pathogenic Species of Rickettsia and Related Organisms

Organism	Disease	Reservoir	Vector	Target Cell	Basic Lesion
Spotted fever group (*Rickettsia*)					
R. rickettsii	Rocky Mountain spotted fever	Wild rodents, dogs	Tick	Endothelial and smooth muscle	Vasculitis
R. australis	North Queensland tick typhus	Wild rodents, marsupials	Tick		
R. sibirica	North Asian tick typhus	Wild rodents	Tick		
R. conorii	Boutonneuse fever	Wild rodents, dogs	Tick		
R. akari	Rickettsialpox	Mice	Mite		
Typhus group (*Rickettsia*)					
R. prowazekii	Epidemic typhus	Man, flying squirrels	Louse		
R. typhi	Murine typhus	Rodents	Flea	Endothelial	Vasculitis
R. tsutsugamushi	Scrub typhus	Wild rodents	Mite		
Others					
Coxiella burnetii	Q fever	Cattle, sheep, goats	—	Monocytes, endothelial cells, macrophages	Granulomas
Rochalimaea quintana	Trench fever	Man	Louse	?	?
Ehrlichia sennetsu	Sennetsu ehrlichiosis	Man	?		
Ehrlichia canis?	Human ehrlichiosis	Dogs	Tick	Monocytes	

to the cell membrane, and multiplying freely in the cytoplasm. Rickettsia of the spotted fever group also replicate in the nucleus. Rickettsial replication causes the death of the cell. There is evidence that lipopolysaccharide from the rickettsia have endotoxic properties. Rickettsial infections begin in the vascular system, following the bite of an arthropod. The basic rickettsial lesion is a vasculitis. The organisms damage capillary endothelial cells resulting in thrombosis, increased permeability, tissue edema, hemorrhage, circulatory failure, and meningoencephalitis.

ROCKY MOUNTAIN SPOTTED FEVER

Rocky Mountain spotted fever (RMSF) is a severe, protean systemic illness caused by *R. rickettsii* and characterized by a rash (Fig 51–1) and increased vascular permeability. *Rickettsia rickettsii* is a small, obligate intracellular bacterium that has antigens in common with the spotted fever group. The organism contains numer-

ous antigenic proteins; the immunodominant antigens are two surface proteins designated as 120 and 155 kilodaltons. The cell wall also contains lipopolysaccharide. The reservoir of *R. rickettsii* is in various species of ticks, to which the organisms are highly adapted.

At least 75% of cases of RMSF occur east of the Rocky Mountains, in the South Atlantic and Middle Western States. States with the greatest number of cases are Oklahoma, North Carolina, Virginia, Arkansas, Missouri, and Kansas. Most of the infections take place in the spring and summer months, with a high incidence in children. Sixty percent to 80% of cases have a history of tick bites.

The incubation period of RMSF ranges from 2 to 14 days, most commonly 7 days. There is an abrupt onset of severe headache, chills, fever, mental confusion, generalized muscle pain and tenderness, nausea, vomiting, and abdominal pain. Conjunctivitis with petechial lesions and photophobia are common symptoms. Thrombocytopenia occurs in up to half of the patients. A characteristic maculopapular or petechial rash

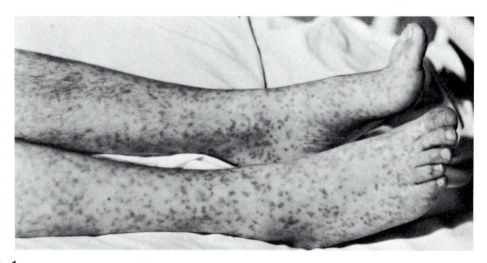

FIG 51–1.
The rash of Rocky Mountain spotted fever consists of generally distributed, sharply defined purpuric macules initially involving the extremities, including the palms and soles, and then spreading to the trunk. (From Binford CH, Connor DH (eds): *Pathology of Tropical and Extraordinary Diseases: An Atlas,* vol 1, Washington, DC, Armed Forces Institute of Pathology, 1976. Used by permission.)

appears on the third day of illness, appearing first on the extremities, palms, and soles, and then spreading to involve the rest of the body. In severe cases, the rash may progress to extensive hemorrhagic and necrotic lesions. After a few days, edema develops, at first periorbitally and then becoming generalized, involving the extremities. Untreated, there may be vascular collapse. Life-threatening complications include encephalitis (28% of cases), involvement of the pulmonary microcirculation (12% of patients have severe respiratory failure), and acute renal failure. The fatality in untreated cases is 15% to 25%, higher in older patients and in those without a history of a tick bite (because of the delay in diagnosis).

Rickettsia rickettsii are introduced as the tick takes a blood meal. The organisms undergo reactivation from a dormant avirulent state to a highly pathogenic form. This reactivation is mediated by the body temperature of the host and possibly nutritional factors, and requires at least 24 hours. (Infection seldom occurs if the ticks are removed within that period.) From the skin the organisms pass, via the lymphatics and bloodstream, to all parts of the body. At each site, rickettsia attach to and enter endothelial cells where they proliferate, causing cell death. Organisms released from dead cells invade vascular smooth muscle cells. The actual mechanism of cell damage is not known; cytotoxicity may be due to cell membrane damage by phospholipase activity. Other pathophysiologic effects are due to activation of both extrinsic and intrinsic pathways of coagulation, platelets, the fibrinolytic system, and possibly inflammatory mediators. The increased vascular permeability leads to tissue edema, hypovolemia, hypoproteinemia, and reduced perfusion of various organs.

The diagnosis of RMSF is essentially clinical and includes a history of tick bite. It must be differentiated from many other infectious and noninfectious illnesses. Immunochemical staining of lesion biopsy material can demonstrate the organisms. Antibodies do not appear until 7 to 9 days after the onset of symptoms and therefore serologic tests are retrospective and only useful in confirming the clinical diagnosis. Historically, the Weil-Felix test was used to detect antibodies that agglutinated certain strains of *Proteus vulgaris*, but this test is insensitive and nonspecific and should not be used for RMSF. A complement fixation test is specific but lacks sensitivity. Recently, indirect fluorescent antibody, indirect hemagglutination, and latex agglutination procedures have become available which are sensitive and specific.

Treatment is with tetracycline or chloramphenicol.

RICKETTSIALPOX

Rickettsialpox is a mild, febrile illness caused by *R. akari*, transmitted by a mite, and characterized by a primary cutaneous lesion and a rash. *Rickettsia akari* is a member of the spotted fever group of rickettsia. The reservoir is in mice, and the infection is transmitted to man by the bite of a mite. The incubation period is 10 to 14 days. An initial skin lesion appears at the site of inoculation together with regional lymphadenopathy. There is a sudden onset of headache, chills, and fever followed in 1 to 4 days by a diffuse, maculopapular, nonpruritic rash. The rash persists for 2 to 8 days, eventually becoming vesicular and crusting over. The diagnosis is clinical. Antibodies detectable by complement fixation or immunofluorescent techniques appear after about 14 days.

Treatment is not necessary.

EPIDEMIC TYPHUS

Epidemic typhus is an acute infectious disease caused by *R. prowazekii* that is transmitted from man to man by the human body louse. *Rickettsia prowazekii* is a member of the typhus group of rickettsia. It is a diplobacillus that reproduces by binary fission and grows in the cytoplasm of infected cells. The organism can be readily visualized in these cells by Giemsa or Gimenez staining. Viable *R. prowazekii* contains a toxin lethal to mice, and a hemolysin, both of which are tightly bound to the organism. The major antigens are a heat-labile protein that is species-specific, and a soluble, heat-stable polysaccharide, identical to that of *R. typhi* and to *P. vulgaris* OX-19.

Epidemic typhus occurs in the cooler regions of Mexico, Central and South America, Africa, and Asia. Outbreaks of epidemic typhus follow wars and other disasters where there is overcrowding and poor hygiene. The disease was widespread in Europe during World War II. Epidemic typhus is transmitted by the bite of the human body louse, *Pediculus humanus*. The reservoir is man. The louse becomes infected by feeding on the blood of a patient with acute typhus fever or recrudescent typhus. Infected lice excrete rickettsia in their feces; humans become infected by rubbing the feces or crushed lice into the pruritic bite wound or into superficial skin abrasions by scratching. Lice die 2 weeks after they become infected, but the rickettsia remain viable in the dead louse for many weeks. In the United States, a reservoir of *R. prowazekii* exists in flying squirrels, and humans have become infected by the bite of fleas, lice, and other ectoparasites.

The incubation period is 1 to 2 weeks, commonly 12 days. There is an abrupt onset of chills, fever, headache, weakness, backache, and myalgia. Conjunctivitis and photophobia are common symptoms. The fever remains high until recovery or until the patient dies. A generalized rash appears on the fifth to the ninth day of illness, at first in the axillae and upper chest, then spreading to the abdomen and rest of the body, sparing the face, palms, and soles. Meningoencephalitis occurs by the end of the first week, progressing in fatal cases to uremia, stupor, and coma. Pneumonia is an important complication of typhus. Pneumonia occurring during the first week of disease is generally rickettsial, but secondary bacterial pneumonia may occur later in the disease. The fever generally resolves by the third week leaving the patient weak, irritable, or apathetic for 2 or 3 months. The mortality of untreated disease may be as high as 40%, especially in patients older than 40 years. Following the introduction of the organisms into the skin, there is a rickettsemia with dissemination to the endothelial cells of small blood vessels, especially of the skin, brain, heart, and kidneys. The resulting increased capillary permeability leads to a loss of plasma, and hemoconcentration. Disseminated intravascular coagulation may occur with peripheral vascular collapse.

Recrudescent typhus (Brill-Zinsser disease) is *R. prowazekii* typhus that recurs after a latent period of 4 to 50 years following the primary attack. The symptoms are less severe and of shorter duration, but patients with Brill-Zinsser disease represent a potential reservoir in a louse-infested population. A vaccine containing inactivated *R. prowazekii* is available for special risk groups.

Although *R. prowazekii* can be isolated from the blood of patients during rickettsemia by inoculation into the yolk sac of chick embryo, or into guinea pigs, serologic methods are often used for diagnosis. Specific antibodies detectable by complement fixation with rickettsial antigens appear by the end of the first week, and continue to rise to the fourth week. The Weil-Felix reaction is not reliable; antibodies are short-lived, and false-negative results are common, especially in Brill-Zinsser disease.

Therapy of typhus is with tetracycline or chloramphenicol.

MURINE TYPHUS

Murine (endemic) typhus is an acute febrile disease caused by infection with *R. typhi*. Murine typhus is primarily a disease of rats; man becomes infected by the bite of the rat flea. *Rickettsia typhi* (formerly *R. mooseri*) is a member of the typhus group of rickettsia and shares common antigens with *R. prowazekii* and *P. vulgaris* OX-19. Murine typhus is worldwide in distribution and occurs where people live in close proximity to large populations of rats or mice and their ectoparasites. Cases in the United States occur in the Southeastern States and along the Gulf Coast. Large numbers of cases have occurred in Hispanics in Texas. The majority of cases occur in late summer and autumn. Transmission to man follows the bite of the rat flea, *Xenopsylla cheopis*, which excretes rickettsia in the feces while taking a blood meal, contaminating the wound. Infection also occurs in cats and other domestic and wild animals, and their ectoparasites, e.g., the cat flea, can serve as a vector for human infection.

The clinical picture of murine typhus resembles that of epidemic typhus, but the disease is milder. The incubation period is 1 to 2 weeks, and the onset is sudden, but the progression of symptoms is more gradual than with epidemic typhus. The rash appears on the third to fifth day of illness, typically first on the abdomen and spreading to the chest, back, and upper extremities. About one third of the patients do not develop a rash. Headache and arthralgia continue throughout the course of the illness which generally lasts 12 to 16 days in the untreated person. Complications are uncommon, and recrudescence does not occur. The mortality is less than 2%.

The diagnosis is made by serologic methods or by recovering the organism. *Rickettsia typhi* can be isolated by injecting the patient's blood intraperitoneally into guinea pigs, which develop fever and scrotal swelling, or by inoculating the chick embryo yolk sac. The serologic methods of choice are complement fixation or microagglutination tests utilizing the common rickettsial antigen. The cross-reacting antibodies to *P. vulgaris* OX-19 develop by the fourth day of disease, and peak around the tenth day.

SCRUB TYPHUS

Scrub typhus (tsutsugamushi disease) is an acute febrile illness caused by *R. tsutsugamushi*, and characterized by a primary cutaneous lesion and a rash. *Rickettsia tsutsugamushi* (formerly *R. orientalis*) is a small gram-negative obligate intracellular parasite that multiplies in the cytoplasm of infected cells. It can be visualized after staining with Giemsa or Macchiavellos stains. Unlike other rickettsia, *R. tsutsugamushi* is immunologically heterogeneous and there are many distinct strains that vary serologically and in their virulence. Scrub typhus occurs primarily in Asia and Australia, and is largely an occupational disease affecting workers in mite-infested scrub, forest, or desert regions.

The reservoir is in infected larval stages of trombiculid mites (chiggers), and is maintained in these arthropods by transovarial passage. Their mites are usually ectoparasites of rats or other small rodents. Man becomes infected by the bite of the larval mite. The incubation period is 8 to 12 days. An ulcer forms at the site of the mite bite and is followed in a few days by the abrupt onset of headache, high fever, profuse sweating, and conjunctival injection. There is tender lymphadenopathy of the regional nodes draining the site of the initial lesion. A rash appears after the first week of illness, initially on the trunk and then extending to the extremities. The rash disappears in a few days. Bronchitis or interstitial pneumonia is common. The fever generally persists for 14 days. The case fatality varies widely from 1% to 60%, according to the virulence of the strain. Recurrent infections are common.

The basic lesion is a disseminated, focal, perivasculitis with damage to the vascular endothelial cells. Diagnosis is primarily serologic.

IgM appears by day 8 of illness and rises rapidly; IgG appears about 5 days later. The Weil-Felix test is widely used; by the ninth day of disease, *P. vulgaris* OX-K agglutinins are positive; OX-2 and OX-19 are negative.

Treatment is with tetracycline or chloramphenicol.

Q FEVER

Q fever (Q for "query" when the etiologic agent was unknown) is a systemic febrile illness caused by infection with *C. burnetii*. *Coxiella burnetii* is a highly pleomorphic coccobacillus that morphologically resembles rickettsia, but differs from them in a number of significant ways: *C. burnetii* does not require an arthropod vector; the organism is resistant to desiccation and other physical and chemical factors and can survive in the environment for long periods; it enters host cells by a passive phagocytic process and replicates in the phagolysosome, resisting lysosomal hydrolases and the low pH; it metabolizes pyruvate and synthesizes enzymes of the Embden-Meyerhof pathway; and the organism does not elicit agglutinins against any of the *P. vulgaris* OX strains. *Coxiella burnetii* exhibits a unique phase variation which is host-induced. In nature or in laboratory animals, the organism exists as a virulent phase I; on repeated passage in embryonated hens' eggs, the organism converts to an avirulent phase II. This phase variation, which is somewhat analogous to the smooth-rough variation of some bacteria, is accompanied by changes in major antigenic components, immunogenicity, resistance to phagocytosis, and physicochemical changes.

Q fever occurs worldwide. The reservoir is in cattle, sheep, goats, and many species of ticks. In occupationally acquired disease affecting farmers, meat and dairy workers, and veterinarians, transmission is via the inhalation of dust contaminated with excreta and fetal and placental tissues and fluids of infected animals. *Coxiella burnetii* is extremely virulent; a single inhaled organism can cause disease. Laboratory infections are common. Sporadic cases may result from the ingestion of unpasteurized milk from infected cows.

The incubation period is 2 to 3 weeks. The onset is sudden with fever spikes to 40° C, severe headache, myalgia, and chest pain. Most patients present with pneumonitis; in others acute hepatitis is the major symptom. More than half of the patients have hepatomegaly, and related bradycardia is characteristic. Symptoms persist for 4 to 7 days and the temperature gradually returns to normal within 15 days. Acute Q fever is rarely fatal. Persistent infection with *C. burnetii* can cause chronic Q fever characterized by endocarditis and liver and kidney involvement. Chronic Q fever is invariably fatal.

Coxiella burnetii has a predilection for the vascular endothelium of arteries, veins, and capillaries, the epithelium of the respiratory tract and the renal tubules, and serosal cells. There is a persistent rickettsemia. The granulomatous nature of the lesion may be due to induction of immune complex phenomena. The diagnosis of Q fever is usually made serologically, by complement fixation, microagglutination, or microimmunofluorescent tests. Complement fixing antibodies to phase II antigen appear by the second week of disease; the more sensitive tests can detect antibody 1 week earlier. The polysaccharide antigen is protective. A heat-killed vaccine is available for persons with an occupational risk.

TRENCH FEVER

Trench fever is a nonfatal, febrile disease caused by infection with *Rochalimaea quintana*. *Rochalimaea quintana* is a gram-negative, rickettsia-like organism that differs from rickettsia in its ability to grow on cell-free media. The organism requires an enriched medium containing horse serum and hematin or erythrocytes, and a moist atmosphere with 5% carbon dioxide. Small colonies appear in the agar surface after 12 to 14 days. A previously uncharacterized rickettsia-like organism closely related to *R. quintana* is thought to be the cause of bacillary angiomatosis and possibly also cat-scratch disease. Endemic foci of trench fever have been detected in Eastern Europe, Mexico, South America, and Africa. The reservoir is man. The disease is transmitted by the body louse, *P. humanus.*

The incubation period is 7 to 30 days. The onset of trench fever may be sudden or slow, with headache, fever, and pain and tenderness in the shins. Splenomegaly is common. Recurrences occur many years after the primary infection. The diagnosis is made by culturing the patient's blood on specially enriched media.

Recently, *R. quintana* has been shown to be a cause of cutaneous vasculitic lesions in HIV-infected patients and to cause angiomatous changes in the liver of these individuals.

EHRLICHIOSIS

Two distinct syndromes are recognized: sennetsu ehrlichiosis, occurring in southwestern Japan, and human ehrlichiosis, occurring in the United States. *Ehrlichia* are rickettsia-like organisms that parasitize peripheral blood leukocytes. *Ehrlichia sennetsu* infects blood monocytes while *E. canis* infects lymphocytes, neutrophils, and monocytes. Sennetsu ehrlichiosis is a mononucleosis-like acute, febrile disease caused by infection with *E. sennetsu.* It is characterized by lethargy, lymphadenopathy, and hematologic abnormalities. The reservoir is man, but the means of transmission is unknown.

Human ehrlichiosis clinically resembles RMSF, except that rash is uncommon. There is malaise and fever, often accompanied by relative bradycardia, headache, nausea, vomiting, abdominal cramps, and myalgia. Most patients develop thrombocytopenia and elevated alanine or aspartate aminotransferase levels. Symptoms last about 7 days. The most common complications are acute respiratory failure, encephalopathy, and acute renal failure. Fatalities have occurred. Human ehrlichiosis is caused by a new strain of *E. canis* or a new, closely related species of *Ehrlichia.*

Diagnosis is made during the acute phase of human ehrlichiosis by visualizing inclusion bodies in Giemsa-stained peripheral blood buffy coat smears. The organisms appear as small dots or clusters in the cytoplasm of leukocytes. Antibodies appear that react with *E. canis* by indirect fluorescent antibody staining.

CHAPTER 52

Viral Exanthems

The viral exanthems are primarily diseases of infancy and childhood. They include varicella (chickenpox), measles, rubella, erythema infectiosum, and roseola. The term **exanthem** is used to describe a rash associated with a systemic illness. Rashes are temporary skin eruptions that may take different forms. Erythematous rashes appear as reddened skin resembling a sunburn that blanches when pressed with the fingers. Petechial rashes consist of small discrete skin hemorrhages. Macular rashes are composed of flat lesions; papular rashes are small, raised nodules. A rash may be described as maculopapular and exhibit both flat and raised lesions. A vesicular rash is characterized by small, elevated, blisterlike lesions filled with clear fluid. Pustular rashes are elevated lesions filled with pus. Rashes may be evanescent and disappear within hours or days with no residua, or lesions may evolve into other forms with eventual crusting, scarring, or desquamation of the skin. The characteristic appearance of a rash and its anatomic distribution and progress provide useful clues to diagnosis. Table 52–1 compares the characteristics of the viral exanthems.

Varicella (chickenpox) is discussed in Chapter 27.

MEASLES

Measles is an acute, highly communicable viral disease, usually seen in children, and characterized by cough, coryza, fever, conjunctivitis, and a maculopapular rash. Measles virus is a member of the Paramyxoviridae family. There is only one serotype. The virions are pleomorphic spheres that consist of a nucleocapsid of linear, negative-sense (−), single-stranded RNA and a coiled helix of three proteins. Surrounding the nucleocapsid is an envelope composed of three additional proteins: a matrix M protein and two glycoproteins that exist as short surface projections (peplomers). One of these glycoproteins (H) mediates the adsorption of the virus to receptors on the cell surface and also is responsible for the hemagglutination reaction. The other glycoprotein (F) mediates the fusion of the virus with the host cell, the penetration of virus into the host cell, and hemolysis. Unlike other paramyxoviruses, measles virus has no neuraminidase.

Prior to widespread immunization, measles was very common in childhood. The reservoir is man. Measles is one of the most contagious infectious diseases. Transmission is by direct con-

TABLE 52–1.
Characteristics of the Viral Exanthems

Disease	Etiology	Incubation (days)	Clinical Characteristics	Rash	Duration
Varicella	Varicella-zoster virus	14–21	Fever, headache, malaise	Maculopapular, becoming vesicular and crusting; appears in crops	Few days–2 weeks
Measles	Measles virus	7–14	Fever, coryza, cough, conjunctivitis, Koplik's spots	Brownish-pink maculopapular; starts on head, spreads to trunk	4–7 days
Rubella	Rubella virus	14–21	Fever, headache, rhinitis, tender posterior auricular lymphadenopathy	Fine, pink, macular, becoming confluent, first on face and neck,	1–3 days
Erythema infectiosum	Parvovirus B19	5–10	Low-grade fever	Maculopapular; starts on face, spreads to extremities and trunk.	1–2 days
Roseola infantum	Human herpesvirus 6 ?	10–15	Mostly infants; high fever that disappears with rash	Diffuse maculopapular on trunk, spreading to face and extremities	1–2 days

tact with respiratory secretions of infected persons or by airborne respiratory aerosols. The incubation period is 7 to 14 days. This is followed by a prodromal phase, with malaise, fever, cough, coryza, conjunctivitis, and photophobia, that lasts a few days. Just prior to the appearance of the rash, Koplik's spots appear, which are pathognomonic of measles. Koplik's spots are small, bluish-white specks on a red areolar base that appear on the buccal mucosa opposite the second molars. Koplik's spots persist for a few days and then slough with the appearance of the rash. The rash is a brownish-pink maculopapular eruption that begins behind the ears and on the forehead and neck, and then spreads to the trunk (Fig 52–1). The rash lasts for about 5 days with the other symptoms persisting for 2 to 5 days.

"Modified" measles is a mild form of the disease seen in infants younger than 1 year with passively acquired maternal antibody or in persons treated with immune gamma globulin. Atypical measles occurs in persons who receive killed measles vaccine. A rash appears peripherally after a brief prodrome of high fever, edema of the extremities, pulmonary infiltrates, and hepatitis. This syndrome is believed to represent hypersensitivity to the measles virus in a partially immune host.

The most common complication of measles is otitis media due to group A streptococci, pneumococci, or *Haemophilus influenzae*. Other frequent complications involve bacterial infections of the lower respiratory tract. Encephalitis occurs in 0.1% of measles cases and varies in severity from mild to fulminant. A rare complication is the development of a fatal neurologic disease—subacute sclerosing panencephalitis (SSPE). This disease of children usually begins 2 to 10 years after a measles infection and is characterized by progressive intellectual deterioration, spasms, seizures, and ataxia ending in death in 6 to 12 months. It is believed that in SSPE the measles virus becomes latent in the brain, to be reactivated later by some unknown

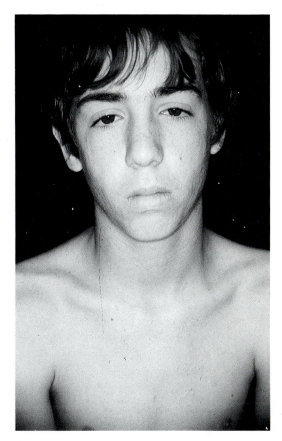

FIG 52–1.
Measles rash. (From Habif TP: *Clinical Dermatology: Color Guide to Diagnosis and Therapy.* St Louis, Mosby–Year Book, Inc, 1985. Used by permission.)

mechanism. Most patients with SSPE have high titers of measles antibody in the cerebrospinal fluid and brain cell inclusions characteristic of paramyxoviruses.

The measles virus enters the body via the upper respiratory tract and replicates locally in the mucosal epithelium and spreads to regional lymphoid tissues. Following a primary viremia in which the virus infects leukocytes, the virus reaches and multiplies throughout the reticuloendothelial system. A secondary viremia takes place (during the prodromal phase) with the virus seeding the skin, conjunctiva, and respiratory tract, resulting in lesions with multinucleated giant cells. Neutralizing and hemagglutination-inhibiting antibodies appear a few days after the onset of the rash and persist for many years. Measles infection also results in the development of cell-mediated immunity.

The diagnosis of measles is often made clinically, especially if Koplik's spots can be seen. Definitive diagnosis depends upon a rise in titer of measles antibody or by recovery of measles virus in cell culture. An attenuated live measles vaccine is highly protective, but must be administered after 12 months of age to yield effective protection, with greatest protection achieved by vaccination after 15 months of age.

RUBELLA

Rubella (German measles) is a mild, febrile disease of children and adults with serious consequences for the developing fetus. Rubella virus is a spherical particle with short projections extending from the envelope. The capsid is icosahedral, with a genome of single-stranded RNA enclosed in a lipoprotein envelope. Rubella virus is a member of the Togaviridae family. The single serotype has been placed in the genus *Rubivirus*.

The reservoir is man. Rubella is a highly communicable disease transmitted by droplets spread by aerosols or by direct contact with the nasopharyngeal secretions of infected persons. The virus is shed from 10 days before the onset of the rash to 15 days after its appearance. Pregnant women can transmit the disease to their fetus. Infants born with congenital rubella shed large quantities of virus in their urine and respiratory secretions for many months after birth.

Acquired rubella is mild and most cases are subclinical, especially in children. Adults may experience several days of malaise, anorexia, fever, rash, and lymphadenopathy involving the posterior cervical, posterior auricular, and suboccipital nodes. The rash is erythematous, appearing first on the face and spreading rapidly to the trunk and extremities, disappearing in 3 to 4 days. Complications are uncommon, but up to one third of women develop arthritis or arthralgia involving the fingers, wrists, or knees.

The main importance of rubella is the risk of fetal damage in the pregnant woman. Congenital rubella can lead to premature delivery, fetal death, or congenital defects that include deafness, mental retardation, and congenital heart disease. The effects on the fetus are related to the time of infection. Maternal viremia may result in limited placental infection or the involvement of many fetal tissues. Fetal infection during the first trimester is the most critical. Rates for congenital anomalies are 50%, 20%, and 4%, respectively, for the first, second, and third months.

The pathogenesis of rubella is not completely understood. Circulating immune complexes have been detected and may explain the rash and arthralgia. In congenital rubella, growth may be compromised by placental and fetal vasculitis.

The diagnosis of rubella is usually made serologically, although virus is readily recovered in cell culture from throat, blood, or stool specimens. A fourfold rise in titer of rubella antibody between acute and convalescent serum specimens is diagnostic, as is the presence of rubella-specific IgM. Immunization with a live attenuated rubella virus is very effective and has prevented major epidemics since its adoption in 1969.

ERYTHEMA INFECTIOSUM

Erythema infectiosum (fifth disease) is a mild illness usually occurring as epidemics in children, and caused by human parvovirus B19. Parvoviruses are very small, nonenveloped icosahedral virions containing one linear, single strand of DNA that is positive (+) in some virions and negative (−) in others. The B19 capsid enclosing the genome is formed of two structural proteins, coded by messenger RNA.

The reservoir of parvovirus B19 is man. Transmission is probably via respiratory secretions. Transplacental transmission can occur in pregnancy. The incubation period is 4 to 12 days. In the usual patient, an erythematous rash appears on the face, giving the "slapped cheek" appearance, and a reticulated, lacelike eruption appears on the trunk or extremities. The rash usually resolves in 3 weeks, but can recur a month later following exposure to hot water, sunlight, or stress. More than half the patients develop arthropathy of the wrist, hand, knee, or ankle. In persons with chronic hemolytic anemia or other conditions requiring maximal red cell production (sickle cell disease, thalassemia, hereditary spherocytosis), B19 infection and lysis of erythrocyte precursor cells can rapidly lead to an acute, life-threatening anemia. Patients with this transient aplastic crisis often have no reticulocytes in their peripheral blood, and they may require blood replacement. Primary B19 infection occurring during pregnancy may cause fetal death. The fetus may develop a persistent infection and anemia leading to extensive edema (hydrops fetalis) and congestive heart failure. Infection with B19 is followed by a viremia. Parvovirus B19 primarily infects erythroid precursor cells in the bone marrow, causing them to lyse. Peripheral blood leukocytes and fetal myocardial cells are also infected. Acute infection can be documented by symptoms of a B19 illness and by IgM antibodies specific for B19.

ROSEOLA INFANTUM

Roseola infantum (exanthem subitum) is an acute febrile illness that typically occurs in children from 6 months to 2 years of age. Recently, human herpesvirus 6 has been implicated as the cause of roseola. The disease occurs most frequently in the spring and fall. The incubation period is about 10 to 15 days. The disease is characterized by high fever that usually lasts from 3 to 5 days, but the child is not particularly ill. Forty-eight hours after the temperature returns to normal, a maculopapular rash appears on the neck or trunk which lasts for a day or so. Complications are uncommon. The diagnosis is based on the characteristic clinical appearance.

CHAPTER 53

Other Viral Agents of Multisystem Disease

Four groups of viruses are considered here: flaviviruses, bunyaviruses, arenaviruses, and filoviruses. All are enveloped RNA viruses. With a few exceptions, the diseases they cause are not seen in the United States. Flaviviruses and bunyaviruses are transmitted by arthropod vectors; direct or indirect contact with the animal reservoir and person-to-person transmission occurs with arenaviruses and filoviruses. The main characteristics of these agents are shown in Table 53–1.

Flaviviruses are small spherical particles with a dense nucleocapsid core surrounded by a glycoprotein envelope. The genome consists of single-stranded, positive-sense (+) RNA. There are only three structural proteins in the virion: a nucleocapsid protein (C), a membrane protein (M), and an envelope glycoprotein (E) present as surface spikes that mediate the absorption of the virus to target cells.

Mosquitoes become infected with flaviviruses when taking a blood meal from a viremic host. The virus enters the epithelial cells of the mosquito and spreads to the salivary glands where replication takes place. The mosquito regurgitates virus-containing saliva into the bloodstream of the next host. The virus circulates in the blood, infecting monocytes, macrophages,

vascular endothelial cells, and the reticuloendothelial cells of liver, spleen, and lymph nodes. A secondary viremia may occur with the seeding of other organs with the virus.

Flaviviruses attach to specific receptors on cell surfaces and enter the cell by endocytosis. The genome and capsid enter the cytoplasm following fusion of the envelope with the endosomal membrane and bind to the ribosome as messenger RNA. Cell death results when viral RNA is synthesized at the expense of ribosomal RNA. Virus is released from the cell by budding from the cell membrane or by cell lysis. Yellow fever and dengue are examples of diseases caused by flaviviruses.

YELLOW FEVER

Yellow fever is an acute viral illness of short duration and varying severity characterized by jaundice, hemorrhage, and renal damage. Yellow fever occurs in tropical areas of Africa Central, and South America. In urban disease the reservoir is man and transmission is by *Aedes* mosquitoes. In jungle yellow fever the mosquitoes transmit the disease to monkeys.

The incubation period is 3 to 6 days. There

TABLE 53–1.

Characteristics of Some Viral Agents

Virus Group	Virion	Diseases	Reservoir	Transmission	Geographic Distribution
Flaviviruses	Enveloped, single-stranded positive-sense RNA	Yellow fever Dengue	Man	Mosquito	South America, Africa Tropical America, Africa, Asia
Bunyaviruses	Enveloped, single-stranded negative-sense RNA	California encephalitis Hemorrhagic fevers	Rodents Various vertebrates	Mosquito, tick, contact with reservoir	Southwest United States Africa, Asia, Middle East, Balkans, USSR
Arenaviruses	Enveloped, two strands of negative-sense RNA	Lymphocytic choriomeningitis Lassa fever	Rodents	Direct/indirect contact with reservoir, person-to-person	West and Central Africa
Filoviruses	Filamentous, enveloped, negative-sense, single-stranded RNA	Ebola-Marburg	?	Person-to-person	Africa

is a sudden onset of fever, headache, backache, nausea, and vomiting. In severe forms, there are chills, hemorrhagic diatheses, and jaundice. Relative bradycardia is common. The case fatality is less than 5%, but is 20% to 50% in patients with jaundice. There is a protective vaccine which should be administered to those travelling to endemic areas.

DENGUE

Dengue is an acute febrile disease caused by a flavivirus: dengue virus types 1, 2, 3, and 4. Dengue is present throughout tropical America, Africa, and Asia. The reservoir is man, and transmission occurs via the bite of *Aedes* mosquitoes. The mosquito becomes infected 8 to 11 days after feeding on a viremic host and remains infective for life. The incubation period is 3 to 15 days, commonly 5 days. Dengue has a sudden onset with fever to 40° C, intense headache, and severe retro-orbital, muscle, and joint pain. A maculopapular or erythematous rash appears 3 to 4 days after the onset of fever, and petechiae may be seen on the palate, feet, legs, or in the axillae. The symptoms are accompanied by leukopenia, thrombocytopenia, and lymphadenopathy. The diagnosis can be made by serologic methods.

Dengue hemorrhagic fever is a more severe form of the disease occurring in Asia. Dengue hemorrhagic fever usually is the result of a second dengue infection in a person with acquired immunity to heterologous dengue virus serotype. The disease is characterized by increased vascular permeability, bleeding diatheses, and disseminated intravascular coagulation, mediated by circulating immune complexes, activation of complement, and release of vasoactive amines.

Bunyaviruses are a large group of serologically related arthropod-borne viruses. They are spherical particles with surface projections. The genome consists of three molecules of negative-

sense (−), single-stranded RNA. The virion contains a capsid protein (N), two glycoproteins (G1,G2) as spikes, and an RNA-dependent RNA polymerase. Bunyaviruses include the agent of **California encephalitis,** a major cause of mosquito-borne encephalitis in the United States, and the agents of a number of hemorrhagic fevers that include **Rift Valley fever, Congo-Crimean hemorrhagic fever,** and **Korean hemorrhagic fever.** Rift Valley fever occurs in Africa and is transmitted by mosquitoes. The incubation period is 3 to 12 days. Congo-Crimean hemorrhagic fever is seen in Africa, the Middle East, the Balkans, and the USSR. It is transmitted by ticks. The reservoir of these diseases is in various vertebrates. Korean hemorrhagic fever is a severe febrile disease with thrombocytopenia and acute renal insufficiency. The incubation period is 9 to 35 days. The initial toxic phase of headache, abdominal and lower back pain, blurred vision, and an erythematous rash on the face and trunk lasts 4 to 7 days, and leads to hypotension and shock. There is an oliguric phase of hypertension, pneumonitis, pulmonary edema, and bleeding that lasts 3 to 10 days, followed in turn by a polyuric phase with stress on fluid and electrolyte balance. The case fatality is 6%. Convalescence is prolonged with weakness lasting for weeks or months. The disease is transmitted by direct or indirect contact with the excreta of rodents.

Arenaviruses are a group of immunologically related enveloped viruses with prominent surface projections of glycoprotein. The genome consists of two single strands of RNA. The reservoir of arenaviruses is in small rodents. Arenaviruses include the agents of lymphocytic choriomeningitis (discussed in Chapter 20) and of Lassa fever. **Lassa fever** is a highly contagious, acute febrile illness found in West and Central Africa. Following an incubation period of 6 to 21 days, there is a gradual onset of fever, headache, pharyngitis, vomiting, and diarrhea, and in severe cases, hemorrhage and shock. The case fatality ranges from 15% to 50%. The reservoir of

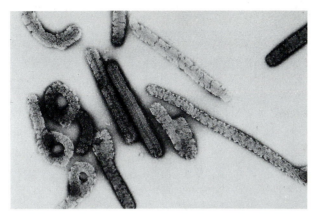

FIG 53–1.
Electron micrograph of Ebola virus. (Courtesy Centers for Disease Control, Atlanta.)

Lassa fever is in wild rodents. Man becomes infected by contact with the excreta of infected rodents. Person-to-person transmission occurs.

Lassa fever can be treated with ribavirin.

Filoviruses include the filamentous antigenically distinct Marburg and Ebola viruses. These enveloped viruses contain a single molecule of linear, negative-sense (−), single-stranded RNA, and five major proteins. The reservoir of these viruses is unknown, and person-to-person transmission occurs. Marburg virus occurs in Kenya and Zimbabwe; Ebola virus is found in Sudan and Zaire. Both viruses produce a similar syndrome, **Ebola-Marburg virus disease.** The incubation period for Marburg virus is 3 to 7 days; it is 2 to 21 days for Ebola virus. The syndrome has a sudden onset of fever, headache, pharyngitis, vomiting, diarrhea, a maculopapular rash, renal and hepatic involvement, and hemorrhage from multiple sites. The case fatality is 90%.

Opportunistic Infections and the Compromised Host

CHAPTER 54

Overview of Opportunistic Infections

Opportunists are microorganisms of low virulence that are generally unable to initiate disease in an intact immunocompetent host. The source of these organisms is most commonly from the indigenous flora, but opportunistic microorganisms may be acquired from the external environment in air, water, food, soil, or plant material. In many cases, the infection is acquired nosocomially from hospital personnel, other patients, or medical devices. Opportunistic infection occasionally results from a massive dose of one of these organisms being introduced into a normal host, but more frequently results from an alteration in host defense mechanisms. Host defenses include the intact skin and mucous membranes and their indigenous flora; the flushing action of secretions such as tears and urine; the phagocytic activity of inflammatory cells; nonspecific humoral substances like complement and interferons; specific immunoglobulins; and cell-mediated immunity (see Chapter 2). Opportunistic infections may be caused by a variety of bacteria, fungi, viruses, or parasites (Table 54–1).

FACTORS PREDISPOSING TO OPPORTUNISTIC INFECTIONS

Structural alterations such as loss of the mechanical barriers of skin and mucous membrane as a result of extensive trauma, burns, or surgery; obstruction associated with tumors, calculi, or congenital abnormalities; or foreign bodies such as sutures, or indwelling devices such as catheters or prostheses, all predispose to opportunistic infection either by facilitating the entry of large numbers of organisms into normally sterile areas of the body, or by interfering with efficient phagocytosis.

A number of underlying diseases may also render the patient susceptible to opportunistic infection. A severe decrease in the number or quality of phagocytic cells may be associated with malignant lymphoproliferative disorders, leukemia, or agranulocytosis associated with bone marrow failure. Diabetes affects the metabolism and bactericidal properties of polymorphonuclear neutrophils. Impairment of the respiratory clearance mechanism is a frequent manifestation of cystic fibrosis. Altered splenic function may follow multiple splenic infarcts in sickle cell anemia or removal of the spleen for trauma, resulting in decreased production of IgG-type antibodies. Decreases or absence of antibodies may be seen in the primary B cell immunodeficiency diseases such as the hypogammaglobulinemias. Diminished cell-mediated immunity is seen in allograft recipients, various malignant disorders, acquired immunodeficiency syndrome, and other primary T cell immunodeficiency diseases.

TABLE 54–1.

Microorganisms Commonly Causing Opportunistic Infections

Bacteria	Viruses
Enterobacteriaceae	Cytomegalovirus
Pseudomonas spp.	Varicella-zoster
Legionella	Herpes simplex
Bacteroides	Respiratory syncytial
Staphylococci	virus
Streptococci	Adenoviruses
Enterococci	*Parasites*
Listeria	*Pneumocystis*
Mycobacterium	*Toxoplasma*
Nocardia	*Cryptosporidium*
Mycoplasma hominis	*Isospora*
	Giardia
	Entamoeba histolytica
	Strongyloides
Fungi	
Candida	
Cryptococcus	
Mucor	
Aspergillus	
Histoplasma	
Coccidioides	

TABLE 54–2.

Conditions Predisposing to Opportunistic Infection

Age—elderly, neonate
Malnutrition
Severe trauma—wounds, burns
Parenteral drug abuse
Diabetes
Neoplastic disease—acute lymphoblastic or myelogenous leukemia, chronic lymphocytic leukemia, Hodgkin's disease, myeloma, solid tumors
Hypogammaglobulinemia
Complement deficiency
Granulocytopenia
Chronic granulomatous disease
Chédiak-Higashi syndrome
Acquired immunodeficiency syndrome
Hospitalization
Indwelling medical devices—vascular and urinary catheters, prosthetic devices
Surgery
Splenectomy
Transplant recipient—bone marrow, solid organ
Immunosuppressive therapy—corticosteroids, cytotoxic drugs
Radiation
Prolonged antimicrobial therapy

Opportunistic infections may also occur as a side effect of certain medical treatments. Radiation and the use of steroids and other immunosuppressive agents result in impaired antibody synthesis and cellular response. The prolonged use of antibiotics may result in suppression of most of the normal indigenous flora with resulting selection, overgrowth, and invasion of more virulent strains (Table 54–2).

Commonly occurring opportunistic infections are urinary tract infection; skin and soft tissue infections, such as burns or surgical wounds; pneumonia; catheter-associated vascular infection; septicemia; gastroenteritis; and infection of indwelling prosthetic devices.

CHAPTER 55

Bacterial Opportunists

Bacteria are the major cause of both fatal and nonfatal infections in the immunocompromised patient. These organisms vary in their pathogenicity. Some species are capable of disease production only in immunocompromised persons; others produce more severe disease in persons with impaired defenses than in immunocompetent persons.

Phagocytic cells, complement, immunoglobulins, and delayed hypersensitivity all have been shown to be important against bacterial invasion. Certain white blood cell defects such as chronic granulomatous disease of children with NADH oxidase and superoxide deficiency, which result in inadequate intracellular killing, are associated with infections from bacteria that produce catalase such as *Staphylococcus aureus*.

Gram-negative infections also occur in these persons and organisms such as *Salmonella* and *Serratia* have been implicated in sepsis and death. White blood cells are essential for protection against *Pseudomonas aeruginosa*. Humoral immunity is extremely important in protection against "classic" bacteria such as *Streptococcus pneumoniae* and *Haemophilus influenzae*, which have capsules that prevent ingestion by white blood cells. Although antibodies are also seen to be protective against *Pseudomonas*, the role of humoral immunity in protection against infection by members of the Enterobacteriaceae fam-

ily, e.g., *Escherichia coli*, *Klebsiella*, is less clear. Patients with agammaglobulinemia, advanced chronic lymphocytic leukemia, or multiple myeloma are particularly susceptible to recurrent episodes of pneumococcal and *Haemophilus* infections. Even loss of immunoglobulins, as occurs with the nephrotic syndrome, predisposes to these infections. The spleen has a special role in clearing the bloodstream of pneumococci and *Haemophilus*. Overwhelming sepsis due to these organisms occurs in asplenic persons.

Patients with deficiencies of lower complement components get infections similar to the agammaglobulinemia patients. These are most often *S. pneumoniae* or *H. influenzae*, or both. Deficiencies of higher complement components, C5–9, predispose to *Neisseria meningitidis* or *N. gonorrhoeae* infection.

Immune lymphocytes exert their protective influence by activation of mononuclear phagocytes—the mobile macrophage and the fixed macrophage of the reticuloendothelial system in liver and spleen. Cellular immunity has been shown to be particularly important in defense against bacterial organisms that can parasitize macrophage cells: *Listeria*, *Salmonella*, *Brucella*, *Mycobacterium tuberculosis*, *Legionella*. The fixed macrophage of the reticuloendothelial system has been shown to be important in clearing organisms which invade from the gut. In patients with chronic hemolysis, such as sickle cell disease or those with hemoglobulinopathies, the liver and spleen macrophages have decreased clearance ability. These patients are particularly prone to salmonella infections.

Bacteria frequently involved in opportunistic infections are shown in Table 55–1. The source of these organisms is usually the indigenous skin or bowel flora but environmental species are also frequently involved. Other bacteria producing infection in immunocompromised patients are *Corynebacterium* species, *Legionella*, and non–*P. aeruginosa* pseudomonads. Aerobic gram-negative bacilli are the most common bacteria involved in opportunistic infections. Two large groups, Enterobacteriaceae (enteric bacilli) and nonfermenters, are included in this category.

ENTEROBACTERIACEAE

Enterobacteriaceae account for approximately 75% of all aerobic gram-negative bacilli recovered from clinical specimens. The species in this family are differentiated by their constitutive enzymes (amino acid deaminases and decarboxylases, urease, etc.) and their ability to utilize various substrates. As fermenters, they can dissimilate glucose via the Embden-Meyerhof pathway. Most species are motile by means of peritrichous flagella.

The antigenic structure of the Enterobacteriaceae includes cell wall, flagellar, and envelope antigens. The cell wall antigens include the common antigen, a polysaccharide-polypeptide complex present in all members of the Enterobacteriaceae. Antibodies to the common antigen are

TABLE 55–1.

Bacteria Frequently Involved in Opportunistic Infections

Immune Defect	Organism
Disturbed integument	*Staphylococcus aureus*
	Pseudomonas aeruginosa
Surgical situations	*S. aureus*
	Group A streptococci
	Bacteroides
	Salmonella
Indwelling prostheses	Coagulase-negative staphylococci
Disturbed neutrophil function	Enterobacteriaceae
	S. aureus
	P. aeruginosa
Immunoglobulin defects	Enterobacteriaceae
	P. aeruginosa
	Group A streptococci
	Streptococcus pneumoniae
	Haemophilus influenzae
Decreased monocyte function	*Listeria monocytogenes*
	Mycobacteria
Impaired cell-mediated function	*Nocardia*
	Salmonella
	Myobacteria
	Listeria

normally present in human serum. The other cell wall constituent is the somatic O antigen, a lipopolysaccharide-mucopeptide complex. When organisms are freshly isolated, the lipopolysaccharides have side chains of 3,6-dideoxyhexoses, each specific for the species. After transfer on laboratory media, the organism dissociates into the rough colonial form in which the species-specific side chains are lost. The lipopolysaccharide moiety is the endotoxin characteristic of gram-negative species. Flagellar or H antigens are protein in nature and are only present in motile species. Envelope (capsular) K antigens are polysaccharides that have a negative charge and a neutral pH. Certain K antigens are associated with virulence, presumably because they interfere with phagocytosis. Virulent strains of *Salmonella typhi* have a specialized K antigen, designated Vi. Antibodies to H and O antigens appear following infection with enterobacterial species.

Identification of the various species of Enterobacteriaceae in the laboratory is based upon their biochemical activities, supplemented by serologic typing of their H and O antigens. Species of Enterobacteriaceae involved in opportunistic infections are listed in Table 55–2.

ESCHERICHIA COLI

Escherichia coli is the organism most commonly recovered from clinical material. It is the etiologic agent of 90% of community-acquired urinary tract infections. Enteropathogenic and enteroinvasive strains are responsible for a significant proportion of infectious diarrheal disease. Extraintestinal invasive diseases caused by *E. coli* include neonatal meningitis, pneumonia, hepatobiliary infections, and abdominal and pelvic abscesses. *Escherichia coli* accounts for 40% of all nosocomial infections. Bacteremic *E. coli* infection has a fatality rate of 26%.

Escherichia coli is antigenically complex. There are at least 155 somatic (O), 100 capsular (K), and 50 flagellar (H) antigens. The invasive capability of *E. coli* has been correlated with its ability to resist killing by fresh normal human serum. Strains resistant to killing by neutrophils and by fresh human serum have a polysaccharide capsule designated as K1. K1 capsule is unique among *E. coli* capsular polysaccharides in its ability to confer resistance to both the bactericidal effects of neutrophils and serum, whereas other capsular polysaccharides only provide protection against serum killing. The K1

TABLE 55–2.

Species of Enterobacteriaceae Causing Opportunistic Infections

Genus	Species
Escherichia	*E. coli*
Citrobacter	*C. freundii, C. diversus, C. amalonaticus*
Klebsiella	*K. pneumoniae K. ozaenae, K. rhinoscleromatis, K. oxytoca*
Enterobacter	*E. aerogenes, E. agglomerans, E. cloacae, E. sakazakii, E. gergoviae*
Serratia	*S. liquefaciens, S. marcescens, S. rubidaea*
Proteus	*P. mirabilis, P. vulgaris*
Morganella	*M. morganii*
Providencia	*P. alcalifaciens, P. stuartii, P. rettgeri*
Edwardsiella	*E. tarda*
Salmonella	*S. choleraesuis, S. enteritidis* serotypes

antigen is a polymer of *N*-acetylneuraminic acid, and has a negative charge, a neutral pH, and is immunologically identical to the capsular material of group B *N. meningitidis.*

The virulence of *E. coli* in extraintestinal invasive disease correlates very strongly with the presence of the K1 antigen. More than 70% of cases of *E. coli* neonatal meningitis are caused by strains with the K1 antigen.

In contrast to the predominance of the K1 capsule in invasive disease, only 10% to 20% of *E. coli* strains recovered from urinary tract infections have this antigen. Other K antigens (K2a and K2c) have been associated with strains causing urinary tract infections, particularly pyelonephritis. Many of the strains of *E. coli* implicated in urinary tract infections possess pili, which provide the means for the attachment of the organisms to the specific receptor sites on host cells within the urinary tract.

KLEBSIELLA

Species of this nonmotile genus often possess a thick mucoid capsule, and are generally resistant to ampicillin and carbenicillin. They are frequently recovered from urinary tract infections, wound infections, from bacteremia, and occasionally, from meningitis. *Klebsiella* is a common cause of nosocomial infections. *Klebsiella pneumoniae* can cause a primary pneumonia (Friedländer's pneumonia) that was most frequently seen in older men, especially those suffering from alcoholism, diabetes, or chronic obstructive pulmonary disease. Within the past decade, *Klebsiella* has accounted for less than 5% of cases of community-acquired pneumonia.

ENTEROBACTER

Most commonly, E. cloacae is the most common nosocomial species, probably secondary to cephalosporin use in hospitals. *E. aerogenes* and *E. hafnia* are recovered from urinary tract infections; *E. gergoviae* has been isolated from wound and urinary tract infections, and *E. sakazakii* has been the agent in some cases of neonatal meningitis. Outbreaks of nosocomial bacteremia have resulted from the administration of intravenous fluids contaminated with *E. cloacae* or *E. agglomerans.*

SERRATIA

Many strains of *Serratia* produce a pink or red pigment. Before the pathogenic potential of these organisms was recognized, they were widely used as tracer or indicator organisms in studies of aerosol dissemination or water supplies. *Serratia* are important causes of nosocomial infections and of serious concern because they are often resistant to most antimicrobial agents. They have caused cases of pneumonia in instances where they have contaminated respiratory equipment, and have also been associated with wound and urinary tract infection, and septicemia.

PROTEUS, MORGANELLA, PROVIDENCIA

These highly motile organisms are often recognized in the laboratory by their characteristic swarming on moist agar plates (rather than forming discrete colonies). All *Proteus* and the closely related *Morganella* species are potent producers of urease, and can grow at an alkaline pH.

Proteus mirabilis causes about 8% of community-acquired urinary tract infections. The organism can split urea to ammonia, resulting in a highly alkaline urine. The high urinary pH predisposes the patient to the formation of urinary calculi by inducing the precipitation of salts normally present in the urine. The alkaline urine also diminishes the efficacy of many antimicrobial agents used in treating urinary tract infections. *Proteus mirabilis* can infect wounds, often in combination with other bacterial species.

NONFERMENTERS

Pseudomonads are widely distributed in soil, water, and plant material. They are obligate aerobes that grow readily on simple laboratory media at room temperature (20° C) or at 35° C. Most species are motile with polar flagella, and are oxidase-positive.

Pseudomonas aeruginosa is the species most frequently encountered in clinical material, and is an important opportunistic pathogen. It is widely distributed in soil and water and is found among the indigenous flora of the skin and the intestinal tract. The organism thrives in moist environments, and is able to utilize a variety of organic compounds as a source of nitrogen and carbon. In the hospital environment, *P. aeruginosa* has been found growing in intravenous fluids and soap solutions. Aqueous solutions of antiseptics, such as quaternary ammonium compounds, e.g., benzalkonium chloride, can support growth of *P. aeruginosa*.

Many strains of *P. aeruginosa* have a capsulelike slime layer external to the cell wall. The slime layer is composed of polysaccharide and protein that may protect the organism from ingestion by phagocytic cells. The cell envelope consists of the cytoplasmic membrane, an intermediate peptidoglycan layer, and an outer cell wall containing lipopolysaccharide. The outer membranes of *P. aeruginosa* contains an iron-binding protein (siderophore). Pili (fimbriae) can be demonstrated in most strains recently isolated from clinical material, but there is no evidence that they play a role in attachment of *P. aeruginosa* to host cells.

Pseudomonas aeruginosa produces a number of extracellular products, some of which play an important role in the virulence of the organism and the pathogenesis of infection. These include exotoxins A, B, and C, proteases, and hemolysins. A major virulence factor is exotoxin A, and adenosine diphosphate (ADP) ribosyltransferase, which resembles diphtheria, cholera, and *E. coli* LT toxins in its mode of action. It is produced by about 90% of *P. aeruginosa* strains isolated from clinical material. Exotoxin A is a single chain polypeptide of 71.5 kilodaltons. It occurs as a proenzyme consisting of an enzymatically active A fragment and an inactive B fragment. The B fragment (45 kilodaltons) appears to play a role in facilitating the binding of the toxin to the mammalian cell; the A fragment (26 kilodaltons) enters the cell and catalyzes the transfer of the ADP ribosyl moiety of NAD to elongation factor 2 (EF-2) resulting in the inactivation of EF-2 halting the assembly of polypeptides into proteins. Exotoxin A is cytotoxic in vitro for polymorphonuclear neutrophils and mononuclear cells, and necrotizing for certain tissues in vivo. The toxin is lethal for a variety of animals including primates, and produces hypotension, shock, clotting abnormalities, decreased cardiac output, and necrosis of liver cells. It is extremely potent; the lethal dose for mice is about 2.5 μg/kg of body weight. The proteases of *P. aeruginosa* may play a role in the pathogenesis of hemorrhagic lesions seen in the skin, cornea, and lungs. One of the hemolysins has phospholipase activity; this enzyme may be involved in the pathogenesis of pseudomonal pneumonia by virtue of its damaging action to alveolar surfactant. The virulence of *P. aeruginosa* can be enhanced by iron compounds which markedly affect the growth rate of the organism, and indirectly by the number of organisms that remain extracellular.

In normal persons, *P. aeruginosa* infection is rare and limited to minor infections such as otitis externa (swimmer's ear). In persons with compromised host defenses, *P. aeruginosa* can cause serious infections that are often difficult to treat. The organism commonly contaminates or colonizes burns, draining sinuses, and decubitus ulcers, and frequently produces severe infections that may progress to ecthyma gangrenosa and septicemia. Rarely, the exudate from abscesses, burns, or wounds infected with *P. aeruginosa* is blue-green in color. Urinary tract infections are common, especially following instrumentation or catheterization with indwelling catheters. Pseudomonal tracheobronchitis, necrotizing bronchopneumonia, occurs in persons with chronic pulmonary disease such as cystic fibrosis. Corneal infections occur following injury or surgery, and in some cases have been associated with the instillation of eye drops contaminated with *P. aeruginosa*. Pseudomonal meningitis is usually secondary to central nervous system trauma or the use of contaminated intrathecal solutions. Subacute bacterial endocarditis due to *P. aeruginosa* is associated with intravenous narcotic usage. In the neonate, *P. aeruginosa* can cause infections of the umbilical stump, otitis media, meningitis, and septicemia. Almost all *P. aeruginosa* infections can progress to septicemia, which has a mortality of 50%.

Resistance to *P. aeruginosa* infection depends upon both the presence of specific antibody and competent phagocytic cells. In the lower respiratory tract, specific IgG and, to a lesser extent, IgA antibodies promote phagocytosis. Bacteremic strains resist killing by complement but not by polymorphonuclear neutrophils. In experimental animals, antibodies to the slime layer protect against pseudomonal infection. Opsonizing antibody directed against the lipopolysaccharide also plays an important role in immunologic defense. The use of a lipopolysaccharide vaccine has been hampered by the accompanying endotoxic side effects. Recently, it has been possible to detoxify the lipopolysaccharide by altering the toxic lipid A moiety by deacylation. This experimental vaccine has prevented *P. aeruginosa* respiratory infections in an intensive care unit, reduced *Pseudomonas*-associated deaths in cancer patients, and provided

protection in animal models of *Pseudomonas* infection.

There is evidence that antibodies to exotoxin A play a protective role in the infected host; most patients with *Pseudomonas* infections produce antibodies to the toxin. Exotoxin A can be converted to toxoid by treatment with formalin, which neutralizes the lethal, cytotoxic, and enzymatic activity of the native toxin. Toxoid-immunized mice are protected against challenge with live *P. aeruginosa*. The protection conferred by antibodies to exotoxin A appears to be additive with that provided by antibodies to the *P. aeruginosa* lipopolysaccharide. In view of the importance of iron to the growth of *P. aeruginosa*, iron-binding proteins such as transferrin probably play an important role in nonspecific resistance to infection.

Xanthomonas maltophilia accounts for approximately 7% of pseudomonads recovered from clinical material. This species has been incriminated in meningitis, septicemia, pulmonary disease, infected wounds, brain abscess, pericarditis, lymphadenitis, and urinary tract infections. Other *Pseudomonas* species such as *P. cepacia* may contaminate or colonize various anatomic sites, and can, under appropriate circumstances, produce opportunistic infections.

Acinetobacter is common in the environment and, when recovered in culture of clinical material with other organisms, usually represents a contaminant or colonizer. In debilitated patients *Acinetobacter* may cause pneumonia, abscesses, pleural effusion, and septicemia. Urinary tract infections are usually associated with the presence of an indwelling catheter.

Flavobacteria are soil and water organisms that are highly virulent for neonates, especially premature infants. The organism has been responsible for outbreaks of septicemia and meningitis in hospital nurseries, and septicemia following cardiac surgery or in association with indwelling arterial catheters. Nonfermenters causing opportunistic infections are listed in Table 55–3.

NOCARDIA

Nocardia are gram-positive filamentous bacteria that show branching. They resemble *Actinomyces* except that *Nocardia* are strict aerobes. The species most commonly involved in human infections—*N. asteroides* and *N. brasiliensis*—are weakly acid-fast. *Nocardia* are commonly present in soil. Growth on artificial media appears in about 2 to 3 days. The colonies are dry and by 7 to 10 days become wrinkled with yellow or red pigment.

Nocardia produce chronic suppurative infections. Three clinical forms of nocardiosis are seen: pulmonary, subcutaneous tissue infections, and central nervous system disease.

Pulmonary infection is most commonly due to *N. asteroides*. The organisms are inhaled with dust or soil. Approximately half of the patients that develop pulmonary nocardiosis have some underlying disease. About 30% of the patients have been treated with steroids or similar immunosuppressive therapy, but the disease also occurs as an opportunistic infection in patients with neoplastic disease. The initial lesion is an acute inflammation with suppuration that de-velops into multiple large, confluent abscesses scattered throughout the lung. The organisms find their way into the bloodstream and establish metastatic abscesses, most frequently in the brain, and to a lesser extent in the spleen, skin, peritoneum, and kidney. Cell-mediated immunity is the most important defense mechanism.

Subcutaneous infection is usually secondary to some minor trauma, such as a splinter or thorn. The most common species in this type of infection is *N. brasiliensis*. Subcutaneous infections are slowly progressive and destructive of muscle and bone. Eventually, sinuses develop which drain pus containing sulfur granules—macroscopic yellow grains composed of a mass of mycelia.

Therapy of nocardia infections is with trimethoprim/sulfamethoxazole.

LISTERIA

Listeria monocytogenes is a short aerobic gram-positive rod, motile at room temperature, catalase-positive, and hemolytic on blood-containing agar media. The organism grows slowly at 5° C, as well as at room temperature (18–20° C) and at 35 to 37° C, on routinely employed

TABLE 55–3.
Species of Gram-Negative Nonfermenters Causing Opportunistic Infections

Genus	Species
Pseudomonas	*P. aeruginosa, P. maltophilia, C. cepacia, P. fluorescens, P. putida, P. stutzeri, P. alcaligenes, P. diminuta, P. pseudoalcaligenes*, IIk group, Ve group
Xanthomonas	*X. cepacia*
Acinetobacter	*A. calcoaceticus* var. *anitratus, A. calcoaceticus* var. *lwoffi*
Flavobacterium	*F. meningosepticum* group II, group III
Kingella	*K. kingae*

laboratory media. *Listeria monocytogenes* is widespread in nature and has been recovered from soil, water, and animal feed. The reservoir is infected domestic and wild mammals, fowl, and man. Up to 5% of normal persons are asymptomatic fecal carriers of *L. monocytogenes*.

Predisposing factors for *Listeria* infection are the extremes of age, malignancy, or immunosuppression. *Listeria monocytogenes* is an intracellular pathogen, surviving and multiplying in nonactivated macrophages. A toxin is produced that resembles streptolysin O that is a virulence factor for the organism.

Transmission is most commonly by ingestion of contaminated food, including vegetables, and cheese and other dairy products. Intrauterine infection can occur during a maternal bacteremic episode. Newborns can also be infected during passage through the birth canal. The incubation period varies from a few days to 3 weeks. About 70% of the patients are immunosuppressed or have a malignancy.

The most common (60%) clinical manifestation of listeriosis is meningoencephalitis, usually occurring in the neonate or immunosuppressed adult. Septicemia may also occur in these patients without any evidence of central nervous system involvement. Intrauterine infection of the fetus can result in spontaneous abortion, stillbirth, or neonatal listeriosis, which can take the form of sepsis, meningitis, or abscesses and granulomas in multiple organs (granulomatosis infantisepticum). Endocarditis and focal infections of skin, eyes, and other organs due to *L. monocytogenes* are uncommon.

CORYNEBACTERIUM AND RELATED ORGANISMS

Corynebacteria are aerobic, nonmotile, gram-positive rods. Several species are part of the normal indigenous flora of the skin and mucous membranes and are often categorized as "diphtheroids," i.e., corynebacteria other than *C. diphtheriae*. Several species have been implicated as etiologic agents of infections in immunocompromised and immunocompetent patients.

Arcanobacterium (Corynebacterium) haemolyticum has been implicated as a cause of acute pharyngitis. About 50% of the patients also have a scarlatiniform rash and lymphadenitis. The organism has also been found to cause chronic skin ulcers, osteomyelitis, brain abscess, and endocarditis. *Corynebacterium ulcerans* has also been recovered from exudated pharyngitis and skin ulcers. *Rhodococcus (Corynebacterium) equi* can cause a necrotizing pneumonia in immunosuppressed patients. *Corynebacterium bovis* has been recovered from ventriculojugular shunt infection, epidural abscesses, and prosthetic valve endocarditis. *Corynebacterium xerosis* has also been recovered from patients with endocarditis, pneumonia, and surgical wound infections in immunocompromised patients. *Corynebacterium jeikeium* (JK) colonizes patients treated with multiple antibiotics and causes sepsis in patients with protracted neutropenia, neoplastic diseases, or who have suffered integumentary disruption.

CHAPTER 56

Fungal Opportunists

Opportunistic fungal infections are most often seen in patients with hematologic disorders; in those who have undergone extensive surgical procedures; in patients receiving high doses of corticosteroid, cytotoxic, or immunosuppressive therapy; and in persons with the acquired immunodeficiency syndrome (AIDS).

The role of humoral and cellular factors in protection of a normal host against fungal infections is a complicated one. The integument and body secretions are major factors in controlling overgrowth of fungi. Normal bacterial flora elaborate substances that retard the proliferation of many fungal species. Local defense mechanisms in the lung act to remove large particles such as fungal spores before they reach the lower parts of the lung. If the fungi enter the alveolar areas they are phagocytosed and cleared by the alveolar macrophages. If the alveolar macrophage system fails, local specific humoral and cell-mediated immunity evolve. The role of neutrophils in fungal infection is not completely established; however, fungal infections (excluding cryptococcoses) are seen in patients with hematologic malignancies, particularly when they are neutropenic.

Fungi such as *Candida*, *Aspergillus*, or the members of the group Phycomycetales (*Mucor*) tend to colonize and infect only in the absence of the normal cutaneous and bacterial defenses.

Certain fungal diseases are widespread, e.g., coccidioidomycosis and histoplasmosis, yet these illnesses rarely result in serious widespread illness in normal patients. In the immunosuppressed patient these fungal infections may reactivate and disseminate, as seen by their frequency in transplant and AIDS patients.

Fungi are eukaryotes with a distinct nucleus, nuclear membrane, and organelles such as mitochondria and endoplasmic reticulum. Most species are free-living in soil and on plant material; a few species are members of the indigenous commensal flora of the body. The cell wall of fungi contains chitin, glucans, and mannans, and the cytoplasmic membrane contains sterols. Fungi grow more slowly than bacteria; some species require several days or weeks before colonies appear. Fungi are strictly aerobic organisms that are able to grow on simple laboratory media at a wide range of temperature (18–37° C). Fungi are resistant to most antimicrobial agents that affect bacteria.

Two forms of fungi occur: yeasts and molds. Yeasts are spherical or ellipsoid cells that reproduce by budding. Molds are filamentous forms that grow by extension and branching of a hyphal element to form a tangled mass called a mycelium. Certain fungi are dimorphic, capable of existing in either the yeast or mold form, depending upon the environmental conditions.

Molds reproduce by various forms of asexual spores that include blastospores, arthrospores, chlamydospores, and conidia. Blastospores are small, round structures that are formed by "pinching" off a hypha. Arthrospores are rectangular and are formed by the segmentation of a hyphal element. Chlamydospores are thick-walled round structures. Conidia are spores borne on a stalk called a conidiophore, and may be large (macroconidia) or small (microconidia).

CANDIDA

Candida species are the most frequent cause of fungal infection in the immunocompromised host. *Candida* are yeasts that are widely found in nature, especially on the surfaces of fruit and grains. Several species are normally present in low numbers in the mouth, lower gastrointestinal tract, and the vagina. Under certain conditions the skin may be colonized with *Candida*. Species commonly recovered from infection include *Candida albicans* (the most frequently involved species), *C. tropicalis*, *C. parapsilosis*, *C. pseudotropicalis*, *C. lusitaniae*, *C. krusei*, and *Torulopsis glabrata*.

Superficial *Candida* infections are those involving the mucocutaneous regions of the mouth, vagina, and esophagus. These infections are seen during pregnancy, in neonates, in women using oral contraceptives, and in patients with diabetes, leukemia, and AIDS. Disseminated *Candida* infection most frequently involves the kidneys (Figs 56–1 and 56–2), but the heart, lungs, and other organs may be involved. Disseminated infections may occur in intravenous drug abusers, patients with indwelling vascular catheters, grafts, prostheses, and in those with leukemia being treated with corticosteroids or cytotoxic drugs.

Candida may enter the bloodstream from the gastrointestinal tract, especially following abdominal surgery, with alterations in the intesti-

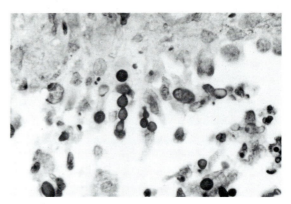

FIG 56–1.
Candida albicans invading kidney.

nal mucosa, and with treatment with multiple antibiotics, which promotes yeast overgrowth. Candidemia may also result from vascular catheters becoming colonized with yeast from the skin. The adhesins of *Candida* are fibrillar peptidomannans that have an affinity for fibronectin on the surface of cells. The yeast phase initiates tissue damage. Environmental factors that inhibit yeast cell division but not growth induce the formation of mycelia, and hyphal elements invade the tissues. Both yeast and hyphal forms are present in the tissues. Toxic and inflammatory reactions are due to the cellular components of the yeast. The initial cellular reaction is polymorphonuclear neutrophilia resulting in the

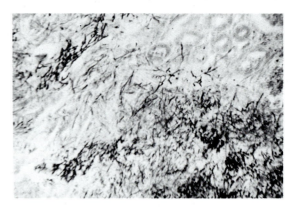

FIG 56–2.
Candida albicans in kidney.

formation of microabscesses. Later, mononuclear cells arrive with granuloma formation.

Both humoral and cell-mediated immunity are important defense mechanisms in *Candida* infection. Polymorphonuclear neutrophils, monocytes, and eosinophils all phagocytose *Candida*. This process becomes more efficient when the organisms are opsonized by antibody and complement. Antibody is not required for killing *Candida*. Lymphocytes are also important in defense against *Candida*. At least 80% of normal persons exhibit delayed-type hypersensitivity to *Candida* antigens.

The diagnosis of superficial *Candida* infection is readily accomplished by visualizing the organism microscopically in material from a mucocutaneous lesion, or by recovering the yeast by culture. Disseminated candidiasis presents a problem, and many serologic tests to detect cell wall polysaccharide, mannan, or other *Candida* antigens have been tested, but all lack sensitivity or specificity.

Candida infection can be treated with amphotericin B or with imidazoles such as ketoconazole or fluconazole.

ASPERGILLUS

Aspergillus is a genus of molds that are widespread in nature, occurring in soil, compost, decaying vegetation, and organic debris. Growth takes place by the elongation and branching of septate hyphal elements to form a mycelium. The organism produces fruiting heads (sporangia) with spores (conidia) which become airborne and are the infective stage. There are several hundred species of *Aspergillus*. The most common species in human infections are *A. fumigatus* and *A. flavus*. Some species of *Aspergillus* produce toxins such as aflatoxin, a powerful carcinogen. These toxins are only produced in vitro and have no role in the pathogenesis of aspergillosis. *Aspergillus* infection usually results from the inhalation of airborne conidia.

The major forms of aspergillosis are allergic bronchopulmonary disease, aspergilloma, and invasive pulmonary disease seen in immunosuppressed patients. Other less common manifestations of aspergillus infection are endocarditis, endophthalmitis, and cerebral infarction. **Allergic bronchopulmonary disease** is characterized by asthma, eosinophilia, and transient pulmonary infiltrates. Allergic *Aspergillus* expansile sinusitis may mimic malignancy. **Aspergilloma** (fungus ball of the lung) may result from chronic allergic pulmonary aspergillosis, or by colonization of preformed cavities resulting from tuberculosis, histoplasmosis, sarcoidosis, or other forms of chronic obstructive pulmonary disease (Fig 56–3). Colonies of *Aspergillus* growing in cavities or bronchi enlarge and though they seldom invade lung parenchyma, they can produce bronchial obstruction. **Invasive pulmonary aspergillosis** is seen in patients with leukemia, lymphoma, recipients of renal, heart, or lung transplants, and others with profound neutropenia. The infection is an acute, rapidly progressive pneumonia.

Aspergillus endocarditis may involve normal or prosthetic cardiac valves during fungemia, or valve replacement surgery. Endophthalmitis can result from a fungemic episode, cataract removal, or trauma to the cornea. Cerebral infarction in immunosuppressed patients results from

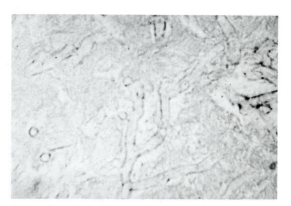

FIG 56–3.
Aspergillus in lung.

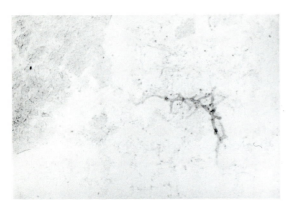

FIG 56–4.
Mucor—low power.

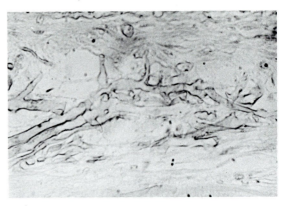

FIG 56–5.
Mucor in sinus.

the cerebral blood vessels becoming occluded by the growth of the fungus disseminated from the lung.

Diagnosis of aspergillosis is made by microscopic examination and culture of tissues. A serologic test for *Aspergillus* galactomannan antigenemia is being studied as a possible test for disseminated disease.

MUCORACEAE

Mucoraceae are molds in the class Zygomycetes (Phycomycetes), organisms associated with soil and plant debris. The fungi grow rapidly at temperatures ranging from 25 to 37° C. The hyphae are broad, irregular, and lack septa (cenocytic) (Fig 56–4). The genera most often involved in human disease are *Mucor* and *Rhizopus,* but other genera sometimes cause infection. Infections with Mucoraceae (mucormycosis) are most often seen in patients with diabetes mellitus, hematologic malignancy, neutropenia, drug addicts, or patients with extensive burns or recipients of organ transplants.

Rhinocerebral mucormycosis occurs most commonly in patients with uncontrolled diabetes and ketoacidosis, but is also seen with leukemia or therapy with corticosteroids or cytotoxic drugs (Fig 56–5). The main symptoms are orbital edema, nasal congestion, and headache. The infection often progresses to orbital cellulitis, and the mortality rate is high. Pulmonary infection begins with fever and pulmonary infiltrates and rapidly disseminates to the liver, intestinal tract, kidneys, brain, and skin. Intestinal infection has been associated with extreme malnutrition, and skin involvement has sometimes been traced to the use of contaminated dressing materials. The fungus usually enters the body by the inhalation of spores which may lodge in the nose or reach the alveoli. Fungal elements invade adjacent tissues and spread, via the bloodstream, to other organ systems. The fungus invades blood vessels resulting in thrombosis. Diagnosis of mucormycosis is based on the demonstration of the organism in tissues and microscopic examination.

CHAPTER 57

Viral Opportunists

There are three major components to the host's defense against viral illness: interferon, antibody, and lymphocytes. Interferon is produced within hours after viral infection. Subsequently, specific antibodies form and ultimately cell-mediated immunity develops. Viruses differ in their inhibition by interferon, susceptibility to neutralization by antibody, and finally in their ability to stimulate and be destroyed by lymphocyte-mediated cellular immunity. Precise analysis of individual host protective mechanisms is not possible, but it appears that deficient cellular immunity is the critical factor in development of serious viral infection in the compromised host. Immunologic deficiency which involves cell-mediated immunity, e.g., thymic dysfunction, lymphoma at an advanced stage, or the leukemias after chemotherapy, predisposes to viral infection. The viruses involved have been primarily of the herpes group, varicella-zoster (VZ), herpes simplex (HSV), and cytomegalovirus (CMV), as well as the measles, vaccinia, and hepatitis viruses. Immunoglobulin-deficient persons may be more susceptible to enterovirus infections such as echovirus 11.

Viruses account for 25% of infections in bone marrow and renal transplant recipients. Varicella-zoster, cytomegalovirus, HSV, and measles viruses are major sources of morbidity in children undergoing chemotherapy for acute leukemia. Other viral infections in this population are those caused by adenoviruses, parainfluenza viruses, rhinoviruses, respiratory syncytial virus, and enteroviruses.

VARICELLA-ZOSTER VIRUS

Varicella (chickenpox) results from the initial infection with VZ virus; zoster is a recrudescence of latent VZ virus infection. In patients with T lymphocyte deficiency or combined T and B cell dysfunction, VZ virus causes more serious disease than in the immunocompetent patient. These patients have a more extensive rash, and prolonged viremia, often with dissemination to the lungs, liver, central nervous system, and other organs. Disseminated varicella is a frequent occurrence in children with profound lymphopenia (less than 500 lymphocytes per cubic millimeter). Primary varicella, usually pneumonia with hepatitis, is the greatest threat to children with leukemia. Zoster is a serious complication in recipients of bone marrow transplants. Immunosuppressed patients often develop hemorrhagic manifestations of VZ virus infection that range from mild purpura with fever to fatal fulminating purpuric disease. The underlying thrombocytopenia may be due to the direct effect of VZ virus in the bone marrow, or immune-mediated destruction of platelets.

HERPES SIMPLEX VIRUS

Compromised patients at risk for severe or even fatal HSV infections include pregnant women, severely malnourished children, and persons who are immunosuppressed by treatment or by disease. The last group includes renal, cardiac, and bone marrow transplant recipients, and patients with leukemia, or solid tumors, and with acquired immunodeficiency syndrome (AIDS). HSV infection in these patients invariably starts as severe mucosal lesions of the oral cavity (gingivostomatitis) which can extend to involve the esophagus. Sustained viremia can lead to dissemination to the liver, adrenals, lungs, and brain.

CYTOMEGALOVIRUS

Cytomegalovirus infection is common in renal and bone marrow recipients, less frequent in acute leukemia. Most CMV infections are asymptomatic, even in patients with leukemia in relapse. Clinical manifestations of CMV infection include esophagitis with ulceration and bleeding, and severe pneumonitis. Cytomegalovirus often causes chorioretinitis, particularly in AIDS patients. Primary CMV pneumonitis in immunodeficient patients is a slowly progressive viral pneumonia with spiking fever, leukopenia, hypoxemia, dyspnea, and cough, and over the next 3 to 4 weeks there is development of he-

patic and ureteral dysfunction. Most of these patients die. In contrast to this primary infection, reactivation of CMV infection in transplant patients is a relatively mild disease.

VACCINIA VIRUS

Vaccinia virus is a laboratory virus originally derived by Jenner for immunization against smallpox (variola). It is not known whether vaccinia virus is a modification of the variola virus, or is derived from the agent of cowpox. Vaccination is the inoculation of humans with vaccinia virus to produce immunity to smallpox.

In practice, a drop of vaccinia virus is placed on the skin which is then multiply scratched or punctured superficially. In nonimmune persons a papule appears at the site after 4 days and evolves through vesicle and pustule over the next 5 days, reaching maximum size by the 12th day. During this period, there may be low-grade fever, headache, and lymphadenitis. The lesion begins to shrink, a scab appears and eventually falls off leaving a scar and immunity to smallpox. A rare but serious complication of vaccination occurring in less than 1 in 100,000 is postvaccinial encephalitis. This usually was seen in infants less than 12 months of age and had a mortality rate of 30% to 40%. Immunocompromised persons inoculated with vaccinia virus can develop a highly fatal progressive vaccinia in which the initial lesion becomes necrotic; the necrosis extends over a period of months to involve skin, bones, and viscera. Smallpox no longer exists in the world, and routine vaccination was discontinued in the 1970s.

CHAPTER 58

Acquired Immunodeficiency Syndrome

In June, 1979, a 32-year-old man presented at a New York City hospital complaining of severe dyspnea, and a persistent, nonproductive cough. He had been in good health until 10 days before his admission to the hospital. Despite 10 days of antibiotic therapy, his symptoms became progressively worse, and an open lung biopsy was performed which revealed the presence of *Pneumocystis carinii* and cytomegalovirus inclusion bodies. Pneumonia due to *P. carinii* is extremely rare in an adult who is immunocompetent. The known causes of immunodeficiency (starvation; extremes of age; hypogammaglobulinemia; malignancy of lymphoreticular or histiocytic tissue; treatment with corticosteroid, cytotoxic, or immunosuppressive drugs) were ruled out.

Over the next several months, 15 additional cases of pneumocystis pneumonia appeared in New York City, all in previously healthy young males who were either homosexuals or intravenous drug abusers. At about the same time, a substantial number of cases of rapidly progressive Kaposi's sarcoma appeared in young, previously healthy male homosexuals. Many of these patients also developed fatal opportunistic infections. Kaposi's sarcoma is usually an indolent skin tumor of elderly males.

By 1981, the Centers for Disease Control recognized that these New York City cases and similar cases in San Francisco, Los Angeles, and Miami, all in male homosexuals or intravenous drug abusers, represented an epidemic of an apparently new and severe form of immunodeficiency now known as acquired immunodeficiency syndrome (AIDS).

AIDS is one end of a clinical spectrum of conditions resulting from infection with the human immunodeficiency virus (HIV). This spectrum ranges from asymptomatic carriage of the virus to the late manifestations of AIDS, including opportunistic infections, malignancy, wasting, and dementia. Intermediate stages, previously referred to as AIDS-related complex (ARC), include a mononucleosis-like syndrome (acute retrovirus syndrome) and persistent generalized lymphadenopathy.

HIV is a retrovirus, a group of enveloped, positive-sense (+) RNA viruses that encode reverse transcriptase (an RNA-dependent DNA polymerase) and replicate via DNA copy of the viral genome which is integrated into the host chromosome and transcribed as a cellular gene.

The first human retrovirus—human T-cell lymphotrophic virus (HTLV-1)—was isolated from patients with adult T cell leukemia or lymphoma. Subsequently, other related tumor viruses (HTLV-2, HTLV-5) have been isolated. This subfamily of retroviruses are now referred to as oncornaviruses.

HIV belongs to a subfamily of retroviruses called lentiviruses, and includes HIV-1 (previously designated HTLV-III/LAV) and HIV-2. HIV-2 is able to cause an infection indistinguishable from AIDS but which may be less pathogenic than HIV-1. Most cases of HIV-2 have occurred in West Africa.

The HIV virion is an icosahedral particle, containing 72 external spikes formed by viral envelope proteins gp120 and gp141. The bilayered lipid envelope contains viral glycoproteins and surrounds a capsid containing two identical positive strands of RNA inside a core of associated RNA polymerase and nucleocapsid proteins (p24, p17, p9, and p7). The genome consists of three structural genes: *gag* (codes for viral core components); *pol* (codes for reverse transcriptase); and *env* (codes for envelope proteins). Additional genes are present and a number of precursor and structural proteins have been identified. These include p55, p24, p17, p15 (core antigen); gp120 (surface attachment glycoprotein); gp160, gp41 (transmembrane glycoprotein); p66, p51 (reverse transcriptase); and p31 (endonuclease). The major cells infected by HIV are CD4 T lymphocytes, and monocytes. The virus also infects brain cells and neurons.

T helper cells (which induce B lymphocytes to produce antibody) and cytotoxic T cells (which kill cells whose antigens they recognize) have a surface glycoprotein marker called CD4. The CD4 molecule is also expressed on the surface of some monocytes and neurons. CD4 is the receptor for HIV.

The HIV gp120 envelope protein binds to a specific epitope (OKT4) of the CD4 cell. The receptor-bound virion enters the cell by virus-mediated membrane fusion involving the gp41 envelope protein. After internalization the HIV virion is uncoated and viral replication is initi-

ated. The reverse transcriptase generates a first-strand DNA copy of the viral RNA. The RNA template is partially degraded by ribonuclease, and a second strand of DNA is synthesized, yielding a double-stranded DNA replica of the viral RNA genome. This DNA replica is then transferred to the nucleus and inserted into the host chromosome by viral integrase. Once integrated, the viral DNA is transcribed as a cellular gene by the host RNA polymerase II. The entire viral genome is transcribed to produce *gag*, *gag-pol*, and *env* messenger RNA (mRNA). Full-length transcripts can be assembled into new virions. After entry into the CD4 cell, HIV may establish a latent infection or the virus kills the cell by several cytopathic effects: accumulation of nonintegrated circular DNA copies of the genome, increased permeability of the plasma membrane, and the formation of syncytia of multinucleated giant cells.

The reservoir of HIV is man. HIV is thought to have originated from primates in Central Africa and to have rapidly become adapted to humans. This introduction of a novel infectious agent into a population that lacked previous immunologic experience with it may explain its devastating consequences. HIV has been isolated from blood, semen, vaginal secretions, saliva, tears, breast milk, cerebrospinal fluid, amniotic fluid, and urine of infected persons. Transmission of HIV is primarily by sexual contact; the sharing of unclean intravenous needles; transfusion of blood and blood products; and perinatally, either in utero or by ingesting the virus with breast milk.

As of May 1991, almost 180,000 cases of AIDS among people of all ages in the United States had been reported to the Centers for Disease Control. By the end of 1991, AIDS will be the second leading cause of death among men 25 to 44 years of age, and is likely to be one of the five leading causes of death among women aged 15 to 44 years in the United States. The World Health Organization estimates that 8 to 10 million adults and 1 million children worldwide are infected with HIV, and that 40 million people may be infected by the year 2000. More than 90% of these people will live in Africa, South-East Asia, Latin America, and the Caribbean. In the United States, 70% of AIDS cases are in homosexual or bisexual males; 17% in intravenous drug abusers; 4% in Haitian and African immigrants; and 1% in patients with hemophilia or recipients of blood transfusions. As the AIDS epidemic has expanded, different populations have become affected. Although homosexual men still account for most AIDS cases, cases associated with intravenous drug use are more common in several northeastern states, and there has been a marked increase among persons exposed to HIV through heterosexual contact. Transfusion-acquired disease has decreased as a result of the testing of blood for HIV.

The incubation of AIDS is unknown. Based on transfusion-acquired disease, the range is 6 months to 10 years. Infection with HIV may result in an acute viral syndrome resembling mononucleosis, with fever, headache, and malaise. This acute phase is followed by an asymptomatic latent period, averaging about 8 years, after which all HIV-infected persons develop clinical signs of AIDS.

Prodromal symptoms are extremely variable and may last a few weeks to several years. Symptoms of weakness, malaise, weight loss, arthralgias, night sweats, generalized lymphadenopathy, oral candidiasis, and local herpes zoster are common. Initial manifestations are either an opportunistic infection, or Kaposi's sarcoma. (Most patients with Kaposi's sarcoma ultimately develop opportunistic infections, but relatively few patients with opportunistic infections develop Kaposi's sarcoma.) Other manifestations include unexplained fever, diffuse pneumonia, chronic diarrhea, and neurologic disorders. Laboratory findings include lymphopenia (less than 1,000 lymphocytes per cubic millimeter; 1,500/mm^3 is normal), a T helper-suppressor ratio of less than 1.0, and hypergammaglobulinemia with elevated IgG and normal IgM.

Common opportunistic infections include *P. carinii* pneumonia; diarrhea due to *Giardia*, *Entamoeba histolytica*, *Cryptosporidium*, *Isospora*, *Salmonella*, or *Shigella*; *Candida* esophagitis; disseminated cytomegalovirus, mucocutaneous herpes simplex; disseminated *Mycobacterium avium-intracellulare* infection; cryptococcal meningitis; and cerebral toxoplasmosis, often with chorioretinitis. Tuberculosis is an early complication of HIV infection, and some patients have had bacteremia due to *Mycobacterium tuberculosis*. Disseminated *M. avium* infection is a late complication. Neoplasms other than Kaposi's sarcoma that occur in AIDS include non-Hodgkin's lymphoma of Burkitt's type associated with Epstein-Barr virus; squamous carcinoma of the tongue or rectum associated with the herpes simplex viruses types 1 or 2.

About 70% of AIDS patients suffer from neurologic abnormalities. Subacute encephalitis due to HIV is the most frequent cause of neurologic dysfunction in AIDS, resulting in progressive cognitive, motor, and behavioral abnormalities in at least two thirds of patients with AIDS. HIV can also cause aseptic meningitis, peripheral neuropathies, and vacuolar myelopathy. Neurologic disease may be the only clinical manifestation of HIV infection.

The pathogenesis of AIDS is complex and poorly understood. One of the most baffling and important aspects of HIV infection is the long interval between the appearance of signs and symptoms, and seroconversion, and the ability of the virus to induce latent and slowly progressive infection. The hallmark of AIDS is a depletion of T4 helper/inducer lymphocytes. Infection of monocytes and macrophages may result in a defect in chemotaxis, and the involvement of alveolar macrophages may explain the high incidence of pneumocystis pneumonia in AIDS patients. High immunoglobulin levels with a poor antibody response to challenge with novel antigen may reflect B cell abnormalities secondary to T cell dysfunction.

Within 2 weeks to 5 months after HIV infection, p24 core antigen can be detected. Antigenemia usually coincides with the initial symptoms of acute infection. The interval between the development of antigenemia and the first appearance of antibody may be as long as 6 to 14 months, and even longer in infants. The first antibodies to appear are the gp160 or gp120 envelope antibodies. These may be detected as early as 2 weeks following the onset of symptoms. Simultaneously, or shortly following the development of the envelope antibodies, p24 core antibody appears. Five to 6 months after the onset of symptoms, antibodies to reverse transcriptase (p66, p51) and endonuclease (p31) can be detected by Western blot technique. Months or years after the appearance of core and envelope antibodies, core antigen may reappear with the concomitant loss of p24 and gp120 antibodies. The reappearance of antigenemia usually coincides with the clinical development of AIDS.

Several types of serologic assays have been developed to facilitate the diagnosis of HIV infection. They include detection of antigenemia by enzyme-linked immunosorbent assay (ELISA); and the identification of various antibodies by ELISA, Western blot, indirect immunofluorescence assay (IFA), radioimmunoprecipitation assay (RIPA), and latex agglutination (LA). The HIV antigen assay provides a more sensitive marker than routine antibody screening during the early stages of infection and for confirming neonatal infection in the presence of passively transferred maternal antibody. HIV antigen assays may also be useful in the diagnosis of persistent infection in seronegative children. The ELISA for HIV antibody is a very sensitive and fairly specific screening method for HIV infection. It is insensitive during the early weeks after infection because of the lack of detectable antibodies. False-positive results in a low-risk population may be due to severe alcoholic liver disease, hematologic malignancies, chronic renal failure, Stevens-Johnson syndrome, and the presence of a variety of autoantibodies. The Western blot technique is a method for analyzing sera for antibodies to specific proteins, and is currently the most sensitive and specific assay for HIV serodiagnosis in common use. The main use of the Western blot is as a confirmatory test for patients testing positive with ELISA. The IFA is a rapid and reliable supplementary test, detecting antibodies to HIV somewhat earlier than ELISA. The RIPA is a research technique limited to laboratories capable of growing HIV in cell culture. The RIPA is slightly more sensitive and more specific than the Western blot, and is useful to resolve indeterminate Western blot results. The LA is an excellent screening method and may prove useful in developing countries lacking the sophisticated equipment and trained technologists to perform ELISA testing.

Culture of HIV is not widely used because the procedure is difficult, requiring fresh human peripheral blood monocytes and frequent assays to detect the virus.

Diagnostic Approach to Infectious Disease

CHAPTER 59

Fever of Undetermined Origin

In 1891 a young physician set up consulting rooms as an eye specialist near Harley Street in London. Patients were very few, so partly to amuse himself, and partly in the hope of supplementing his meager income, he began writing detective stories. The character of his detective-hero was suggested to him by his student memories of Dr. Joseph Bell of the Edinburgh Infirmary, whose diagnostic intuition astounded his patients and students. The fictional detective, whose associate and confidante was a physician, had the remarkable ability to observe details usually overlooked, and by a logical process deduce the details of the crime and the identity of the criminal. English literature owes a debt of gratitude to those ophthalmic persons who stayed away from the office of Dr. A. Conan Doyle, providing him with the leisure to write the fascinating adventures of the immortal Sherlock Holmes and Dr. Watson.

Fever without an apparent cause represents one of the most challenging aspects of medicine. The diagnostic enigma presented by such patients can often only be solved by a Holmsian approach—the observation of details (signs, symptoms, laboratory tests) usually overlooked, and the logical deduction of the underlying disease process. The satisfaction derived from solving the puzzle ranges from effecting the recovery of a dying patient, to the fun of saying "Elementary, Watson" to one's colleagues and students.

Fever is a hallmark of disease recognized since ancient times by physician and patient alike. Healthy people keep their core body temperature within 1.0 to 1.5° C of normal (37° C) throughout the day. All energy from oxidation of food is converted into heat since not all energy from food can be converted to adenosine triphosphate (ATP). There is an obligatory heat production as a result of circulation, respiration, secretion of urine, etc. Involuntary heat production occurs with muscular activity. If extra heat is needed to maintain the core body temperature, it can be generated by shivering in skeletal muscle. Body heat is produced mainly in skeletal muscles and in the liver during metabolism. Body heat is continually dissipated at the surface through the skin and lungs by the usual methods of convection, conduction, and radiation. The autonomic nervous system varies the blood supply to the periphery, permitting heat loss by convection and radiation. Blood flow through the cutaneous vessels in the arms and legs regulates temperature. Increase or decrease of vaso-constrictor tone by adrenergic mechanisms causes heat loss, and the increase of vasocon-strictor tone causes heat retention.

The "normal body temperature" is about 98.6° F (37° C), but the normal temperature may range from 97° F to 99.6° F. In all people there is a diurnal variation in body temperature with the maximum levels reached in the late after-noon or early evening, and a low point at 3 to 5 A.M. People who work at night have a reversal of this circadian temperature pattern.

The anterior hypothalamus is central to the regulation of body temperature. Neural struc-tures supply the information to the hypothala-mus. Specific sensory receptors supply the skin, and there are thermoreceptors in the spinal cord. The content of sodium and calcium in the cerebrospinal fluid alters thermoregulation. Thermoregulation can also be altered by many drugs that affect neurotransmitters.

Central nervous system (CNS) lesions in-volving the hypothalamus can cause inability to regulate temperature. Persons with high cervical transections of the spinal cord have difficulty regulating temperature. In very hot weather, temperature elevation can occur, and in some patients, there will be complete loss of thermo-regulation resulting in the syndrome of heat stroke. Elevated temperature is seen with hy-permetabolic states such as pheochromocytoma and thyrotoxicosis as well as in strenuous exer-cise. Skin diseases such as ichthyosis prevent sweating so the core body temperature can rise rapidly.

Fever is defined as a temperature above 100.5° F (37.8° C). In fever, as distinct from the hyperthermic syndromes—heat stroke, malig-nant hyperthermia, neuroleptic malignant syn-drome,—the normal regulatory mechanisms are intact. The normal hypothalamic thermoregula-tory center, however, is perturbed resulting in a new elevated "set point." Fever is not always pathologic. So-called physiologic fever is seen following a heavy meal; exercise often raises the

temperature to 100° F, and temperatures as high as 103° F may be seen in babies who are dehy-drated from poor water intake or excessive fluid loss. Psychogenic fever (up to 100° F) is often seen immediately following admission to the hospital; subsequent temperatures are normal.

Virtually all infections can produce fever in humans. Fever begins with the release of endo-genous pyrogens into the circulation after an in-fectious, immunologically mediated, or inflam-matory event. The endogenous pyrogens reach the hypothalamic thermoregulatory centers via the arterial blood supply and arachidonic acid is liberated. Arachidonic acid is metabolized to prostaglandin E_2 (PGE_2), and the hypothalamic thermostat is raised to a higher level. This new setting of the CNS thermostat signals various ef-ferent nerves, particularly sympathetic fibers in-nervating peripheral blood vessels. The result-ing vasoconstriction initiates heat conservation. The subjective feeling of "cold" causes the indi-vidual to seek a warmer environment. Heat loss is decreased and heat production increased by the behavioral changes. The efforts to increase temperature continue until the temperature of the blood supplying the hypothalamus matches the elevated set point.

Endogenous pyrogens in the periphery do not penetrate the blood-brain barrier. There is a vascular network close to the preoptic or ante-rior hypothalamus which has a minimal barrier. Either the endogenous pyrogen or PGE_2 and other prostaglandins produced by the endothe-lial cells of this area induce a neurotransmitter-like substance that acts to raise the set point. One of the most important endogenous pyrogens is interleukin-1 (IL-1). Human $IL-1_\beta$ and $IL-1_\alpha$ are about 17 kilodaltons molecular weight. Many different cells produce IL-1. These are mononu-clear phagocytes, such as peripheral blood monocytes, lung and peritoneal macrophages, synovial macrophages, splenic and Kupffer mac-rophages, and Hodgkin's lymphoma cells. Other sources have been keratinocytes, Langerhans' cells, gingival exudate cells, astrocytes and glial cells, and renal mesangial cells. There are many inducers of IL-1 production (Table 59–1) including microbial agents, microbial products, antigens, and inflammatory agents. Endotoxin is the most potent inducer of IL-1. Other factors that are endogenous pyrogens are tumor necrosis factor (cachectin) and interferons. Like IL-1, tumor necrosis factor can act directly on the hypothalamus. It also can act as an inducer of IL-1. Inter-

feron-α produces fever and like the other two substances acts on hypothalamic tissue to increase PGE_2 levels. Interferon-β is a weak pyrogen, and interferon-γ also may cause fever. Interleukin-1 seems to increase body temperature and activate lymphocytes simultaneously. There is induction of cytotoxic T cells and an effect on B cells due to upregulation of T helper cells so that at elevated temperatures B cells make more antibody. Antipyretics function by altering prostaglandin synthesis so that PGE_2 is not produced. Figure 59–1 diagrams the steps in fever production.

Temperature elevation has been associated with the effects of the several phases of the immune response. Specific immunologic responses are generally enhanced in the setting of temperature elevation within the physiologic range but not the supraphysiologic range (greater than 104° F). Although fever appears to be associated with enhanced immune function, a direct connection between the beneficial effect of fever on the outcome of infectious disease has not been demonstrated, but indirect evidence supports an overall beneficial effect on host defense mechanisms.

TABLE 59–1.
Inducers of Interleukin-1 Production

Microorganisms
  Viruses
  Bacteria
  Spirochetes
  Yeasts
Microbial products
  Endotoxins from gram-negative bacteria
  Peptidoglycans from all bacteria
  Exotoxins from staphylococcal and streptococcal pathogenic strains
  Yeast polysaccharides
Inflammatory agents
  Bile salts
  Etiocholanolone
  C5a
  Silica
  Urate crystals
Antigens (via antibody or lymphokine production)
  Microbial antigens (e.g., old tuberculin, staphylococcal proteins, others)
  Nonmicrobial antigens (e.g., ovalbumin, penicillin, human serum albumin, bovine gamma globulin)
  Alloantigens (in the mixed leukocyte reaction)
Plant lectins
  Phytohemagglutinin
  Concanavalin A
Lymphokines
  Colony-stimulating factor
  Macrophage-activating factor(?)
Other inducers
  Bleomycin
  PolyI:C
  Muramyl dipeptide

CLINICAL PATTERNS OF FEVER

Fever patterns have been characterized as intermittent—peak elevations in the evening with return to normal in 1 day; remittent—the temperature does not return to baseline but is elevated persistently, although the fluctuation is 2 to 3° F; and sustained—elevated with little variation. Although these patterns have been associated with particular diseases, this association has been overemphasized. Age may greatly affect the degree of fever. Children under 5 years old may have temperature elevations to 104° F due to a trivial viral illness. Adults over 70 years old may have minimal fever even though they have a severe bacterial or mycotic infection. Temperatures above 106° F, except when due to

PATHOGENESIS OF FEVER

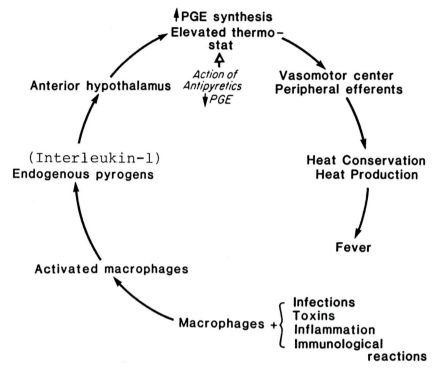

FIG 59–1.
Mehcanism of fever production. PGE_2 = prostaglandin E_2. (Modified from Dinarello CA, Cannon JG, Wolff SM: *Rev Infect Dis* 1988; 10:168.)

encephalitis or meningitis, usually are not the result of infection. Fever can be seen with viral illness—dengue, influenza, or fungemia due to *Candida*. Hence, assumptions as to the cause of a fever cannot be based on the fever profile or the presence of chills. Each fever must be elevated individually.

Prolonged fever is rarely due to organic disease in people who are feeling well, working, gaining or maintaining their weight, and who have no anemia or localizing signs. Prolonged psychogenic fevers often respond to small doses of sedatives or tranquilizers, but not to aspirin; the reverse is true in fever due to infection. Febrile episodes of short duration are almost always due to infection; prolonged fevers are frequently noninfectious. It is critical to determine if a fever is due to infection.

The clinical setting is extremely important in making a decision. A patient who develops a fever after a blood transfusion may be different from a patient who has a sudden chill with production of blood-streaked sputum. The gradual development of a low-grade fever after a myocardial infarction is viewed as a result of the disease, whereas a sudden fever or spike to 102° F in the same patient requires a different evaluation since it could mean infection due to some procedure performed on the patient, e.g., an intravenous (IV) site infection or a urinary tract infection.

The approach to initiation of therapy must be individualized. A patient who appears to be in septic shock requires a different approach than a patient with suspected *Streptococcus mutans* endocarditis of the mitral valve. An agranulocytic patient will die of his infection before cultures return. Fever with a generalized cutaneous eruption in late July could be measles, a drug reaction, or be due to Rocky Mountain spotted fever. The approach to the problem of fever is similar to that employed in other diseases. Occupational exposure, foreign and domestic travel, exposure to animals, immunizations, exposure to drugs, and illness in the community must be determined. During the physical examination there should be particular attention paid to cutaneous lesions. Examination for lymph nodes, enlargement of abdominal organs, and areas of point tenderness often are helpful. Laboratory tests such as the complete blood count, urinalysis, erythrocyte sedimentation rate, chemistry profile; and above all, cultures and Gram stains of body fluids that are accessible to diagnostic sampling; serologic studies and skin tests; as well as chest films may provide a diagnosis.

FEVER OF UNKNOWN ORIGIN

Fever of unknown origin (FUO) has been arbitrarily defined as a fever present for 3 weeks. This eliminates a host of self-limiting causes of fever. This may be an overly rigid definition in view of the ability to rapidly perform many tests which range from blood counts to whole body scans, and was established in the 1960s before many of today's tests were available. The major causes of unexplained fever in the United States have been infections—40%; neoplastic disease—20%; collagen-vascular disease—15%; miscellaneous disorders account for some 15%; and ultimately 10% are never diagnosed (Table 59–2). The frequency of infection as a cause of FUO is much higher in developing countries and the so-called miscellaneous rare category must always be considered in patients from these areas and in patients who have traveled to such areas.

Infections should always be considered first in the evaluation of the FUO. Infections can be divided into systemic and localized illness as noted in Table 59–2. Tuberculosis, primarily miliary, and infective endocarditis are major causes of FUO. Pulmonary involvement is not usually seen when tuberculosis presents as an FUO. The skin tests for tuberculosis, as well as other skin tests, are often negative. Anemia and either leukopenia or leukocytosis may be present. Hepatic involvement may be indicated by elevation of alkaline phosphatase and alanine aminotransferase (ALT, SGPT): a liver biopsy may yield the diagnosis. Presentations of endocarditis vary, but it is important to realize that the blood cultures may be initially negative if the patient is infected with fastidious organisms such as *Haemophilus parainfluenzae* or *Cardiobacterium.*

Miscellaneous infections frequently are difficult to diagnose, since routine cultures and laboratory studies are negative. Only if the physician thinks of the disease and orders the proper serologic studies or performs a biopsy can he make the diagnosis. This is particularly true for diseases such as brucellosis, toxoplasmosis, histoplasmosis, psittacosis, and Q fever. However, since many people have had exposure to these organisms a positive serologic test does not make a diagnosis and one must be cautious in attributing an unexplained fever to a rare illness if the only evidence is a serologic titer.

Localized infections in and about the liver are often occult. A history of trauma or of previously unexplained right upper quadrant pain may be the only clues. Liver enlargement and tenderness are frequently absent. Elevation of the diaphragm, particularly if there is a pleural effusion, should suggest a subphrenic abscess. Isotope scans of the liver and the liver-lung scan are extremely helpful as are ultrasound studies, computed tomography (CT), and magnetic resonance imaging.

The diseases which cause prolonged fever in children are somewhat different from those seen in adults. Children have more viral, inflamma-

TABLE 59–2.

Diagnostic Categories of Fever of Undetermined Origin

I. Infections
   A. Systemic
      1. Tuberculosis (miliary)
      2. Infective endocarditis (subacute)
      3. Miscellaneous infections: cytomegalovirus infection, toxoplasmosis, ·
         brucellosis, psittacosis, gonococcemia, chronic meningococcemia,
         disseminated mycoses (e.g., histoplasmosis, candidiasis)
   B. Localized
      1. Hepatic infections
         a. Liver abscess, cholangitis
      2. Other visceral infections
         a. Pancreatic, tubo-ovarian abscesses; empyema of gallbladder;
           precholecystic abscess
      3. Intraperitoneal infections
         a. Subhepatic, subphrenic, paracolic, appendiceal, pelvic, other
           abscesses.
      4. Urinary tract
         a. Pyelonephritis, renal carbuncle, perinephric abscess
         b. Prostatic abscess
II. Neoplasms (lymphoma)
III. Collagen-vascular disease
IV. Less common causes
   A. Granulomatous disease (other than that due to known infectious agents)
   B. Inflammatory bowel disease
   C. Pulmonary embolization
   D. Drug fever
   E. Factitious fever
   F. Hepatic cirrhosis with active hepatocellular necrosis
   G. Miscellaneous uncommon diseases (familial Mediterranean fever,
      Whipple's disease, etc.)
   H. Undiagnosed

tory, and miscellaneous causes of fever. Children are more likely to have protracted viral infections and the common infections are less likely to have tuberculosis and occult abscesses. The age of the child is helpful since two thirds of prolonged fever in children under 6 years of age are caused by infections, while collagen-inflammatory disorders are more often seen as causes of fever in older children.

In addition to the careful history, physical examination, and usual laboratory tests, biopsy with appropriate culture has been a helpful method in the diagnosis of FUO, particularly liver biopsy. Therapeutic trials have been more misleading than helpful except in cases such as tuberculosis in which drugs with specific activity against mycobacteria alone are used and in which the response usually is seen within 2 weeks. The availability of gallium scans, technetium 99m scans, ultrasound, and CT scans may give a diagnosis or suggest an area in which biopsy will more likely yield a diagnosis.

Rarely, a patient will cause an apparent elevation of body temperature by manipulating the thermometer. Most often such patients are associated with the hospital environment, e.g., a nurse, physician, or member of a medical person's family. The easiest way to detect factitious fever is to use one of the new instant thermometers or determine the temperature of fresh voided urine. There is no way a patient can alter the bladder urine temperature. Oral and rectal readings, however, may be falsified even with an attendant at hand. Lack of a normal diurnal variation should suggest that the fever may not be "real."

CHAPTER 60

Using the Diagnostic Microbiology Laboratory

WHAT TO EXPECT FROM THE MICROBIOLOGY LABORATORY

Appropriate testing can often determine if an infection exists, its cause, and, in many cases, the drug or drugs most likely to effect a cure. Clinical situations may be those where the diagnosis is obvious but the cause remains to be determined (meningitis, pneumonia, urinary tract infection, etc.), or where the diagnosis is uncertain, as in unexplained fever. There are numerous clinical situations in which the microbiology laboratory can provide information that is extremely useful in establishing a diagnosis and determining treatment. Most of these situations involve infectious diseases. Additionally, the microbiology laboratory can provide valuable data for the surveillance and epidemiologic investigation of nosocomial infections. The effective utilization of the microbiology laboratory depends upon three fundamental principles: (1) obtaining the right specimen, (2) providing clinical information to the laboratory, and (3) interpreting the results of the laboratory tests.

Figure 60–1 illustrates how a clinical problem can result in tests being ordered by the physician and specimens and information sent to the laboratory for analysis, and the results returned to the physician who makes the diagnostic or therapeutic decisions.

There are two approaches that the laboratory can use to document an infection: directly, by demonstration of the microorganism itself; or indirectly, by demonstrating antibodies typical of that infectious agent and thus inferring that the agent was or is present. In both approaches, it is essential to collect the right specimen, provide clinical information to the laboratory, and correctly interpret the laboratory results.

SPECIMENS

Selection of the appropriate specimen is generally governed by what has come to be known as Sutton's law.* One samples the anatomic site or organ system indicated by the signs

*Willie Sutton was a notorious (and highly successful) bank robber in the 1960s. His eventual capture attracted many newsmen and reporters, one of whom asked the dapper prisoner, "Willie, why do you only rob banks?" The succinct reply, "That's where the money is," has become a classic statement of going directly to the source.

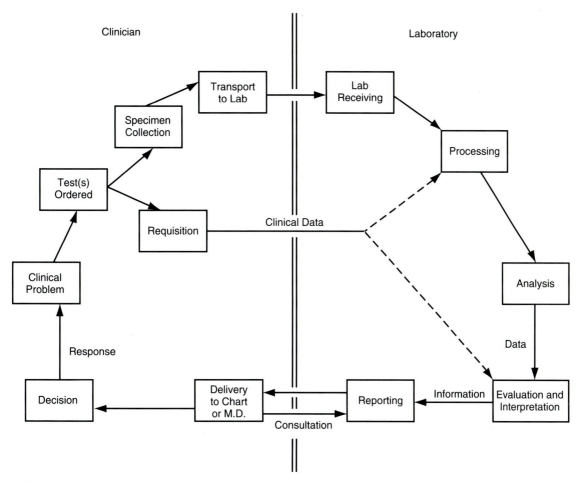

FIG 60–1.
Interaction between the microbiology laboratory and the clinician with particular reference to information transfer.

and symptoms. In situations where a lesion or suspected organ cannot be sampled directly (meninges, endocardium), samples are obtained of the body fluid that drains or circulates over the lesion (cerebrospinal fluid, blood). Where normally sterile sites such as blood or tissue are being sampled, any microorganism that is recovered is suspected of being the causative agent of the infection. If the area being cultured is one that is normally inhabited by organisms, then potential pathogenic species are sought among the indigenous flora.

The timing of specimen collection is impor-

tant and is determined by the stage of the disease. For example, blood cultures obtained when a septicemic patient is having a shaking chill, or when fever is increasing, are more likely to be positive than if taken at other times.

One of the biggest problems in obtaining representative cultures of normally sterile areas is avoiding contamination from the environment and from the patient himself. Every effort must be made to keep the sample free of indigenous organisms by using aseptic (sterile swabs, syringes, etc.) and antiseptic techniques.

Unless media are inoculated at the bedside,

transportation of the specimen to the laboratory requires that conditions be maintained that assure the viability of the organisms while minimizing growth. Replication of the organisms during transport may be undesirable in situations where quantitation is significant, e.g., urine, or when indigenous organisms or contaminants could overgrow, mask, or suppress the etiologic agent. If anaerobes are a consideration, the specimen must be protected from atmospheric oxygen. Some species are adversely affected by chilling, whereas others survive best when refrigerated. In some cases, non-nutritive transport media may be employed to maintain the viability of the organisms.

BACTEREMIA

Bacteremia, the presence of bacteria in the blood, may be a transient phenomenon or associated with a disease process. Transient bacteremias occur regularly when mucous membrane having a commensal flora is disturbed. Thus, transient bacteremia may occur following vigorous brushing of the teeth or other dental manipulations, during menstruation or parturition, or following manipulation of the genitourinary tract, such as catheterization. Transient bacteremias are asymptomatic and are terminated within 15 to 20 minutes with the removal of bacteria from the blood by the reticuloendothelial system.

Bacteremia may also occur with systemic diseases such as pneumonia, meningitis, or cardiovascular infections. Cardiovascular infections include endocarditis, an infection of the endocardium and heart valves; and sepsis (septicemia), a disease caused by the presence of pathogenic microorganisms and their toxic products in the blood.

The diagnosis and treatment of bacteremia depends upon the identification of the organism in the patient's blood; consequently, blood cultures are an extremely important procedure. In-

dications for blood cultures are intravascular infections (sepsis, endocarditis), and infections with a bacteremic phase (pneumonia, meningitis, abdominal and pelvic abscesses, osteomyelitis, typhoid fever, brucellosis, etc.). In suspected sepsis, two blood cultures should be taken immediately or during a shaking chill—one from each arm—before starting antimicrobial therapy. In subacute endocarditis, three cultures should be taken randomly throughout the day for 2 consecutive days.

Blood is obtained by venipuncture following scrupulous skin preparation at the puncture site. This involves the use of iodine, which should not be removed until the procedure has been completed. Ten to 20 mL of blood should be removed from adults and distributed into aerobic and anaerobic bottles or vials each containing 30 to 50 mL of a rich broth and 10% carbon dioxide. A nontoxic anticoagulant such as sodium polyanethol sulfonate must be used; citrate, fluoride, or ethylenediamine tetraacetic acid (EDTA) is unsuitable. One or two blood cultures taken from different sites during a chill or temperature spike are usually adequate to document septicemia before initiating treatment.

The quantity of blood has a direct bearing on the probability of recovering the pathogen. With small children, 1 to 2 mL of blood distributed in two vials of 10 mL of broth are satisfactory. The blood should be kept at room temperature during transport to the laboratory. Blood culture bottles are incubated in the laboratory and are monitored for growth by visual inspection, blind subculture, or staining, or any combination of these, or by radiometric technique.

Organisms commonly involved in endocarditis are: the viridans group of *Streptococcus*, enterococci, *Streptococcus bovis*, *Staphylococcus aureus*, *Staphylococcus epidermidis*, *Candida albicans* and other fungi, gram-negative bacilli, *Streptococcus pneumoniae*, *Streptococcus pyogenes* (group A), and *Corynebacterium* sp. (especially with prosthetic valves). Organisms commonly involved in sepsis are listed below in the approximate order of frequency with which they occur.

Adults: *Escherichia coli* (or other gram-negative bacilli), *S. aureus*, *S. pneumoniae*, *Bacteroides*, *S. pyogenes* (group A), *S. epidermidis*, *Neisseria meningitidis*, *C. albicans*, *Neisseria gonorrhoeae*, other *Candida* species.

Children: *S. pneumoniae*, *N. meningitidis*, *Haemophilus influenzae*, *S. aureus*, *S. pyogenes* (group A), *E. coli* (or other gram-negative bacilli).

Newborn infants: *E. coli* (or other gram-negative bacilli), *Streptococcus* group B, *Listeria monocytogenes*, *S. aureus*, *S. pyogenes* (group A), enterococci, *S. pneumoniae*.

CENTRAL NERVOUS SYSTEM INFECTIONS

Common central nervous system infections include encephalitis, brain abscess, and meningitis. Infectious encephalitis is invariably viral in etiology; brain abscess and meningitis are frequently caused by bacteria.

In order to establish a diagnosis of bacterial meningitis, it is essential to examine the cerebrospinal fluid (CSF). Following careful preparation of the skin site with iodine, a lumbar puncture is performed and CSF is aseptically removed. In adults, 1 or 2 mL should be collected in a tube for chemical determination; 0.5 to 1.0 mL in a second tube is adequate for a cell count and differential; and at least 3 to 5 mL should be collected in a third sterile tube for bacteriologic examination. This last tube should be kept warm (body temperature) and should reach the laboratory as soon as possible. CSF is normally clear, sterile, and seldom contains more than five mononuclear cells per cubic millimeter. The protein concentration is normally 15 to 45 mg/100 mL and the glucose is about half of the blood sugar level. In bacterial meningitis, the CSF may be cloudy and contain many polymorphonuclear leukocytes. Usually the protein

is elevated and the sugar content is reduced. Bacteria may be seen on a Gram stain.

Organisms commonly involved in meningitis include: *N. meningitidis*, *H. influenzae* (in children), *S. pneumoniae*, *Streptococcus* group B (infants less than 2 months old), *E. coli* (or other gram-negative bacilli), *S. pyogenes* (group A), *S. aureus* (with endocarditis or after neurosurgery, brain abscess), *Mycobacterium tuberculosis*, *Cryptococcus neoformans* and other fungi, *Listeria monocytogenes*, enterococci (neonatal period), and *Leptospira*.

OTHER NORMALLY STERILE BODY FLUIDS AND TISSUES (PERICARDIAL, SYNOVIAL, BONE MARROW, BIOPSY, ETC.)

Scrupulous skin preparation with iodine (see Blood cultures) is essential. The fluid should be sent to the laboratory in a sterile plastic screw-cap tube and kept at room temperature. If a biopsy specimen is very tiny, a small amount of sterile saline can be added.

ABSCESSES AND DEEP CLOSED BODY AREAS

Since such specimens often contain anaerobes, they are best sampled by aspiration with a sterile syringe following skin preparation with iodine. Any air bubbles are expressed from the syringe, the needle protected with a rubber stopper, and the syringe sent to the laboratory. Alternatively, a special anaerobic specimen collector may be used. Any of the organisms involved in bacteremia or wound infections may also be involved in these sites.

WOUNDS AND BURNS

Swabs rolled over the surface are unsatisfactory and usually reproduce skin flora. Medication and superficial detritus should be removed with alcohol or sterile saline. Using a sterile curette or skin punch, obtain a sample from the edge or depth of the wound. Place the specimen in a sterile tube for transport.

The most common organisms in wounds and burns are: *S. aureus, S. pyogenes, Pseudomonas aeruginosa,* other gram-negative bacilli, and anaerobes.

RESPIRATORY INFECTIONS

UPPER RESPIRATORY INFECTIONS

Upper respiratory infections include pharyngitis, sinusitis, and otitis media (infection of the middle ear). A wide variety of bacteria occur normally in the nasopharynx of healthy persons. Bacteria commonly found in the mouth and pharynx include α-hemolytic and nonhemolytic streptococci, staphylococci, *Neisseria,* corynebacteria (diphtheroids), and *Haemophilus* species. Occasionally, members of the coliform group and other species are encountered.

Most cases of pharyngitis are caused by viruses or mycoplasma; 10% to 25% are due to β-hemolytic streptococci (usually group A). Middle ear and sinus infections are often caused by *S. pneumoniae, H. influenzae,* or *Moraxella.*

Throat cultures are essential to establish the diagnosis of streptococcal pharyngitis, as well as to confirm a clinical diagnosis of diphtheria. Sheep blood agar is regularly used as the culture medium, since it supports good growth of most of the principal pathogens and aids in identifying those that produce alpha or beta hemolysis, e.g., pneumococci and β-hemolytic streptococci. Sheep erythrocytes contain NADase, which inhibits the growth of *Haemophilus hemolyticus*— a normal commensal which could be confused with hemolytic streptococci. For *H. influenzae,* horse blood agar or chocolate blood agar is used. *Corynebacterium diphtheriae* requires special media that are not routinely inoculated.

The major purpose of a throat culture is to detect the presence of group A streptococci. A heavy growth of group A streptococci in a throat culture from a patient with pharyngitis is indicative of streptococcal pharyngitis. A few colonies of group A streptococci can sometimes be recovered from persons with viral pharyngitis or from those who are asymptomatic and represent the carrier state.

To take a throat culture, use a dry, sterile swab. The areas of the throat to be swabbed are the posterior oral pharyngeal wall and both tonsillar areas, irrespective of whether or not the tonsils have been removed or are atrophied. Wipe the same swab gently across all of these areas. If pus is present in any of the lymphoid crypts, gently squeeze some onto the swab. Do not let the swab touch the tongue or other parts of the mouth. Place the swab in a tube containing a transport medium such as Stuart's or Amies. The use of charcoal-coated swabs or transport media containing charcoal should be avoided. A transport medium is important as cotton fibers are toxic to some bacteria, and others do not survive desiccation.

Organisms commonly involved in otitis media or sinusitis include: *S. pneumoniae, H. influenzae, S. pyogenes, Moraxella catarrhalis,* and less commonly, *S. aureus* and anaerobes.

LOWER RESPIRATORY INFECTIONS

Expectorated sputum is obtained from a deep cough, preferably on arising in the morning. Patients who have difficulty raising sputum can be assisted by postural drainage, thoracic percussion, the inhalation of warm saline aerosols, mucolytic agents, and combinations of these aids. Saliva and nasopharyngeal secretions are not satisfactory. Children under 8 years of age have difficulty raising sputum and a nasopharyngeal swab is an adequate substitute. Twenty-four-hour pooled sputum specimens are highly contaminated by the overgrowth of oropharyngeal flora and should not be used. Sputum specimens should be sent to the laboratory promptly. If anaerobes are being considered, expectorated sputum is unsatisfactory. Bronchoscopy specimens obtained with a rigid-tube bronchoscope are no better than expectorated sputum. (*Caution:* Most local anesthetics contain bacteriostatic agents.) If an anaerobic infection is a possibility, or if the patient is unable to raise sputum, then fiberoptic bronchoscopy, transtracheal aspiration, percutaneous transthoracic aspiration, or open lung biopsy should be considered.

Common organisms that may cause pneumonia include: respiratory viruses, *Mycoplasma pneumoniae*, *S. pneumoniae*, *H. influenzae*, anaerobic streptococci, *Bacteroides*, *S. aureus*, *Klebsiella* (or other gram-negative bacilli), *Legionella pneumophila*, *S. pyogenes* (group A), *Rickettsia*, *Mycobacterium tuberculosis*, *Pneumocystis carinii* (a protozoan), fungi, *Legionella micdadei* (*L. pittsburgensis*), and *Chlamydia psittaci*.

Lung abscesses may be due to: anaerobic streptococci, *Bacteroides*, *S. aureus*, *Klebsiella* (or other gram-negative bacilli), *S. pneumoniae*, fungi, *Actinomyces*, and *Nocardia*.

GASTROINTESTINAL INFECTIONS

Gastrointestinal infections are generally manifested by the presence of diarrhea, and may be caused by a variety of bacteria, viruses, or protozoa. In diarrheal disease caused by bacteria, the causative organisms are invariably present in the stool, and consequently stool culture is an important part of the diagnostic workup. It is important to know the particular agent responsible for the infection, since the need for therapy and the antimicrobials employed depend upon the etiologic agent.

Specimens for culture may be obtained by picking up a small (pea-sized) portion of the evacuated stool with a cotton swab. Alternatively, a cotton swab may be inserted into the rectum. Swabs containing fecal material should be placed in a non-nutritive transport medium to prevent dehydration during the trip to the laboratory. Upon arrival in the laboratory, stool specimens are plated on a variety of selective-differential media designed to recover and partially identify particular bacterial species. Microscopic examination of a methylene blue-stained smear of the feces for the presence of inflammatory cells (WBC) is a valuable procedure.

Bacteria commonly causing diarrheal diseases include: *Campylobacter fetus* subsp. *jejuni*, *Salmonella* species, *Shigella* species, *E. coli*, *Clostridium perfringens*, *Yersinia enterocolitica*, *Vibrio parahaemolyticus*, and *Vibrio cholerae*.

URINARY TRACT INFECTIONS

Urinary tract infection is one of the most common bacterial diseases and proper management requires an understanding of the numbers and kinds of bacteria involved. Most urinary tract infections result from ascending infection by organisms introduced through the urethra.

With the exception of the terminal portion of the urethra, which has normal commensal bacteria, the urinary tract and bladder urine are normally sterile. Infections are usually associated with bacterial counts of 100,000 (10^5) or more organisms per milliliter of urine (significant bacteriuria). This is because urine is an excellent culture medium for most uropathogens, and growth occurs in the urine itself in vivo, resulting in high counts in untreated infections. In contrast, normal urine usually contains less than 1,000 organisms per milliliter in properly collected and transported specimens. These organisms represent urethral commensals and contamination from the external genitalia. Since bacteria continue to grow in the urine, it is essential that the specimen be cultured within 2 hours after voiding. Otherwise, the specimen must be refrigerated or preserved with boric acid.

Quantitation of bacteria in urine may be accomplished by plating several dilutions of the urine or by using a calibrated loop to deliver a known volume of urine to the surface of one or more plates. A simple and rapid method is the microscopic examination of a Gram stain of uncentrifuged urine. If bacteria are seen with the oil immersion lens, this means that there are at least 10^5 organisms per milliliter. Alternatively, a dip slide coated with agar may be dipped into the urine and incubated.

Ninety percent of the bacteria involved in urinary tract infections are gram-negative bacilli. The most common organism is *E. coli*; other species include *Klebsiella, Enterobacter, Proteus, Pseudomonas,* and *S. saprophyticus.* Enterococcal infections (enterococci) are frequent in patients with obstructive uropathy or following manipulation of the urinary tract. *Staphylococcus aureus* and *S. epidermidis* are occasionally involved in urinary tract infections. Two species are occasionally recovered from the urine of patients with complicated or chronic infections; the recovery of three or more species usually suggests improper collection or transport of the specimen.

The laboratory diagnosis of urinary tract infections depends on the demonstration of significant bacteriuria and the identification of the organism(s). The laboratory is often called upon to determine the antibiotic susceptibility of the uropathogen(s). Voided urine specimens are obtained after cleaning the external genitalia with soap and water. Females must separate the labia with their fingers while voiding. The specimen may be collected in a clean Dixie cup or sterile tube. Voided urine specimens are always contaminated with urethral and (in females) vaginal flora. These organisms grow rapidly in urine at room temperature and can result in spuriously high bacterial counts and obscuration of the pathogen if the specimen is not cultured promptly. If the urine specimen cannot be cultured within 2 hours of voiding, it should be cultured immediately on a commercially available agar-coated dip slide. Alternatively, the specimen may be preserved for 24 hours by refriger-

ation, or by the addition of 0.9% boric acid. Urine obtained by catheter, cytoscopy, or bladder aspiration is collected in a sterile plastic tube and sent promptly to the laboratory.

GENITAL SPECIMENS FOR SEXUALLY TRANSMITTED DISEASES

In males, urethral exudate or prostatic expressate may be collected on a swab. Rectal and pharyngeal cultures should also be taken from homosexual males. With females, cervical and rectal sites should be cultured. Pharyngeal swabs should also be taken if there is a history of oral-genital contact. A selective medium for the gonococcus (Martin-Lewis or NYC) should be inoculated immediately and sent to the laboratory. If chlamydial cultures are to be performed, the swab can be placed in a special transport medium (2-sucrose phosphate with glutamate).

The organisms most commonly involved are: *N. gonorrhoeae, Chlamydia trachomatis,* and *Ureaplasma.*

PROVIDING CLINICAL INFORMATION

It is essential that pertinent clinical information accompany the specimen. Specifically, laboratory personnel must be told what the specimen is, how it was obtained, and what the clinical problem is. If a special organism such as *Legionella,* or a group of organisms, e.g., fungi, is suspected, this must also be stated. This information will determine how the specimen is processed. Many organisms require special media or environments not routinely employed. Some examples are: *Bordetella pertussis, Haemophilus ducreyi, Legionella, Francisella tularensis, Leptospira, Corynebacterium diphtheriae,* mycoplasma, etc.

The clinical information will also affect the interpretation of results. For example, 100 *E. coli* organisms per milliliter of voided urine is of no significance in a male being evaluated for pyelonephritis, but could be very significant in a female with symptoms of a bladder infection.

LABORATORY PROCEDURES TO DEMONSTRATE MICROORGANISMS

In many cases the organism is apparent on microscopic examination. Wet mounts can reveal parasites such as *Trichomonas vaginalis*, and an India ink preparation of CSF may reveal *Cryptococcus neoformans*. Parasites such as plasmodia may be visualized by examination of a Giemsa-stained smear of peripheral blood.

Gram-stained direct smears should always be made of body fluids including CSF, tissues, biopsies, aspirates, eye specimens, urethral exudate, and all purulent material. Direct examination of Gram stains of stool, sputum, wounds, and urine may also be helpful under certain circumstances. Acid-fast stains of sputum concentrates may reveal acid-fast bacilli. Fluorescent microscopic examination of specimens stained with specific antibody conjugates can detect *Legionella*, *B. pertussis*, bacteroides, group A streptococci, and other organisms. When clinical specimens are to be cultured, the nature of the specimen and the organism sought must be considered. The importance of this information accompanying the specimen has previously been mentioned.

Specimens from normally sterile body sites are planted on rich media such as blood and chocolate agar. As previously noted, certain organisms require specialized media. Selective media containing substances that inhibit particular groups of bacteria are usually employed when culturing specimens from body sites with an indigenous flora. MacConkey agar will permit the growth of most nonfastidious gram-negative bacilli while inhibiting the growth of gram-positive bacteria. Colistin-nalidixic acid (CNA) agar permits the growth of streptococci, enterococci, most strains of staphylococci, and other gram-

positive species, and inhibits the growth of most gram-negative bacteria. Selective media are often made differential so that the colonies of one genus appear different from the colonies of other genera. An example of this is the addition of lactose and a pH indicator to media used to culture stool specimens. Colonies of lactose-fermenting organisms appear in a different color than nonlactose fermenters such as *Salmonella* or *Shigella*.

Conditions of incubation vary. Some species require an anaerobic atmosphere or one with a higher carbon dioxide content (gonococci, meningococci, *Brucella*, etc.). A few organisms need temperatures higher or lower than the normal body temperature of 35 to 37° C. Slow-growing organisms such as mycobacteria or many fungi require many days or weeks of incubation.

A more recent approach to demonstrating a pathogen in clinical material is direct antigen detection. These methods have the advantages of rapidity and not requiring that the organism be viable. Direct antigen detection may be accomplished by counterimmunoelectrophoresis, in which the specimen and known antisera are placed in adjoining holes on an agar-coated slide and a current passed through the agar for 30 to 40 minutes. Antibody and antigen, if present in the specimen, are brought into contact in the agar and form a band of precipitation. Several antibodies may be run simultaneously.

Simpler, faster, and more sensitive methods of antigen detection are coagglutination and latex agglutination. With these techniques, suspensions of staphylococci (coagglutination) or latex particles are sensitized by coating them with specific immunoglobulin. These suspensions clump immediately when brought into contact with clinical material containing the homologous antigen. These methods have been most effective in detecting carbohydrate capsular material in CSF and urine.

A newer, highly specific technique for the identification of microorganisms is the nucleic acid probe method. The specimen is heated to denature microbe-specific DNA or RNA, mixed with the probe (single-stranded nucleic acid tagged with an isotope or fluorescent dye), and tested for hybridization. The technique can be made extremely sensitive with amplification by the polymerase chain reaction.

ANTIMICROBIAL SUSCEPTIBILITY TESTING

The purpose of in vitro susceptibility testing is to determine the suitability of various antimicrobial agents for treating a particular infection. The selection of an antibiotic requires a physician's judgment and must involve a consideration of the inhibitory activity and the pharmacologic characteristics of the agent. While the in vitro susceptibility of the etiologic agent is of prime importance, other factors must also be considered. These include the pharmacokinetics of the agent (route of administration, protein binding, tissue levels at the infection site, and toxicity), host factors (allergy, renal function), and the cost of the drug.

Bacteria that are routinely tested are those that are the probable etiologic agents of the infection and which show significant strain variation in their susceptibility to antibiotics. These include *S. aureus*, Enterobacteriaceae (*E. coli*, *Klebsiella*, etc.) and *Pseudomonas* species. *Staphylococcus epidermidis*, group D streptococci, and anaerobes should also be tested when recovered in pure culture from a normally sterile site. *Haemophilus influenzae* and *N. gonorrhoeae* should be tested for β-lactamase. *Streptococcus pneumoniae* should also be tested for penicillin susceptibility. *Haemophilus influenzae* may also be tested for chloramphenicol acetyltransferase to determine susceptibility to chloramphenicol. Species that are uniformly susceptible or resistant to antibiotics, e.g., group A or B streptococci, should not be routinely tested. Obvious contaminants or indigenous species recovered from sites they normally inhabit should not be tested. It is neither practical nor useful to test bacterial isolates against all available antibiotics. Drugs routinely tested are those appropriate to the treatment of infections due to the particular isolate. Drugs should be selected and reported that have acceptable in vitro test accuracy and reliable interpretive criteria, conform to clinical experience, and have the best cost-benefit ratio. It is not necessary to test every member of each drug class. Although pharmacologic differences may exist among members of a class of drugs, susceptibility is usually the same as the class representative.

Qualitative in vitro testing is commonly done by disk diffusion such as the Kirby-Bauer method. A pure culture of the organism is diluted to a standardized concentration and uniformly seeded over the surface of an agar culture plate. Paper disks containing antibiotics are placed on the agar surface, and following 18 to 20 hours of incubation, the plate is examined for zones of incubation around the disks. The diameter of each zone is measured. The organism is considered "susceptible" to a drug when the zone diameter exceeds an established value which varies for each drug, and "resistant" when the zone diameter is less than that value.

Quantitative methods involve the determination of the minimum inhibitory concentration (MIC) or the minimum bactericidal concentration (MBC) of a drug. The MIC is the lowest concentration of a drug that will inhibit the growth of the organism tested. The MIC is determined by making serial dilutions in broth of each drug. A standardized inoculum of the organism is added to each dilution, and following 18 hours of incubation, the tubes are examined for evidence of growth. The highest dilution (lowest concentration) of the drug that prevents growth is the MIC. The MBC is the lowest concentration of a drug that kills the organism. The MBC is determined in the same way as the MIC, except that following incubation each dilution is subcultured to an agar plate. The highest dilution (lowest concentration) of the drug that results in a 99% decrease in the number of colonies is the MBC. The MBC of most isolates is slightly higher than the MIC. Organisms showing a wide disparity between their MIC and MBC are said to be tolerant. MICs and MBCs are reported in micrograms per milliliter. In order to correctly interpret MIC-MBC values, the physician also needs to know the drug levels that can be achieved at the infection site. If a drug can reach a tissue level of at least eight times the MIC or MBC at the infection site, it is a potentially effective drug. In immunosuppressed patients, at least 16 times the MIC should be achieved for a drug to be considered. This multiple of the MIC-MBC is the inhibitory quotient (IQ) and is calculated by dividing the determined MIC or MBC into the achievable drug level at that anatomic site. An IQ of zero indicates that the MIC cannot be achieved and the drug is a poor therapeutic choice.

In vitro determination of susceptibility does not reflect the conditions at the site of infection which determine the interaction between host, microbe, and drug. Failure of susceptibility tests to predict the outcome of therapy may be due to emergence of drug resistance during treatment, impaired contact between drug and microorganism, antagonism between two drugs, inactivation of penicillins by β-lactamase-producing indigenous flora, impairment of normal host defense mechanisms, or testing an organism other than the etiologic agent. In certain situations (*Salmonella typhi* and aminoglycosides; enterococci and cephalosporins) in vitro susceptibility does not correlate with therapeutic efficacy for reasons that are not understood. Therapeutic failure is common in infections treated with antimicrobial agents to which the infecting organism is found to be resistant by in vitro testing; therapeutic success in patients treated with drugs to which the organism is susceptible is only moderately good and cannot be assured.

SEROLOGIC TESTING

The etiology of an infection may be inferred by detecting the presence, or a rise in titer of certain antibodies. Whenever possible, specific antibodies are looked for using a variety of techniques that include agglutination, hemagglutination, neutralization (toxins and viruses), precipitin, complement fixation methods, enzyme-linked immunosorbent assay (ELISA), and radioimmunoassay.

There are two main limitations of serologic methods of diagnosis: the patient may be seen early in the disease before antibody synthesis occurs; or conversely, a high titer of antibody may reflect an antecedent infection unrelated to the present clinical problem. Despite these limitations, the serologic approach is often valuable in situations where the pathogenic microorganisms cannot be demonstrated by visualization, culture, or direct antigen methods.

Blood for antibody studies should be collected in tubes without any anticoagulant. An "acute" specimen should be obtained as early as possible in the disease and a "convalescent" specimen obtained 7 to 10 days later. In many cases, single specimens are useless because a rise in antibody titer cannot be ascertained.

INTERPRETING MICROBIOLOGY LABORATORY RESULTS

Laboratory results must be evaluated in the light of the clinical problem. A knowledge of the distribution and composition of the indigenous flora is helpful. It is also useful to become familiar with the agents commonly involved in infections of the various organ systems.

PART XIV

Antimicrobial Therapy

CHAPTER 61

Chemotherapy of Infectious Diseases

Chemotherapeutic agents in the form of poultices and other substances date back to ancient times in China and Egypt, and in Peru, where cinchona bark was used to treat malaria. Our modern chemotherapy really dates to the work of Paul Ehrlich in Germany, who at the turn of the century sought to discover agents to treat syphilis and African sleeping sickness. The enunciation of a concept that it is possible to find chemicals that are nontoxic to man but which will inhibit parasites was the goal of Ehrlich's research. Beginning with Alexander Fleming's discovery in 1929 of penicillin, and with Gerhard Domagk's discovery of the effectiveness of Prontosil, the forerunner of sulfa drugs, an enormous number of natural products from nature have been found and synthetic substances have been synthesized in the laboratory. We have learned a great deal about chemotherapeutic agents in the past several decades and are at present able to understand precisely what these agents inhibit and what structure-function relationships are important for their activity.

Antimicrobial targets can be separated into groups on the basis of their site of action (Table 61–1). For example, there are inhibitors of bacterial and fungal cell wall synthesis, compounds that destroy cytoplasmic membranes, inhibitors of nucleic acid synthesis, and inhibitors of ribosomal function (Fig 61–1). They may be further characterized as being inhibitors of growth, i.e., bacteriostatic, or as agents which actually kill the microorganisms, i.e., bactericidal.

INHIBITION OF BACTERIAL CELL WALL SYNTHESIS

Both gram-positive and gram-negative bacteria have cell walls whose synthesis is amenable to destruction or inhibition by a variety of different agents. Gram-positive organisms have cell walls that contain peptidoglycan as their main component. Gram-negative bacteria have cell walls that contain peptidoglycan, but they are surrounded in addition by an outer lipopolysaccharide lipoprotein layer that contains channels of protein and phospholipid. All of the agents which attack bacteria at the cell wall site do so by interfering with peptidoglycan synthesis.

323

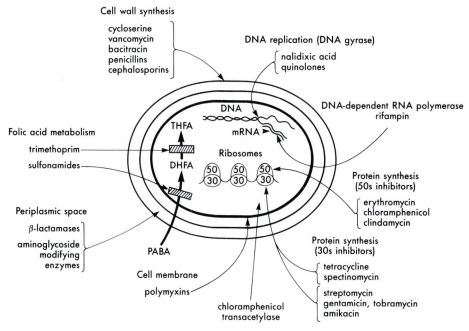

FIG 61–1.
Antimicrobial sites of bactericidal or bacteriostatic action on microorganisms. The five general mechanisms are: (1) inhibit synthesis of cell wall; (2) damage outer membrane; (3) modify nucleic acid/DNA synthesis; (4) modify protein synthesis (at ribosomes); and (5) modify energy metabolism within the cytoplasm (at folate cycle). (From Wingard LE, Brody TM, Larner J, et al (eds): *Human Pharmacology: Molecular to Clinical.* St Louis, Mosby–Year Book, 1991. Used by permission.)

The most important antibacterial agents are the β-lactam compounds that interfere with the third stage of cell wall synthesis which involves the polymerization of subunits and the attachment of growing peptidoglycan to the old cell wall. Enzymes referred to as transpeptidases create peptide bonds between D-alanyl amino acids in a pentapeptide that is attached to N-acetylglucosamine. In recent years these enzymes have been referred to as penicillin-binding proteins (PBPs). β-Lactam antibiotics essentially undergo an acylation reaction with the transpeptidases. β-Lactam antibiotics include penicillins, cephalosporins, carbapenems, and monobactams (Fig 61–2). The PBPs of gram-positive and gram-negative bacteria differ, as do those in anaerobic species. The effect that a particular β-lactam antibiotic has upon a mi-

croorganism depends upon the specific PBPs to which it binds. Binding to certain PBPs may cause immediate swelling and rupture of cells, whereas binding to other PBPs, particularly those in gram-negative organisms, may produce long filaments which eventually die. An agent such as the compound oxacillin, which inhibits gram-positive species such as staphylococci and streptococci, does not inhibit gram-negative organisms, primarily because of its low affinity for the enzymes involved in gram-negative bacterial cell wall synthesis but also because it fails to reach the PBPs. Conversely an agent such as aztreonam, a monobactam, inhibits only gram-negative organisms since it does not bind to the PBPs of gram-positive or anaerobic species.

Vancomycin is an important antimicrobial agent that binds to the D-alanine–D-alanine ter-

TABLE 61–1.

Classification of Antimicrobial Agents by Mechanism of Action*

Mechanism of Action	Agent
Inhibition of synthesis of cell wall	Penicillins
	Cephalosporins
	Monobactams
	Carbapenems
	Vancomycin
	Bacitracin
	Cycloserine
	Fosfomycin
Damage of cytoplasmic membrane	Polymyxins
	Polyene antifungals
	Imidazoles
Metabolism of nucleic acid	Quinolones
	Rifampin
	Nitrofurans
	Nitroimidazoles
Protein synthesis	Aminoglycosides
	Tetracyclines
	Chloramphenicol
	Macrolides
	Clindamycin
	Spectinomycin
	Mupirocin
Modification of energy metabolism	Sulfonamides
	Trimethoprim
	Dapsone
	Isoniazid

*Modified from Wingaard LE, Brody TM, Larner J, et al (eds): Human Pharmacology: Molecular to Clinical. St Louis, Mosby–Year Book, 1991.

mini of the growing peptidoglycan and prevents the interaction of muramidases with the glycan chain. Vancomycin has a large molecular weight and cannot cross the outer wall of gram-negative bacteria. Thus it inhibits only gram-positive organisms and rare gram-negative species that have a weak outer wall such as some *Neisseria* species.

There are several other agents that interfere with cell wall synthesis at different stages. These agents, however, are infrequently administered in the United States. Bacitracin is a peptide antibiotic that only inhibits gram-positive bacteria. It interacts with a long chain alcohol and prevents transfer of the muramyl peptide from the precursor nucleotide to the growing peptidoglycan chain. Cyclosporine is a compound that is structurally similar to D-alanine–D-alanine and binds to the enzymes that make D-alanine. Fosfomycin blocks an enzyme, phosphoenolpyruvate, which is involved in the early cell wall synthesis of the uridine diphosphate (UDP) building blocks of the peptidoglycan backbone.

ANTIMICROBIAL AGENTS AFFECTING CYTOPLASMIC MEMBRANES

There are a number of antimicrobial agents that produce a disorganization of the lipoprotein membrane which surrounds most bacterial organisms. Unfortunately, these agents have proved to be of minor clinical importance owing to their toxicity. The polymyxins, polymyxin B, and colistiethate, are octapeptides that inhibit gram-negative bacteria by binding to phospholipids on the cytoplasmic membrane of the bacterial cell with a resulting disorganization of the membrane, loss of permeability, and death of the cell.

INTERFERENCE WITH DNA FUNCTION

Rifampin is an antimicrobial agent that inhibits DNA-directed RNA polymerase by binding to one of its four subunits and interfering with the initiation process for production of messenger RNA. Quinolones interfere with DNA replication by binding to the enzyme DNA gyrase that is involved in opening and reuniting DNA strands during replication. Examples of such compounds are ciprofloxacin, ofloxacin, and norfloxacin. Other agents which affect DNA synthesis are the nitroimidazoles such as metro-

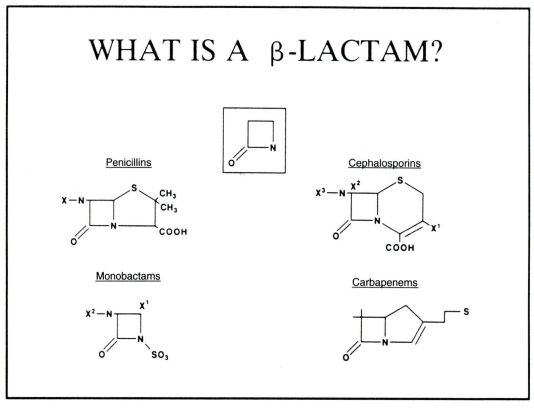

WHAT IS A β-LACTAM?

Penicillins

Cephalosporins

Monobactams

Carbapenems

FIG 61–2.
The composition of a β-lactam. (From Wingard LE, Brody TM, Larner J, et al (eds): *Human Pharmacology: Molecular to Clinical.* St Louis, Mosby–Year Book, 1991. Used by permission.)

nidazole which after being metabolized in the bacteria bind to DNA and produce strand breakage in DNA.

ANTIMICROBIAL INHIBITORS OF RIBOSOME FUNCTION

There are a number of antimicrobial agents which inhibit the function of ribosomes. These agents bind to specific proteins in the ribosome unit and can act either in a bactericidal or bacteriostatic manner. Aminoglycoside antibiotics such as gentamicin bind to specific proteins in the 30s ribosomal subunit but to some extent also to proteins in the 50s ribosomal subunit.

Aminoglycosides basically kill bacteria by causing the formation of nonfunctional initiation complex as well as causing misreading of messenger RNA. Tetracyclines also bind to 30s ribosomes, but the binding is transient in contrast to the permanent binding of the aminoglycosides. Thus tetracyclines are bacteriostatic agents.

A number of important agents interfere with ribosomal function at the 50s ribosomal subunit. Chloramphenicol inhibits gram-positive and gram-negative bacteria by inhibiting a peptidyltransferase enzyme. Macrolides such as erythromycin impair both peptidyltransferase reactions and the translocation of amino acids. Clindamycin has a form of action similar to erythromycin.

DRUGS THAT INHIBIT PRECURSORS OF DNA

Sulfonamides and trimethoprim interfere with folate metabolism in bacteria by blocking the biosynthesis of tetrahydrofolate which acts as a precursor of DNA, RNA, and bacterial cell wall amino acids (Fig 61–3). Sulfonamides block the conversion of pteridine and *p*-aminobenzoic acid to dihydrofolic acid by inhibiting the enzyme pteridine synthetase, whereas trimethoprim inhibits dihydrofolate reductase.

AGENTS ACTIVE AGAINST FUNGI

The membranes of fungi contain sterols similar to the sterols present in many mammalian cells. Polyene antibiotics bind to fungal sterols altering their normal configuration and thereby causing loss of normal permeability. The polyenes such as amphotericin B produce a hole in the fungal membrane allowing loss of the contents of the fungus (Fig 61–4). Amphotericin B is a fungicidal agent. Other agents of the imidazole class, such as ketoconazole, clotrimazole,

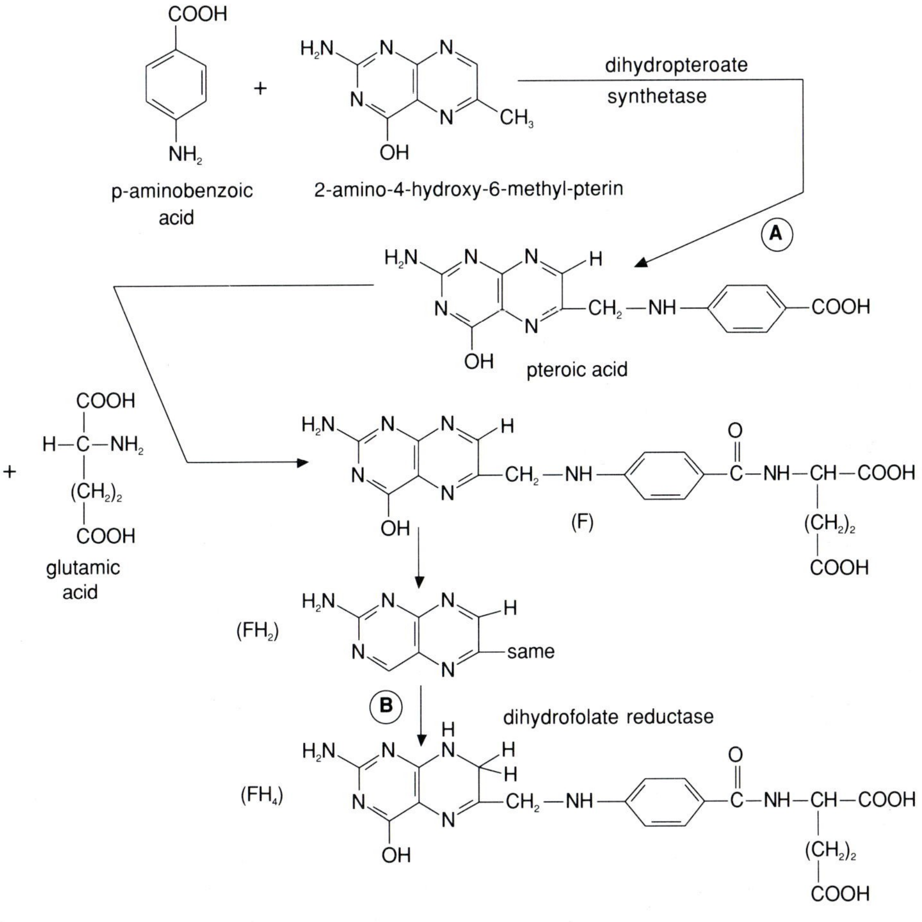

FIG 61–3.
Bacterial synthesis of folic acid *(F)* and reduction to dihydrofolate (FH$_2$) and tetrahydrofolate (FH$_4$), *A* and *B* are sites of drug action. (From Wingard LE, Brody TM, Larner J, et al (eds): *Human Pharmacology: Molecular to Clinical.* St Louis, Mosby–Year Book, 1991. Used by permission.)

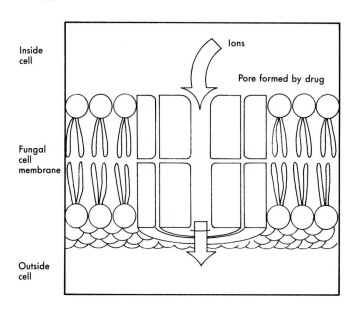

FIG 61–4.
Action of polyene agents such as amphotericin whereby pores are formed in the fungal cell membrane through which K^+ and MG^{++} can leak out of the cell. (From Wingard LE, Brody TM, Larner J, et al (eds): *Human Pharmacology: Molecular to Clinical.* St Louis, Mosby–Year Book, 1991. Used by permission.)

and fluconazole, which inhibit the incorporation of subunits into ergosterol, damage the fungal cell membrane and are not fungicidal but fungistatic. Other antifungal agents can interfere with DNA synthesis in fungi, but only one of these, 5-fluorcoytosine, has proved to be clinically useful.

ANTIVIRAL AGENTS

The effective antiviral agents are those that interfere with purine and pyrimidine synthesis or with the conversion or utilization of nucleotides. Acyclovir and gancyclovir are nucleoside analogues which alter the activity of thymidine kinase and DNA polymerase of DNA viruses. The compound **zidovudine** is an agent that inhibits retroviral human immunodeficiency virus type 1 (HIV-1) replication by interfering with the viral RNA-dependent DNA polymerase (reverse transcriptase).

ANTIMICROBIAL AGENTS AGAINST MYCOBACTERIA

The precise mode of action of agents that inhibit mycobacteria is not fully established. Isoniazid affects the synthesis of lipids, nucleic acid, and the mycolic acid of the cell wall of mycobacteria. It is bactericidal. Pyrazinamide is an analogue of nicotinamide which also inhibits mycobacterial growth in a bactericidal manner, but its exact mechanism of activity has not been established.

BACTERIAL AND FUNGAL RESISTANCE TO ANTIMICROBIAL AGENTS

Unfortunately, bacteria have proved to be particularly clever at developing resistance to each new antimicrobial agent that has been synthesized or found in nature. Bacterial resistance may be the result of a chromosomal change or be due to the presence of extrachromosomal DNA that is transmissible, namely plasmid resistance. Plasmid resistance is found in virtually all bacteria and is a potent way for dissemination of resistance throughout a country or through a smaller unit such as a hospital. The use of antimicrobial agents acts as a strong selective pressure for the selection of organisms that are resistant either on the basis of chromosomal or plasmid-mediated mechanisms.

The basic mechanisms of antimicrobial resistance are: the development of altered receptors for antimicrobial agents; lower concentration of antimicrobial agent within the cell, either due to prevention of entry or to efflux, destruction, or modification of an agent; and finally, development of resistant metabolic pathways. Bacteria have the potential to have all of these mechanisms and hence be resistant to many classes of agents simultaneously (Table 61–2).

RESISTANCE BASED ON ALTERED RECEPTORS

Altered PBPs are an important mechanism of resistance of bacteria to β-lactam antibiotics. Currently throughout the world there are major problems with *Staphylococcus aureus* organisms which synthesize a new PPB, PPB2a, which does not bind any β-lactam and permits synthesis of a cell wall. These organisms are called methicillin-resistant *S. aureus* (MRSA). β-Lactam resistance due to altered PBPs has also been encountered in enterococci, *Neisseria gonorrhoeae*, and *Streptococcus pneumoniae*.

Resistance of macrolides has been a modest problem in staphylococci and streptococci. It is due to the methylation of the adenine nucleotides in 23S RNA, thereby decreasing the affinity of drugs such as erythromycin or clindamycin for the ribosomes of these organisms. Production of a new DNA-directed RNA polymerase with poor affinity for rifampin prevents binding and produces resistance. The resistance of sulfon-

TABLE 61–2.

Major Resistance Mechanisms

Mechanisms	Drugs
Modification of target enzyme or receptors	
Penicillin binding proteins (PBPs)	β-lactams
Altered DNA gyrase	Quinolones
Methylated 23SRNA	Macrolides, clindamycin
Altered DNA-directed RNA polymerase	Rifampin
Dihydropteroate synthetase	Sulfonamides
Dihydroreductase	Trimethoprim
N-acyl-D-alanyl-D-alanine	Glycopeptides
Prevention of access to target (decreased uptake or efflux)	
Altered porin channels	β-lactams, quinolones
Membrane energy source lacking	aminoglycosides
Efflux	Tetracycline, quinolones
Inactivating Enzymes	
β-lactamases	β-lactams
Chloramphenicol transacetylase	Chloramphenicol

amides and trimethoprim is based on synthesis of new enzymes involved in folate synthesis which have a reduced affinity for these compounds. Similarly resistance to the fluoroquinolones can be caused by production of an altered DNA gyrase subunit A.

DECREASED ENTRY OF DRUGS

Tetracycline resistance in bacteria is related to the efflux of the drug from the bacteria because of synthesis of a new protein in the organisms. The resistant bacteria bind less tetracycline and hence protein biosynthesis is not inhibited. Staphylococci and some of the gram-negative organisms can be resistant to fluoroquinolones because the compounds cannot, in the case of gram-negative organisms, enter the cell adequately or, in the case of *S. aureus*, they are pumped out of the bacterial cell.

MODIFICATION OR DESTRUCTION OF ANTIMICROBIAL AGENTS

One of the most important mechanisms of resistance to β-lactams is that due to β-lactamases which hydrolyze the β-lactam nucleus. β-lactamases are present in gram-positive and gram-negative bacteria, both anaerobes and aerobic species. Synthesis of β-lactamases may be either chromosomally or plasmid-mediated (Table 61–3). Resistance to chloramphenicol is on the basis of an enzyme chloramphenicol transacetylase which aceylates the hydroxyl

group of the chloramphenicol structure. Aminoglycosides may undergo modification due to acetylation of amino groups or phosphorylation or adenylation of the hydroxyl groups. These modified aminoglycosides bind less well to ribosomes, and the modified aminoglycoside fails to cause production of a protein which normally moves the compounds into the bacteria.

SELECTION OF ANTIMICROBIAL AGENT

As discussed in earlier chapters, the identification of the infecting microorganisms, bacterial, viral, fungal, or parasitic, is critical to the appropriate utilization of an antimicrobial agent. A number of factors impact on the selection of an agent. These include the age factor since removal of agents from the body frequently is by renal elimination which undergoes marked change with age. Allergy to certain classes is an important factor, particularly for the β-lactam agents. Certain genetic factors, the pregnancy state of a patient, and the antimicrobial site of infection will markedly influence selection of a drug, as will the host defenses present or absent in the particular patient.

In some infections it is critical to have a bactericidal compound, whereas in others, a bacteriostatic agent may prove to be just as effective. Meningitis is an example of an infection in which bactericidal action is necessary and in which it is necessary to achieve concentrations of the antimicrobial agent at least eight- to tenfold above the MBC within the spinal fluid. Infection of heart valves, endocarditis, is another infection in which bactericidal agents are necessary. Endocarditis is an infection that illustrates the concept that therapy must be for a prolonged period owing to the hidden nature of the microorganisms and their protected status in a vegetation.

It should be realized that antimicrobial drug therapy in the presence of a foreign body is fre-

TABLE 61–3.
Bacteria Which Contain β-Lactamases

Species	Frequency (%)
Gram-positive	
Staphylococcus aureus	95
Staphylococcus epidermidis	90
Bacillus species	Most
Clostridium	Rare
Enterococci	1
Gram-negative	
Haemophilus influenzae	10–35
Neisseria gonorrhoeae	5–75
Moraxella catarrhalis	70
Neisseria meningitidis	<0.1
Escherichia coli	10–60
Klebsiella species	100
Pseudomonas aeruginosa	100
Enterobacter, Citrobacter, Serratia, Providencia, etc.	90
Bacteroides tragilis	70–90

quently ineffective even though the agents will kill the microorganism in the test tube. Microorganisms can adhere to foreign body material and cover themselves with a glycoprotein which isolates the bacteria from the action of antimicrobial compounds.

Some microorganisms are able to survive within the cells that ingest them. Examples of such organisms are mycobacteria, *Legionella,* and salmonella. If antimicrobial agents do not penetrate into phagocytic cells, infections due to these organisms will not be cured even though the organisms in vitro are inhibited by the compounds.

ANTIMICROBIAL COMBINATIONS

Antibiotics may be used in combination for a variety of different infections discussed in this book. Currently, the most common use of combinations of antimicrobial agents is to treat life-threatening or polymicrobial infections. Synergy or enhanced antibacterial activity is achieved with certain agents, e.g., β-lactams and aminoglycosides against enterococci or *Pseudomonas aeruginosa,* but in many situations it is difficult

to demonstrate true synergistic action of compounds. Whether combinations of drugs truly prevent the emergence of resistant bacteria except in the case of mycobacterial infection remains an area of controversy.

PROPHYLAXIS WITH ANTIMICROBIAL AGENTS

In certain situations antimicrobial agents are used to prevent bacterial or fungal infections. Use of antimicrobial agents at the time of certain surgical procedures has been shown to prevent postoperative wound infections. Antibiotics of the β-lactam class administered to patients with structural lesions of the heart when undergoing dental or surgical procedures will prevent bacterial endocarditis. Oral antibiotics will frequently prevent infection in neutropenic patients if organisms are eliminated from the gastrointestinal tract. Prophylactic antibiotic use, however, should always be extremely well thought out to avoid the disadvantages of toxic reactions or increased risk of superinfection due to a more resistant flora.

Index